History and Pathology of Vaccination

HISTORY AND PATHOLOGY

OF

VACCINATION

HISTORY AND PATHOLOGY

OF

VACCINATION

VOL. I.

A CRITICAL INQUIRY

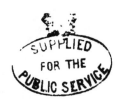

BY

EDGAR M. CROOKSHANK, M.B.

PROFESSOR OF COMPARATIVE PATHOLOGY AND BACTERIOLOGY IN, AND FELLOW OF,
KING'S COLLEGE, LONDON.

AUTHOR OF PAPERS ON THE ETIOLOGY OF SCARLET FEVER; ANTHRAX IN SWINE;
TUBERCULOSIS AND THE PUBLIC MILK SUPPLY; AND THE HISTORY AND
PATHOLOGY OF ACTINOMYCOSIS; IN REPORTS OF THE AGRICULTURAL
DEPARTMENT OF THE PRIVY COUNCIL, ETC.
AUTHOR OF A MANUAL OF BACTERIOLOGY, ETC.

LONDON

H. K. LEWIS, 136, GOWER STREET, W.C.

1889

PREFACE.

IN this Preface I have thought it necessary to lay before the profession, the circumstances which have led to the production of these volumes.

I had devoted myself for some time to pathological researches in connection with the communicable diseases of man and the lower animals, when the discovery of an outbreak of Cow Pox, in 1887, led me to investigate the history and pathology of this affection. At that time I accepted and taught the doctrines, in reference to this disease, which are commonly held by the profession, and are described in the text-books of medicine.

In endeavouring to discover the origin of this outbreak, it was proved beyond question that the cows had not been infected by milkers suffering from Small Pox. This fact, together with the clinical characters of the disease in the cows, and in the milkers infected from the cows, and the certainty, that I had to deal " not with an infectious disease like cattle-plague or pleuro-pneumonia, but with a

disease which is communicated solely by *contact*,"
convinced me that the commonly accepted descriptions
of the nature and origin of Cow Pox were purely
theoretical.   As the natural Cow Pox had not been
investigated in this country for nearly half a century,
it was obvious that a much neglected field of comparative pathology had been opened up for further inquiry.

My interest in this subject was further stimulated
by Sir James Paget, who very kindly examined one
of the milkers casually infected from the cows, and
while so doing drew my attention to a copy of Dr.
Creighton's work on Cow Pox and Vaccinal Syphilis,
then just published.   The question naturally arose,
whether my observations supported or refuted the
conclusions arrived at by Dr. Creighton as the result
of his historical researches.

While attending at the National Vaccine Establishment of the Local Government Board, I was unable
to obtain any exact details, clinical or pathological,
of the source of the lymph which was employed
there.   From my experience of this and other
vaccination stations, I found that both official and
unofficial vaccinators were completely occupied with
the *technique* of vaccination, to the exclusion of
any precise knowledge of the history and pathology
of the diseases from which their lymph stocks had
been obtained.   Thus, at this early stage of my
investigation, I felt that what Ceely said, in 1840,

was still true: "The imperfect knowledge which we at present possess on many points connected with the natural history of the *variolæ vaccinæ*, and the numerous and formidable impediments to the improvement and extension of that knowledge, demand the continuance of vigilant, patient, and diligent inquiry."

In January, 1888, while I was studying the literature of the subject at the Library of the Royal College of Surgeons, Mr. Baily, the librarian, to whom I am indebted for much courteous assistance, was engaged in re-cataloguing the Library. He found a parcel of MSS., which he thought might prove of interest to me. It contained letters from Hunter to Jenner, and a manuscript which was thought to be the MS. of Jenner's *Inquiry*. On carefully perusing it, I discovered that it differed in many respects from the published *Inquiry*; it was, in fact, *Jenner's Communication to the Royal Society*. I was so struck by the contents of this paper, and the small amount of evidence upon which Jenner had first ventured to propose the substitution of Cow Pox inoculation or *vaccination* for the old system of Small Pox inoculation or *variolation*, that I was induced to carefully look into the life of Jenner and the early history of vaccination, as contained in Baron's Biography, and in the correspondence and articles on the subject in contemporary medical and scientific periodicals

Now that the value of Jenner's MS. and the interest attached thereto, have been pointed out, it has been carefully preserved, and entered in the catalogue of the Library, and may be consulted by any one desiring to do so. From a letter, dated 1877, which will be found in the parcel, it will be seen that Hunter's letters and Jenner's MS. were given to Sir James Paget, by a lady into whose - possession they had passed on the death and , by the will of her cousin, the late Colonel Jenner, son of Dr. Jenner. On June 4th, 1879, Sir James Paget wrote to Mr. [now Sir John] Simon, President of the College, presenting the MSS. to the Library of the College. The MSS. appear to have remained in a drawer until they were brought to light under the circumstances which I have just related.

I gradually became so deeply impressed with the small amount of knowledge possessed by practitioners, concerning Cow Pox and other sources of vaccine lymph, and with the conflicting teachings and opinions of leading authorities, in both the medical and veterinary professions, that I determined to investigate the subject for myself. From antiquarian booksellers in Paris, Berlin, and in this country, I succeeded in a very short time in obtaining a large number of works dealing with the early history of vaccination.

They at the same time forwarded many works on Small Pox inoculation, and thus my interest was aroused in this subject also, and its bearing upon the history and pathology of vaccination was soon apparent.

In February, 1888, I resolved to consult the leading authorities in France, and to obtain, if possible, the history both of the Bordeaux Lymph, and of the outbreaks of Cow Pox which had been met with in that country during the time that the disease was supposed to be extinct in this.

I take this opportunity of thanking M. Hervieux for much information, and for his kindness in affording me opportunities for observing the system of public vaccination in Paris.

To M. Cagny, I cannot sufficiently express my indebtedness both for introductions to his colleagues, and for presenting me with a copy of the work of Auzias - Turenne containing his classical essays on Cow Pox and Horse Pox.

From Paris, I proceeded to Bordeaux where Dr. Layet and M. Baillet received me with the greatest courtesy, and afforded me every opportunity of obtaining information concerning the Municipal Vaccination Service; and we discussed the details of the recent outbreaks of Cow Pox which they had observed. I also succeeded in obtaining, through the kindness of Dr. Dubreuilh, a full account of the " spontaneous " outbreak which was the source of a recent official[1]

---

[1] *Report of the Medical Officer of the Local Government Board.* 1882. p. iv.

stock of vaccine lymph now employed in this country, though abandoned at the Animal Vaccine Station at Bordeaux.[1] At Toulouse, at the Veterinary School, I was able to obtain further information about the nature, clinical characters, and origin of Cow Pox and Horse Pox. M. Peuch, the distinguished Professor of Veterinary Pathology, furnished me with the details of his remarkable investigations into Horse Pox, and has since granted me permission to reproduce the coloured plates illustrating this subject. M. Peuch's researches and observations will be of the greatest value in bringing to light a disease of the horse which is still unrecognised by practical veterinarians in this country.

I also had the opportunity of studying the clinical characters, and the results of inoculation of Sheep Pox.

At Montpellier, I visited the Vaccine Establishment of M. Pourquier, and obtained from him some interesting information. On returning to Paris, I was most kindly received by M. Chauveau, who discussed with me the affinities of Cow Pox, and showed me the beautiful and valuable drawings which had been prepared for the Report of the Lyons Commission, but unfortunately had been withheld from publication owing to the expense that would have been entailed.

---

[1] *British Medical Journal.* July 14th, 1888.

On returning to England, I renewed my investigations in Gloucestershire, Wiltshire, and Dorsetshire. I obtained additional information with reference to cases of Cow Pox in this country, and fully realised that the belief that this disease is extinct in England has resulted from the determined and often successful attempts which are made by farmers (for obvious reasons) to conceal outbreaks when they occur. I also followed up the history of Mr. Jesty, by visiting Worth Matravers in the Isle of Purbeck, and obtaining all the local information possible.

Lastly, for reference to some works, copies of which I have not hitherto succeeded in obtaining, I have availed myself of the British Museum and our medical libraries.

The difficulty in gaining access to these works is no doubt the reason why the originals have been so little read. It would hardly be possible for the practitioner with but little time at his disposal, and, if in the country, without access to many medical libraries, to undertake such an inquiry; but I trust that the system which has been followed in this work of giving copious extracts will induce others to study the original authorities. All the selections from Jenner's correspondence have been drawn from Baron's Biography, with the exception of one letter, which was obtained for me by Mr. W. K. Dale.

I desire to thank him; and also the owner for permission to reproduce it in fac-simile. The essays composing the second volume have been reprinted with the object of affording references in a handy form.

My best thanks are due to Mr. James Ceely for approving of the proposal to reprint his brother's classical papers, and to Mr. Badcock for granting me permission to reprint his pamphlet.

In conclusion, I desire to thank Messrs. W. K. Dale and E. F. Herroun for their assistance in passing the proof sheets through the press. Messrs. Vincent, Brooks, Day, & Son are to be congratulated upon the success with which they have reproduced the coloured plates.

EDGAR M. CROOKSHANK.

24, MANCHESTER SQUARE, W.,
   April 1889.

CONTENTS OF VOL. I.

LIST OF PLATES.

Reduced fac-simile of an engraving by W. Say, from the original painting by M. W. Sharp.

The engraving bears the following inscription :—

"To the President, Vice-Presidents, Treasurers, Trustees, and Medical Officers of the Original Vaccine Institution.

"This print of Mr. Benjamin Jesty, from a picture in the possession of the Institution, is respectfully inscribed by their devoted Servant, Willm. Say.

"Mr. B. JESTY, Farmer of Downshay, Isle of Purbeck, æt. 70, who inoculated his Wife and Two Sons for the Vaccine Pock in 1774, from his cows, at that Time disorder'd by the Cow Pock, and who subsequently from the most rigorous Trials have been found unsusceptible of the Small Pox. Having rationally set the Example of Vaccine Inoculation from his own knowledge of the Fact of Unsusceptibility of the Small Pox after casual Cow Pock in his own Person and in that of others, and from knowing the harmlessness of the Complaint. To commemorate the Author of these historical truths the Vaccine Institution have procured this portrait." (Extract from the Minutes of the Original Vaccine Institution, Broad Street, Golden Square.)

"SARAH NELMES, a dairymaid at a Farmer's near this place [Berkeley], was infected with the Cow Pox from her master's cows in May 1796. She received the infection on a part of the hand which had been previously in a slight degree injured by a scratch from a thorn. A large pustulous sore and the usual symptoms accompanying the disease were produced in consequence. The pustule was so expressive of the true character of the Cow Pox, as it commonly appears upon the hand, that I have given a representation of it in the annexed plate. The two small pustules on the wrists arose also from the application of the virus to some minute abrasions of the cuticle, but the livid tint, if they ever had any, was not conspicuous at the time I saw the patient. The pustule on the forefinger shows the disease in an earlier stage. It did not actually

"JOHN BAKER, a child of five years old, was inoculated March 16th, 1798, with matter taken from a pustule on the hand of Thomas Virgoe, one of the servants who had been infected from the mare's heels. He became ill on the 6th day with symptoms similar to those excited by Cow Pox matter. On the 8th day he was free from indisposition.

"There was some variation in the appearance of the pustule on the arm. Although it somewhat resembled a Small Pox pustule, yet its similitude was not so conspicuous as when excited by matter from the nipple of the cow, or when the matter was passed from thence through the medium of the human subject.

"This experiment was made to ascertain the progress and subsequent effects of the disease when thus propagated. We have seen that the virus from the horse, when it proves infectious to the human subject, is not to be relied upon as rendering the system secure from variolous infection, but that the matter produced by it upon the nipple of the cow is perfectly so. Whether its passing from the horse through the human constitution, as in the present instance, will produce a similar effect, remains to be decided. This would now have been effected, but the boy was rendered unfit for inoculation from having felt the effects of a contagious fever in a workhouse, soon after this experiment was made."—(*Jenner.*)

This plate "represents large vesicles which formed on the cheek of my eldest son on the 5th day of the eruption. The face was much swollen, and the skin of a deep crimson colour. On the temple there is a large pustule, which has all the genuine characters of the Small Pox pustule. The depression in the centre was very obvious; and between this and the outer angle of the eye, and also above the eye-brow, there are several pimples of different sizes and forms, some of which never passed beyond the first or inflammatory stage."— (*Monro.*)

"Here my researches were interrupted till the spring of the year 1798, when from the wetness of the early part of the season, many of the farmers' horses in this neighbourhood were affected with sore heels, in consequence of which the Cow-pox broke out among several of our dairies, which afforded me an opportunity of making further observations upon this curious disease.

"A mare, the property of a person who keeps a dairy in a neighbouring parish, began to have sore heels the latter end of the month of February 1798, which were occasionally washed by the servant men of the farm, Thomas Virgoe, William Wherret, and William Haynes, who in consequence became affected with sores in their hands, followed by inflamed lymphatic glands in the arms and axillæ, shiverings succeeded by heat, lassitude and general pains in the limbs. A single paroxysm terminated the disease ; for within twenty-four hours they were free from general indisposition, nothing remaining but the sores on their hands.

"William Summers, a child of five years and a half old, was inoculated the same day with Baker [see description of Plate III., E. M. C.], with matter taken from the nipples of one of the infected cows, at the farm alluded to. He became indisposed on the 6th day, vomited once, and felt the usual slight symptoms till the 8th day, when he appeared perfectly well. The progress of the pustule, formed by the infection of the virus, was similar to that noticed in Case XVII. [James Phipps, E. M. C.], with this exception, its being free from the livid tint observed in that instance.

"From William Summers the disease was transferred to WILLIAM PEAD, a boy of eight years old, who was inoculated March 28th. On the 6th day he complained of pain in the axilla, and on the 7th was affected with the common symptoms of a patient sickening with the Small-pox from inoculation, which did not terminate, till the 3rd day after the seizure. So perfect was the similarity to the variolous fever that I was induced to examine the skin, conceiving there might have been some eruptions, but none appeared. The efflorescent blush around the part punctured in the boy's arm was so truly characteristic of that which appears on variolous inoculation, that I have given a representation of it. The drawing was made when the pustule was beginning to die away, and the areola retiring from the centre."—(*Jenner.*)

PLATE VI. INOCULATED HORSE POX, AFTER TRANSMISSION THROUGH THE COW. Case of Hannah Excell. (*JENNER*)
following Plate V.

"April 5th. Several children and adults were inoculated from the arm of William Pead [see description of Plate V.].

"HANNAH EXCELL, an healthy girl of seven years old, and one of the patients above mentioned, received the infection from the insertion of the virus under the cuticle of the arm in three distinct points. The pustules which arose in consequence so much resembled, on the 12th day, those appearing from the insertion of variolous matter, that an experienced Inoculator would scarcely have discovered a shade of difference at that period. Experience now tells me that almost the only variation which follows consists in the pustulous fluid remaining limpid nearly to the time of its total disappearance, and not as in the direct Small-pox becoming purulent."—(*Jenner.*)

PLATE VII. INOCULATED COW POX AND INOCULATED SMALL POX. (*BALLHORN AND STROMEYER*) *facing p.* 288

This plate was produced by Ballhorn and Stromeyer. *Traité de l'inoculation vaccine,* 1801. [It illustrates the results of cultivated vaccine and the ordinary results of a direct inoculation of Small-pox. In this case the appearances are strikingly dissimilar, but Adams selected a mild variety of Small-pox, called the pearl sort, and succeeded by cultivation on the human subject in producing appearances indistinguishable from ordinary vaccination.—E.M.C.]

Showing the progress of the variolation experiment on the fifteenth day.

" The variolous vesicle at its maximum of development with a large central crust; it had a florid glistening appearance. The vaccine vesicles of the seventh day were also at their greatest development, had slight central crust, and were surrounded, like the variolous vesicle, with a small pale areola."—(*Ceely.*)

The whole history of this experiment is as follows :—

" *Experiment first.*—Red and white sturk, thin skin, gentle, well bred :— Made seven punctures, and introduced fourteen points, charged half their length, near the left side of the vulva and below it. Inserted two setons, charged with Small-pox virus from the same subject, at the same time.

" *Fifth Day.*—Two or three of the punctures tumid, all closed with brown plugs ; setons tumid.

" *Sixth Day.*—Some punctures tumid.

" *Seventh Day.*—Less tumid.

" *Eighth Day.*—Still less so ; setons passive, dry, adherent.

" *Ninth Day.* - No material alteration, and therefore *vaccinated* on the *right side* of the vulva, in seven punctures, with fifth, sixth, and seventh day lymph, on fourteen points, from a young child ; and *below* the vulva, in four punctures, with eight points.

" *Tenth day* of variolation, *second* of vaccination : Some of the variolated punctures hard and elevated ; but *one*, near the margin of the vulva, has assumed the form and appearance of the vaccine vesicle ; it is nearly circular, has an elevated margin, and a small crust in the depressed centre. By gently removing the central irregular crust, and carefully puncturing the cuticle from under which this appears to have exuded, lymph was obtained, and thirty-eight points were scantily charged in the course of an hour. Vaccinated punctures on the right side, rather red and elevated.

" *Eleventh day* of variolation, *third day* of vaccination : The circular indurated intumescence, forming the margin of the vesicle, somewhat flattened and diminished. Vaccine punctures more red, larger, and more elevated. *Evening :* more crust in the centre of the Small-pox vesicle ; margin less elevated. Vaccine vesicles advancing.

" *Twelfth day* of variolation, *fourth day* of vaccination : Margin of the Small-pox vesicle more elevated and red ; central crust darker ; two of the other variolous punctures more tumid, but without lymph, still merely tubercular. Vaccinated punctures more tumid and inflamed.

" *Thirteenth day* of variolation, *fifth day* of vaccination : Small-pox vesicle more inflamed, nearly as florid as the mucous membrane of the vulva, which has lately assumed a bright rose colour. Every puncture made for the vaccine lymph (five days since) effectual, vesicles of different forms and sizes being now apparent. Charged some points from them.

" *Fourteenth day* of variolation, *sixth* of vaccination : Small-pox vesicle has less marginal induration, seems flatter, and crust partially loosened. Vaccine vesicles, some partly subsiding, some a little pustular, others still red, and all surrounded by indurated borders.

"*Fifteenth day* of variolation, *seventh* of vaccination: Small-pox vesicle enlarging; crust larger; indurated elevated margin of the vesicle quite circular, red, and glistening towards the centre. Vaccine vesicles larger and more elevated. Took from them more lymph.

"*Sixteenth day* of variolation, *eighth* of vaccination: Small-pox vesicle diminished; crust increased and loosening. Vaccine vesicles also diminished, some rather pustular; crusts brown and pale yellow, some crusts abraded partially, others loose.

"*Seventeenth day* of variolation, *ninth* of vaccination: Small-pox vesicle has scarcely any redness on its border; crust remaining. Vaccine vesicles diminishing, and covered with blackish brown crusts within their circular or oval margins, which are much flattened.

"*Eighteenth day* of variolation, *tenth* of vaccination: Small-pox vesicle very much flattened. Vaccine vesicles equally so, covered with black crusts of different sizes.

"*Twenty-fifth day* of variolation, *seventeenth* of vaccination: Scar of Small-pox vesicle apparent; it is deep, wrinkled, and of a pale rose colour. Scars of the vaccine vesicles differ only in being smaller, less deep, and have more induration around them."—(*Ceely.*)

Plate IX. NATURAL COW POX. (*CEELY*) . . *facing p.* 348

" Fig. 1 exhibits the disease at the end of the second week. It shows vesicles with central crusts, acuminated vesicles, imperfectly desiccated vesicles, and vesicles further advanced in desiccation. The teat raw and swollen from the injuries sustained during milking.

"Fig. 2. The teat of a cow, with a fairer skin, exhibiting perfect cicatrices, cicatrices with secondary crusts, raw and imperfect cicatrices, and a crust still adherent on the base of the teat."—(*Ceely.*)

Plate X. PHAGEDÆNIC ULCERATION IN NATURAL COW POX. (*CROOKSHANK*). . . . . . *facing p.* 350

Reproduced from the original water-colour drawing of a case from Wiltshire. This animal had been selected by the farm bailiff as one of the severest cases, and was sent to London for the purpose of an investigation. Subsequently the farm was visited, and in the affected herds some cases of equal severity were found.

"In a few cases the condition was most distressing, both to the cow and to the observer. In such cases the teats were encrusted with huge dark brown or black crusts, which, when roughly handled by the milker, were broken and detached, exposing a bleeding, suppurating, ulcerated base. Such ulcers varied in size, from a shilling to a florin, and in form were circular, ovoid, or irregular. Weeks afterwards, when the animals had recovered, the sites of these ulcers were marked by irregular scars. (*Crookshank.*)

Plate XI. CASUAL COW POX. Case of Joseph Brooks, a milker. (*CEELY*) . . . . *facing p.* 358

" This plate is referred to in Vol. II., p. 475; it represents the casual vaccine on the right temporo-frontal region of Joseph Brooks, with recedent areola. With the exception of being rather more florid, it very much resembles the vaccine vesicle on the white skin of the cow's udder, and, like that, yielded lymph only from its centre, and that slowly and scantily, after the removal of the central crust."—(*Ceely.*)

"This plate is referred to in Vol. II., p. 476; it represents the casual vaccine vesicles on the thumb and finger of the same individual, on the same day as that of the preceding plate."—(*Ceely.*)

"This plate is referred to in Vol II., p. 491; it represents the casual vaccine vesicles on the hand and thumb of the same individual. . . . The vesicle on the thumb is still flat on the surface; but the centre is more discoloured, yet without any visible depression; the central crust has increased. The vesicle on the hand is much more depressed in the centre, and the bases of both vesicles are more elevated."—(*Ceely.*)

Fig. 1. "The vesicle on the back of the hand, irregularly puffed at its margin, puckered and depressed at its centre, where the slough is visible."

Fig. 2. "The ulcer on the back of the hand, deep, and not yet granulating, surrounded with a well-defined, elevated, and indurated border."

Fig. 3. "The vesicle on the thumb, with a portion of slough visible through an opening in the bluish or slate-coloured centre, the margin partially vesicated, the base flatter and duller."

Fig. 4. "The ulcer on the thumb not very deep, and granulating." —*Ceely.*

"John Harding, the bailiff's son, also milked the cows. He had a sore on the upper lid of his right eye and on his left hand. In both cases he had been previously scratched by a cat, and the scratches were inoculated from the cow's teats. The right hand also had been inoculated. The eruption broke out a fortnight ago. His hands were swollen, red, and hot. He felt very poorly and went to bed. Little spots like white blisters appeared on the back of his right hand. His mother remarked that they "rose up exactly as in vaccination." Thick dark brown scabs formed. He was very ill for two or three days, but did not send for a doctor. He had painful lumps at the bend of his arm and in the armpit. He gave up milking, and had not taken to it since.

"On examining him the thick crusts on his right hand were identical with the stage of scabbing in ordinary vaccination. The scabs fell off in about three weeks to a month, and left permanent depressed scars."— (*Crookshank.*)

" This case was pointed out to me on the occasion of my visit on December 2nd, and is the only one in which I was fortunate enough to see the eruption in its early stages. The case was of such extreme interest that I took the lad to London on the following day.

" The history of this boy is as follows. He had taken the place of one of the other milkers who had vesicles on his fingers and had been obliged to give up milking. After the seventh time of milking he noticed a small pimple on his right cheek. This occurred on Sunday, November 27th. The pimple became larger, and, as he expressed it, 'rose up like a blister.'

"On December 2nd, the date of my visit, there was a large depressed vesicle with a small central yellowish crust and a tumid margin, the whole being surrounded by a well-marked areola and considerable surrounding induration.

"After making a coloured drawing of the eruption (fig. 1), I punctured the tumid margin, and collected clear lymph in a number of capillary tubes.

" After this I raised the central incrustation, and pointed out to the Inspectors of the Agricultural Department who were present the crater-like excavation, from which lymph welled up and trickled down the boy's cheek.

" On the following day the crust had reformed, and was studded with coagulated lymph. The areola became more marked, and on pricking the margin of the vesicle the contents were slightly turbid.

" From this day the surrounding infiltration increased enormously, the whole cheek was inflamed, and the eyelids so œdematous that the eye was almost closed. There was enlargement of the neighbouring lymphatic glands. The crust which had reformed, thickened day by day, and on December 9th, when I took the boy to Sir James Paget, there was a thick reddish-brown or mahogany-coloured crust, still bearing the character of central depression, surmounting a reddened, elevated, and indurated base. (Fig. 2.)

" From this date the surrounding induration gradually diminished. The crust changed in colour from dark-brown to black, and finally fell off on December 15th, leaving an irregular depressed scar. This scar, when seen several months afterwards, was found to be a permanent disfigurement.

"Thus the eruption appeared on the fourth day after exposure to infection, and allowing two days for incubation, the vesicle was at its height on the seventh or eighth day, and a typical tamarind-stone crust fell off on the twenty-first day after infection, leaving a depressed, irregular cicatrix."—(*Crookshank.*)

Figs. 1, 2, 3, represent the thumb of William Plowman. See also description of the preceding plate.

"A vesicle also formed on the thumb of the left hand. Two days after the pimple appeared on his cheek, the lad says that he noticed a pimple on his thumb, and this, on my visit on December 2nd, presented a greyish flattened vesicle, about the size of a sixpence. On the following day its vesicular character was much more marked, and a little central crust had commenced to form. (Fig. 1.) On the Sunday, especially towards the evening, the margins became very tumid, giving it a marked appearance of central depression. On Monday, December 5th, I punctured the vesicle at its margin with a clean needle, and filled a number of capillary tubes from the beads of lymph which exuded.

"On Wednesday, December 7th, suppuration had commenced ; the vesicle contained a turbid fluid, and the areola was well marked. (Fig. 2.) On December 9th the crust had assumed a peculiar slate-coloured hue, and, on pressing it, pus welled up through a central fissure. (Fig. 3.) The areola had increased, and there was considerable inflammatory thickening. The lymphatic glands in the armpit were enlarged and painful. Though there was deep ulceration, which left a permanent scar, the ulceration did not assume quite so severe a character as in some of the other milkers."

Fig. 4. Case of William Hibbert, junr.

"William Hibbert, a milker, states that he had both hands bad about a month ago. First the index finger of the left hand, and then the right hand on his knuckle and between the first and second fingers.

"He says that it came up like a hard pimple, and the finger became swollen and red. After a few days it 'weeped out' water and then matter came away. Both his arms were swollen, but his left arm was the worst.

"About a fortnight after, he noticed 'kernels' in his armpits, which were painful and kept him awake at night. His arms became worse, he could not raise them, and he had to give up milking. He also had had a 'bad place' on the lower lip.

"On examination, I found that the axillary glands were still enlarged and tender."—(*Crookshank.*)

"Roseola vaccina; an efflorescence which commonly appears in a congeries of dots and small patches, as here represented, but is sometimes diffuse; like the variolous rash it usually occurs at the same time with the areola, and around the inoculated part."—(*Willan.*)

"Fig 1. Result of an inoculation, made on January 13th, at half past nine in the morning, with pus collected at the margin of the prepuce. Drawing made at ten o'clock. Tumefaction of the tissues is already observable, and, in the centre, the puncture of the lancet is surrounded by a slight reddish areola almost limited to the swollen parts.

"Fig. 2. Drawing made on the same day at four o'clock in the afternoon. The inoculated spot is more elevated; the areola is more deeply coloured.

"Fig. 3. Drawing made on January 14th, at nine o'clock in the morning. The swollen parts are sharply circumscribed, and have a deep red colour at the base. A greyish point at the summit corresponds with the puncture of the lancet. . . . The inflammatory areola has, comparatively speaking, extended considerably.

"Fig. 4. Drawing made on the same day at four o'clock in the afternoon. The pustule has developed; the greyish spot noticed in the morning has become quite black, and forms a small gangrenous eschar, and around it the epidermis is raised up by pus.

"Fig. 5. Drawing made on the 15th, at ten o'clock in the morning. All the parts of the pustule have advanced in equal proportion.

"Fig. 6. Drawing made on the 16th, at ten o'clock in the morning. A general advance. There is an irregularity at the periphery of the pustule, from which a small quantity of pus has escaped during the night, and in the centre the gangrenous eschar is depressed, and appears to be adherent to the underlying parts.

"Fig. 7. Drawing made on the 17th, at ten o'clock in the morning. A general advance. The pustule has ruptured at several points, and appears to be almost free from pus.

"Fig. 8. Drawing made on the 18th, at ten o'clock in the morning. A general advance, with the exception of the inflammatory areola, which appears less intense. On raising the irregular slough which covers the ulcer resulting from the inoculation, a red base marked with yellowish points is disclosed. At the edges, a whitish margin is seen formed by the elevated epidermis." (*Traité complet des Maladies Vénériennes*, Plate III., Figs. 2-8. Paris 1851.)

HISTORY AND PATHOLOGY

OF

VACCINATION.

CHAPTER I.

HISTORY OF SMALL POX INOCULATION IN FOREIGN COUNTRIES.

THE practice of Small Pox inoculation is one of very great antiquity. It had been found by experience that a person was not, as a rule, seized with Small Pox a second time; but when, and how, the method of artificially inducing the disease was discovered, or where this preventive treatment was first employed, is quite unknown. It has been suggested, not unnaturally, that as the Arabian physicians were acquainted with the nature and treatment of Small Pox, they were probably the first to whom it occurred to produce the disease by inoculation. Avicenna, who is said to have lived at Bokhara, on the east coast of the Caspian Sea, has been credited with this discovery; and it was supposed that the practice was carried by Tartar and Chinese traders to Surat, Bengal, and China, and by the

I

Mahommedan pilgrims to Mecca. But, according to Woodville,[1] there is little or nothing to support this theory, for there is no evidence that the Circassians, or any of the inhabitants of the countries near the Caspian Sea, had practised the art of inoculation longer than those of other nations; and D'Entrecolles had remarked that the Tartars were ignorant of this treatment in 1724.

There were equally conflicting opinions in Constantinople as to the origin of inoculation. It was said by some to have been introduced from the Morea by an old woman, and by others to have been imported from Circassia, where it was supposed to have been first employed. Dr. Mead[2] was in favour of the latter view.

" I have often wondered how such a notion could come into the heads of people almost quite ignorant of what relates to physic. For, as far as I have been able to find out by inquiry, this was the invention of the Circassians, the women of which country are said to excel in beauty; upon which account it is very common, especially among the poorer sort, to sell young girls for slaves to be carried away into the neighbouring parts. When therefore it was observed that they who were seized with this distemper were in less danger both of their beauty and their life the younger they were, they contrived this way of infecting the body that so the merchandise might bring the greater profit."

In Circassia.—De la Motraye,[3] in 1711, saw the

---

[1] Woodville, *The History of the Inoculation of the Small-Pox*, p. 35. 1796.

[2] *Medical Works of Dr. Richard Mead*, vol. ii., p. 143. 1765.

[3] De la Motraye, *Travels through Europe, Asia, and into Part of Africa*, vol. ii., p. 75. 1723.

operation performed upon a Circassian girl four or five years old. The girl, after being purged with dried fruit, was carried to a boy about three years old, who had caught the natural Small Pox, and whose pocks were *ripe*. An old woman performed the operation ; for women of advanced age exercised the practice of physic in Circassia. The manner of inoculating the disease was thus described :—

" She took **three needles** fastened together, and prick'd first the pit of the stomach ; secondly, directly over the heart ; thirdly, the navel ; fourthly, the right wrist ; and, fifthly, the ankle of the left foot, till the blood came. At the same time, she took some matter from the pocks of the sick person, and applied it to the bleeding part, which she covered, first, with *angelica* leaves dri'd, and after with some of the youngest lamb-skins ; and having bound them all well on, the mother wrapped her daughter up in one of the skin coverings, which, I have observed, compose the *Circassian* beds, and carried her thus packed up in her arms to her own home ; where (as they told me) she was to continue to be kept warm, eat only a sort of pap made of cummin flower, with two-thirds water and one-third sheep's milk, without either flesh or fish, and drink a sort of tisan, made with *angelica, bugloss* roots, and *licorish*, which are all very common throughout this country ; and they assured me that with this precaution and *regimen*, the Small Pox generally came out very favourably in five or six days."

In Constantinople.—The first publication in England giving a description of the custom of inoculating or ingrafting the Small Pox, was written by Kennedy,[1] a surgeon :

" I rather more particularly take notice here of the way or

[1] Kennedy, *An Essay on External Remedies*, p. 153. London, 1715.

manner of giving the Small Pox, to show or confirm how easily distempers or contagious corpuscles or malignity (as well as medecines) may be communicated to the blood. This of giving or ingrafting the Small Pox was practised in the *Peloponnesus* (now called the *Morea*), and, at this present time, is very much used both in *Turkey* and *Persia*, where they give it in order to prevent its more dismal effects by the early knowledge of its coming, as also probably to prevent their being troubled with it a second time. This method of the *Persians* is to use the *Pock* and matter dried into powder, the which they take inwardly; but the common way now used in *Turkey*, and more particularly at *Constantinople*, is thus : they first take a **fresh and kindly Pock** from some one ill of this distemper, and having made **scarifications** upon the forehead, wrists, and legs, or extremities, the matter of the Pock is laid upon the foresaid incision, being bound on there for eight or ten days together; at the end of which time, the usual symptoms begin to appear, and the distemper comes forward as if naturally taken ill, though in a more kindly manner and not near the number of *Pox*. During this time, or from the scarifications being made, the patient is closely confined to his room, so as in no way to be exposed to the air ; and the regimen or diet during the whole time of confinement is altogether from flesh, and one kept mostly to water-gruel. By this very regular way of living, the distemper or *Pock* comes out more kindly and less dangerous ; since it is very probable that most of the malignity is increased and augmented by the irregularities committed in their diet or their manner of living some few days before the malady appears—which, when it comes naturally, cannot be so well seen or known how to prevent its worst symptoms, so as when given after this manner. Whilst as yet there, I was credibly inform'd, both by the physicians and merchants, that of the number of two thousand which had then lately undergone that method, there were not any more than two who died, their deaths being altogether attributed to their want of care; for, having been scarified, and the Small Pox applied to the part, the symptoms not appearing so soon as commonly or as they expected, they went abroad, exposing themselves to the open air, which struck the distemper or malignity to the centre, or more inwardly, and was the occasion of their death.

" *Dr. Janoin*, a *Grecian*, who resides there, had taken or followed this same method with his two sisters, a little before my arrival at *Constantinople.* The greatest objection commonly proposed is, whether or not it hinders the patient from being infected a second time. But in answer to this, it is advanced that we do rarely or never find any to have been troubled with this distemper twice in the same manner, or the same fulness of malignity. For when it happens the second time it generally proves that commonly called the Bastard or Hog Pox, which is empty or skinny, and very little matter or malignity contained in it.

"So that it is presumed to be some seminal matter, in the very *Embrio* or Parent, and only makes its appearance by some proper accident, medium, or means of air, aliment, contact, or the like, varying according to our different natures and constitutions.

" But, however, my intention here is not with a design to introduce this practice into these parts ; though the veracity of what I have advanced is not to be doubted, since there are several merchants or gentlemen who, having lived there, that know it to be a truth : we in *Britain* probably being more timorous and fearful of our lives in this case, because of the great mortalities which so frequently accompany this distemper with us ; though of this method, as those who practise it assert, or maintain it to be, it need be no more minded than giving or taking the *Itch.*"

The practice among the Turks was more fully described by Dr. Emanuel Timoni, and communicated by Dr. Woodward to the Royal Society.[1]

"The writer of this ingenious discourse observes, in the first place, that the *Circassians, Georgians*, and other *Asiaticks* have introduc'd this practice of procuring the Small Pox by a sort of inoculation, for about the space of forty years among the *Turks* and others at *Constantinople.*

---

[1] Woodward, *Phil. Trans.*, 1717, vol. xxix., for the years 1714, 1715, 1716, pp. 72-4.

"That although at first the more prudent were very cautious in the use of this practice; yet the happy success it has been found to have in thousands of subjects for these eight years past has now put it out of all suspicion and doubt; since the operations having been perform'd on persons of all ages, sexes, and different temperaments, and even in the worst constitution of the air, yet none have been found to die of the Small Pox; when at the same time it was very mortal when it seized the patient the common way, of which half the affected dy'd. This he attests upon his own observation.

"Next he observes they that have this inoculation practised upon them are subject to very slight symptoms, some being scarce sensible they are ill or sick; and, what is valued by the fair, it never leaves any scars or pits in the face.

"The method of the operation is thus:—Choice being made of a proper contagion, the matter of the pustules is to be communicated to the person proposed to take the infection, whence it has metaphorically the name of insition or inoculation.

"For this purpose they make choice of some boy or young lad, of a sound healthy temperament, that is seized with the common Small Pox (of the distinct, not flux sort), on the twelfth or thirteenth day from the beginning of his sickness; they, with a needle, prick the tubercles (chiefly those on the shins and hams), and press out the matter coming from them into some convenient vessel of glass, or the like, to receive it. It is convenient to wash and clean the vessel first with warm water. A convenient quantity of this matter being thus collected is to be stopped close and kept warm in the bosom of the person that carries it, and as soon as may be, brought to the place of the expecting future patient. The patient, therefore, being in a warm chamber, the operator is to make several little wounds with a needle in one, two, or more places of the skin till some drops of blood follow, and immediately drop out some drops of the matter in the glass, and mix it well with the blood issuing out; one drop of the matter is sufficient for each place prick'd. These punctures are made indifferently in any of the fleshy parts, but succeed best in the muscles of the arm or radius. The needle is to be a 3-edg'd surgeon's needle; it may

likewise be perform'd with a lancet. The custom is to run
the needle transverse and rip up the skin a little, that there may
be a convenient dividing of the part, and the mixing of the
matter with the blood more easily perform'd; which is done
either with a blunt . stile or an ear-picker. The wound is
cover'd with half a walnut shell or the like concave vessel, and
bound over, that the matter be not rub'd off by the garments;
which is all removed in a few hours. The patient is to take
care of his diet. In this place, the custom is to abstain wholly
from flesh and broth for twenty or twenty-five days. This
operation is performed either in the beginning of the winter
or in the spring. . . . It was observ'd in a year when the
common Small Pox was very mortal, that those by incision
were also attended with greater symptoms. Of fifty persons,
who had the incision made upon them almost in the same
day, four were found in whom the eruption was too sudden,
the tubercles more, and symptoms worse. There was some
suspicion that these four had caught the common *Small Pox*
before the incision was made. It is enough for our present
purpose that there was not one but recovered after the
incision; in these four the *Small Pox* came near the confluent
sort. At other times the inoculated are distinct, few, and
scattered; commonly ten or twenty break out; here and there one
has but two or three, few have 100. There are some in whom
no pustule rises, but in the places where the incision was
made, which swell up into purulent tubercles; yet these have
never had the Small Pox afterwards in their whole lives, tho'
they have cohabited with persons having it."

Another account of the Byzantine method of
inoculation was published by Dr. Pylarini,[1] who
described the operation as it was performed in his
presence upon four sons of a Greek nobleman, by an
old woman who had long practised inoculation. The

---

[1] Pylarini, *Phil. Trans.*, 1716, vol. xxix., p. 393.

variolous matter was inserted into a number of punctures made on the forehead, cheeks, chin, and also on both wrists.

In Turkey in Asia.—Dr. Russell[1] gave evidence of a similar practice among the Arabs. In 1726, Dr. Patrick Russell, physician at Aleppo, wrote a letter to his brother, who presented it to the Royal Society.

"About nine or ten years ago, while on a visit at a Turkish Harem, a lady happened to express much anxiety for an only child who had not yet had the Small Pox; the distemper at that time being frequent in the city. None of the ladies in the company had ever heard of inoculation; so that having once mentioned it, I found myself obliged to enter into a detail of the operation, and of the peculiar advantages attending it. Among the female servants in the chamber was an old Bedouin, who having heard me with great attention, assured the ladies that my account was upon the whole a just one, only that I did not seem so well to understand the way of performing the operation, which she asserted should be done not with a lancet but with a needle; she herself had received the disease in that manner, when a child; had, in her time, inoculated many; adding, moreover, that the practice was well known to the Arabs, and that they termed it buying the Small Pox.

"In consequence of this hint, I set about procuring more particular information from the Arabs of this place; and the result of my inquiry was that the practice of inoculation had been of long standing among them. They, indeed, did not pretend to assign any period to its origin; but those of seventy years old and upwards remembered to have heard it spoken of as a common custom of their ancestors, and made little doubt of its being of as ancient a date as the disease itself. Their manner of operating is to make several punctures in some fleshy

·   Russell, *Phil. Trans.*, vol. lviii., pp. 140-50.

part, with a needle imbued in variolous matter taken from a
favourable kind of pock. They use no preparation of the body ;
and the disease communicated in this way being, as they aver,
always slight, they give themselves little or no trouble about
the child in the subsequent stages of the distemper.

"This method of procuring the disease is termed buying the
Small Pox on the following account. The child to be inoculated
carries a few raisins, dates, sugarplums, or suchlike ; and showing them to the child from whom the matter is to be taken,
asks how many pocks he will give in exchange. The bargain
being made, they proceed to the operation. When the parties
are too young to speak for themselves, the bargain is made by
the mothers. This ceremony, which is still practised, points out
a reason for the name given to inoculation by the Arabs ; but
by what I could learn among the women, it is not regarded as
indispensably necessary to the success of the operation, and is,
in fact, often omitted."

Dr. Russell found that the same custom prevailed
among the Eastern Arabs, not only at Bagdad and
Mousul, but in Bassora. At Mousul, the appearance of Small Pox was announced by a public crier,
so that those who wished might have their children
inoculated.

"In Armenia, the Turkoman tribes as well as the Armenian
Christians have practised inoculation since the memory of man ;
but, like the Arabs, are able to give no account of its first
introduction among them. . . .

"At Damascus, and all along the coast of Syria and Palestine,
inoculation has been long known. In the Castravan mountains
it is adopted by the Drusi as well as the Christians.

"Whether the Arabs of the desert to the South of Damascus
are acquainted with this manner of communicating the Small
Pox, I have not hitherto been able to learn ; but, a native of
Mecca, whom I had occasion to converse with this summer,
assured me that he himself had been inoculated in that city. . . .

"In the different countries above-mentioned, inoculation is performed nearly in the same manner. The Arabs affirmed that the punctures might be made indifferently in any fleshy part. Those I have had occasion to examine, have all (a very few excepted) had the mark between the thumb and the fore-finger.

"Some of the Georgians had been inoculated in the same part, but most of them on the fore-arm. Of the Armenians, some had been inoculated in both thighs, but the greater part (like the Arabs) bore the marks upon the hand. Some of the Georgian women remembered that rags of a red colour were chosen in preference for the binding up the arm, a circumstance of which I have been able to discover no trace among the Arabs."

In Africa.—Mr. Colden[1] thought that inoculation originated in Africa. The negroes in Senegal, whenever the Small Pox visited them, inoculated their children on the arm. The inoculated abstained from animal food, and drank freely water acidulated with the juice of limes.

In other parts of Africa a similar custom existed. Here also it was called *buying the Small Pox*, and there was a superstition that inoculation would be of no avail, unless the person from whom the variolous matter was taken, received a piece of money or some other article in exchange.

The practice of inoculation in Tripoli, Tunis, and Algiers was described by Cassem Aga,[2] ambassador in England in 1728.

---

[1] Colden, *Med. Obs. and Inq.*, vol. i., p. 228.

[2] Scheuchzer, *An Account of the Success of Inoculating the Small Pox*, p. 61; *A Paper relating to the Inoculation of the Small-Pox as it is practised in the Kingdoms of Tripoli, Tunis, and Algier*. Written in Arabic by His Excellency Cassem Aga, Ambassador from Tripoli, F.R.S. Done into English from the French of Mr. Dadichi."

"My opinion being asked relating to the inoculation of the Small
Pox, I will mention in a few words what I know of it. If any one
hath a mind to have his children inoculated, he carries them to one
that lies ill of the Small Pox at the time when the pustules are
come to full maturity. Then the surgeon makes an incision on
the back of the hand between the thumb and forefinger, and puts
a little of the matter squeezed out of one of the largest and fullest
pustules into the wound. This done, the child's hand is wrapp'd
up with a handkerchief to keep it from the air, and he is left to his
liberty till the fever arising confines him to his bed, which commonly happens at the end of three or four days. After that, by
God's permission, a few pustules of the Small Pox break out upon
the child. All this I can confirm by a domestic proof; for my
father carried us, five brothers and three sisters, to the house of a
girl that lay ill of the Small Pox, and had us all inoculated the
same day. Now he that had most of us all, had not above twenty
pustules. Otherwise this practice is so innocent and so sure that
out of a hundred persons inoculated not two die; whereas, on the
contrary, out of a hundred persons that are infected with the
Small Pox the natural way there die commonly about thirty. It
is withal so ancient in the kingdoms of *Tripoli*, *Tunis*, and *Algiers*,
that nobody remembers its first rise; and it is generally practised
not only by the inhabitants of the towns, but also by the wild
Arabs."

Dr. Shaw,[1] also, has given an account of the practice
of inoculation in Barbary. According to his description
the variolous pus was applied to a slight wound.

"The inoculation of them is performed by making a **slight
wound** upon the fleshy part of the hand betwixt the thumb and
the forefinger. The person who is to undergo the operation
receives the infection from some friend or neighbour who hath a
favourable kind, and who is entreated to sell two or three of his
pustules for the same number of nuts, comfits, or suchlike

[1] Shaw, *Travels and Observations relating to Several Parts of
Barbary and the Levant*, p. 265. 1738.

trifles. This they call purchasing of the Small Pox ; and among
the *Jews*, the purchase alone I was told, without inoculation, was a
sufficient preparative for the infection.

"However, it is in no great repute in those parts of *Barbary* or
the *Levant* where I have been ; most people esteem it to be a
tempting of Providence, and the soliciting a distemper before
Nature is disposed to receive it. Accordingly they tell a number
of stories to discourage the practice ; particularly of a beautiful
young lady who purchased only a couple of pustules.   It
happened indeed she had no more than were paid for ; but the
misfortune was, they fell upon her eyes, and she was blind by
the experiment."

In India.—Inoculation, according to tradition, was
a most ancient custom in India. We are indebted to
Holwell [1] for full details of the practice.

"Inoculation is performed in Indostan by a particular tribe of
Brahmins, who are delegated annually for this service from the
different colleges of Bindoobund, Eleabas, Banaras, etc., over all
the distant provinces ; dividing themselves into small parties of
three or four each, they plan their travelling circuits in such wise
as to arrive at the places of their respective destination some
weeks before the usual return of the disease ; they arrive commonly in the Bengal provinces early in February, although they
some years do not begin to inoculate before March, deferring it
until they consider the state of the season, and acquire information of the state of the distemper. . . .

"The inhabitants of Bengal, knowing the usual time when the
inoculating Brahmins annually return, observe strictly the regimen
enjoined, whether they determine to be inoculated or not ; this
preparation consists only in abstaining for a month from fish,
milk, and ghee (a kind of butter made generally of buffalo's milk) ;
the prohibition of fish respects only the native Portuguese and
Mahomedans who abound in every province of the empire.   When

---

[1] Holwell, *An Account of the Manner of Inoculating the Small Pox
in the East Indies*, pp. 8-19. 1767.

the Brahmins begin to inoculate, they pass from house to house and operate at the door, refusing to inoculate any who have not, on a strict scrutiny, duly observed the preparatory course enjoined them. It is no uncommon thing for them to ask the parents how many pocks they chuse their children should have. Vanity, we should think, urged a question on a matter seemingly so uncertain in the issue; but true it is that they hardly ever exceed or are deficient in the number required.

"They inoculate indifferently on any part; but, if left to their choice, they prefer the outside of the arm, midway between the wrist and the elbow for the males; and the same between the elbow and the shoulder for the females. Previous to the operation, the operator takes a piece of cloth in his hand (which becomes his perquisite if the family is opulent), and with it gives a dry friction upon the part intended for inoculation for the space of eight or ten minutes, then with a small instrument he wounds, by many slight touches, about the compass of a silver groat, just making the smallest appearance of blood; then opening a linen double rag (which he always keeps in a cloth round his waist), he takes from thence a small pledgit of cotton charged with the variolous matter, which he moistens with two or three drops of the Ganges water, and applies it to the wound, fixing it on with a slight bandage, and ordering it to remain on for six hours without being moved; then the bandage to be taken off, and the pledgit to remain until it falls off itself.

"The cotton which he preserves in a double callico rag is saturated with matter from the inoculated pustules of the preceding year; for they never inoculate with fresh matter, nor with matter from the disease caught in the natural way, however distinct and mild the species. . . . Early on the morning succeeding the operation, four collons (an earthen pot containing about two gallons) of cold water are ordered to be thrown over the patient, from the head downwards, and to be repeated every morning and evening until the fever comes on (which usually is about the close of the sixth day from the inoculation), then to desist until the appearance of the eruptions (which commonly happens at the close of the third complete day from the commencement of the fever), and then to pursue the cold bathing as before through the course of the disease, and

until the scabs of the pustules drop off. They are ordered to open
all the pustules with a fine sharp-pointed thorn as soon as they
begin to change their colour, and whilst the matter continues in a
fluid state. Confinement to the house is absolutely forbid, and the
inoculated are ordered to be exposed to every air that blows ; and
the utmost indulgence they are allowed when the fever comes on,
is to be laid upon a mat at the door ; but, in fact, the eruptive
fever is generally so inconsiderable and trifling as very seldom to
require this indulgence. Their regimen is ordered to consist of
all the refrigerating things the climate and season produce, as
plantains, sugar-canes, water-melons, rice, gruel made of white
poppy-seeds and cold water, or thin rice gruel for, their ordinary
drink. These instructions being given, and an injunction laid on
the patients to make a thanksgiving Poojah, or offering to the
goddess on their recovery, the operator takes his fee, which from
the poor is a *pund of cowries*, equal to about a penny sterling, and
goes on to another door down one side of the street, and up on the
other ; and is thus employed from morning till night, inoculating
sometimes eight or ten in a house."

In China.—D'Entrecolles[1] ascertained from a
medical work in Pekin, that inoculation encountered
strong opposition in China. The author of the book
is said to have lived in the latter part of the dynasty
of *Ming ;* hence Woodville concluded that inoculation in China had not been practised two hundred
years.[2] In India, on the other hand, it seems from
tradition to have been a custom from time immemorial.
The methods employed in the two countries were
so entirely different, that it is scarcely probable that
they derived their information at the same time or

[1] D'Entrecolles, *Lettres Edif. et Curieuses*, p. 10. 1718.
[2] Woodville, *loc cit.*, p. 54.

from the same source. The Chinese, who called it *sowing the Small Pox*, took from two to four dried pustules or scales, between which they placed a small portion of musk. The scales were kept in a jar for several years; but if it were necessary to resort to recent pustules, it was thought advisable to correct the " acrimony of the matter " by exposing it to the steam of an infusion of the roots of scorzonera and liquorice. Sometimes they employed scales which had been dried, powdered, and made into a paste. The whole was wrapped up in cotton and introduced into the patient's nostril. Woodville pointed out that this method probably accounted for the want of success in China, for if the matter produced the same result as inoculation, a troublesome inflammation of the Schneiderian membrane ensued, and if this did not take place, the variolous effluvia being inhaled into the lungs, would produce the natural Small Pox.

In France. — According to tradition, inoculation had long been practised by the peasants in different parts of France, but more especially in Auvergne and Perigord. Dr. Boyer, who wrote in 1717, was the first writer who noticed inoculation. Six years after- . wards, the success of inoculation in England was published in Paris by Dr. de la Coste, and the result was a declaration by the principal doctors of the Sorbonne, that, for the benefit of the public, it was lawful to make trials of this practice. Shortly after this, Dr. Hecquet published a thesis entitled *Raisons de doute contre l'inoculation*, and this, together with the reports of the failures in Boston, U.S.A., and the great mortality of the natural Small Pox in London, which was attributed to the new practice, soon brought inoculation into disrepute in France, and the proposed experiments were abandoned. In 1752, attention was again paid to this subject, owing to a publication of Dr. Butini of Montpelier, and two years later, M. de la Condamine read a paper on the advantages of inoculation before the Royal Academy of Sciences in Paris; but it was not until 1755 that the practice was really introduced into France. M. Turgot inoculated a child four years old, and M. Chastellux, aged twenty-one, also submitted to the operation. Dr. Hosty, who, at the request of the French Minister, had been attending the Small Pox and Inoculation Hospitals in London, on his return reported favourably of inoculation, and this report had immense effect in promoting it in France. In 1756, the family of the Duke of Orleans, and very many persons of high rank, were inoculated by different physicians, and in 1758, the practice was introduced into most of the large towns. In 1760, Angelo Gatti settled in Paris. His patients had so few pustules that it was said that he diluted the virus. Reports of failures excited general alarm, and led to a violent controversy. A very fatal outbreak of Small Pox in

Paris, in 1763, was attributed partly to inoculation, and the practice was prohibited. In 1768, the faculties of physic and theology decided that it ought to be permitted, and it was again resorted to in the provinces as well as in the principal towns.

In Spain.—Inoculation was not extensively adopted until 1771, although it had been introduced there forty-two years previously. Dr. Miguel Gorman came to England to learn the Suttonian method, and returned to Madrid in 1772, where he operated on the nobility, and gave great satisfaction.

In Italy.—According to M. de la Condamine, inoculation had been secretly practised by the people of Naples from time immemorial; it was reported that nurses often inoculated the infants entrusted to their care, without the knowledge of their parents, usually by rubbing the palm of the hand with '*fluid variolous matter recently taken from a pustule.*' It had not only been adopted by the peasants, but was practised by the Marchese Buffalini. During the violent outbreak of Small Pox in 1754, inoculation was introduced into Rome by Peverini. Considerable opposition was encountered, but, in 1755, M. de la Condamine was in Rome, and succeeded in overcoming this, and, in about t en years, the practice was established in nearly all the large towns in Italy.

In Germany and Austria.—Inoculation was first

performed in Hanover in 1724. Mr. Maitland operated on H.R.H. Prince Frederick, and afterwards on
eight children of a baron. These cases were successful, and led to the establishment of the practice in that
kingdom. It was not generally adopted in Germany
and Austria, owing to the opposition of Haen of
Vienna, although his publication was answered by
Condamine, Tissot, and, later, by Tralles. But in
1768, some of the Imperial family were inoculated by
Dr. Ingenhousz, and shortly afterwards an Inoculation
House was established in Vienna by the Emperor.
In Berlin, the practice was soon discountenanced, for
Meckel inoculated his children, and on repeating the
experiment on others had three deaths, two being in the
family of a baron. Dr. Muzell inoculated six children,
of whom three died, and the three who recovered were
much disfigured. In 1774, Dr. Baylies inoculated
seventeen persons; one death occurred, which, in
order to silence an unfavourable report, was attributed
to a "putrid fever, of which the eruption was only
symptomatic." In 1775, inoculation was encouraged
by Royalty, and physicians from the provinces were
summoned to Berlin to be instructed by Dr. Baylies.
But as no one would submit to the operation, his
Majesty was obliged to utilise the children in the
orphan houses.

In Holland.—Inoculation was introduced, in 1748, by
Dr. Tronchin, who first operated on one of his sons, and

then on a number of persons, including some of high rank. Divines and physicians recommended inoculation, but it was not very generally adopted until 1746, when Morand and others practised it at Amsterdam.

In Denmark.—A countess was inoculated in 1754, and in 1758, two Inoculation Houses were established by the King, at Copenhagen, and in 1760 the Royal Prince was inoculated with success.

In Sweden.—The first trial was made in 1754. It made rapid progress in this country, for Dr. Schulz, a pupil of Dr. Archer, gave such a favourable report of the practice in London, that several Inoculation Houses were established.

In Switzerland.—Inoculation was introduced into Switzerland from Geneva, where it was first employed in 1751. In this country it was first performed in Lausanne by a lady who inoculated her own child, and this encouraged many to follow her example.

In Russia.—Inoculation was reported to have been practised at an early date in parts of the Russian Empire, but it was unknown at St. Petersburg in 1768, when it was introduced there and at Moscow by Dimsdale, who had been summoned to St. Petersburg to inoculate the Empress. Further details of Dimsdale's practice in Russia will be found in the description of the method of inoculation which he employed.[1]

---

[1] *Vide* p. 71.

In America.—In 1721, Small Pox visited this country after *an absence of nineteen years.* The Rev. Cotton Mather copied the accounts of inoculation given by Timoni and Pylarini in the *Philosophical Transactions of the Royal Society*, and sent them to the practitioners of Boston. 'Dr. Zabdiel Boylston[1] was induced to inoculate his child, and two of his negro servants, and in six months he had inoculated 244 persons.

It may be interesting to note that out of these 244 cases, in six there was no effect at all, and six died in consequence of the inoculation, but the deaths were attributed to other causes.

" And as to those who died under Inoculation, I would observe that Mrs. Doxwell, we have great reason to believe, was infected before. Mr. White thro' splenetic delusions, died rather from abstinence than the Small Pox. Mrs. Scarborough and the Indian girl died of accidents by taking cold. Mrs. Wells and Searle were persons worn out with Age and Diseases, and very likely these two were infected before."

The true explanation is to be found in the method which Boylston not only employed in his own cases, but also recommended to other inoculators.

"Take your Medicine or Pus from the **ripe pustules** of the Small Pox of the distinct kind, either from those in the natural way, or from the inoculated sort, provided the person be otherwise healthy and the matter good. . . .

[1] Boylston, *An Historical Account of the Small Pox inoculated in New England upon all Sorts of Persons, Whites, Blacks, and of all Ages and Constitutions.* 1726.

" My way of taking it is thus: Take a fine cut, sharp tooth-pick (which will not put the person in any fear, as a Lancet will do many), and open the Pock on one side, and press the Boil, and scoop the matter on your quill, and so on."

Boylston's experiments, and particularly his fatal cases, excited a great deal of opposition to inoculation, and many pamphlets were published both in defence of, and against, the practice. But the following manifesto gave a severe check to his operations :—

"*At a meeting by Public Authority in the Town-house of* Boston, *before His Majesty's Justices of the Peace and the Select-Men; the Practitioners of Physick and Surgery being called before them concerning* Inoculation, *agreed to the following conclusion :*—

" A Resolve upon a Debate held by the Physicians of *Boston*, concerning Inoculating the Small Pox, on the twenty first day of *July*, 1721. It appears by numerous Instances, That it has prov'd the Death of many Persons soon after the Operation, and brought Distempers upon many others, which have in the End prov'd fatal to 'em.

" That the natural tendency of infusing such malignant Filth in the Mass of Blood, is to corrupt and putrify it, and if there be not a sufficient Discharge of that Malignity by the Place of Incision or elsewhere, it lays a Foundation for many dangerous Diseases.

" That the Operation tends to spread and continue the Infection in a Place longer than it might otherwise be.

" That the continuing the Operation among us is likely to prove of most dangerous Consequence.

" *By the Select-Men of the Town of* Boston, *July* 22d.

" The Number of Persons, Men, Women, and Children, that have died of the Small Pox at *Boston*, from the middle of *April* last (being brought here then by the *Saltertuda's* Fleet) to the 23rd of this instant *July* (being the hottest and the worst Season of the Year to have any Distemper in), are, *viz.*,

2 Men Strangers, 3 men, 3 Young Men, 2 Women, 4 Children,
1 Negro Man, 1 Negro Woman, and 1 *Indian* Woman, 17 in
all ; of those that have had it, some are well recovered, and
others in a hopeful and fair Way of Recovery."

Boylston expressed his disapproval of this report
upon the cases of natural Small Pox.

"It is a thousand pities our Select-Men made so slight and
trifling a Representation of the Small Pox, that had always
prov'd so fatal in *New England*, as they seem to have done
in this Advertisement."

It would appear from this, that in order to make
converts to inoculation, it was necessary to keep alarming accounts of the natural Small Pox, before the eyes
of the public.

In 1764, Small Pox again visited Boston, and
three thousand persons were inoculated successfully;
and this result was attributed to the administration of
mercurials and antimony in the course of treatment
preparatory to the operation.

On the other hand, Inoculation was so unsuccessful in Philadelphia, that, in 1750, there was a strong
feeling in favour of abandoning it.

During the temporary decline of Inoculation in
England, it was progressing rapidly in South America.
A Carmelite missionary near the Portuese colony
of Para inoculated the Indians, who were being carried
off in large numbers by the Small Pox, in 1728 and
1729; another missionary on the banks of the Rio

Niger and some Portuguese inhabitants followed his example.

In 1738, Small Pox was imported into South Carolina by a cargo of slaves from Africa, and Mr. Mowbray, a surgeon, introduced Inoculation. He was followed by Dr. Kirkpatrick and others, so that before long, about a thousand persons were inoculated, eight of whom died in consequence. These fatal cases were subsequently alluded to by Dr. Kirkpatrick,[1] but the account is of little value, for, as Dr. Woodville says, " from the very defective statement given of the eight unsuccessful cases, the reader is unable to profit by a recital of them." In the island of St. Christopher, a planter inoculated three hundred of his slaves without a single loss.

[1] Kirkpatrick, *Essay on Inoculation.* 1743.

CHAPTER II.

HISTORY OF INOCULATION IN GREAT BRITAIN AND IRELAND.

In Wales.—When the Eastern method of preventing Small Pox was introduced into London, and especially when members of the Royal family were inoculated, this subject became a topic of general conversation ; the news spread into the country, and it then became known that a similar practice had long been employed in South Wales. As in the East, it was called *buying the Small Pox.* In Pembrokeshire, according to Dr. Perrot Williams,[1] the inhabitants had carried on this custom from time immemorial.

"In order to procure the distemper to themselves, they rub the matter taken from the pustules, when ripe, on several parts of the skin of the arms, etc., or prick those parts with pins or the like, first infected with the same matter. And notwithstanding they omit the necessary evacuations, such as purging, etc., yet, as I am inform'd, they generally come off well enough ; and what's remarkable, I cannot hear of one instance of their having the Small Pox a second time.

"A learned and very ingenious gentleman of this country told me not long since that about twenty years ago, when at school,

---

[1] Williams, *Phil. Trans.*, 1722, p. 263.

he and several of his schoolfellows (how many I don't exactly remember) infected themselves at the same time, from the same person, and that not one of them miscarry'd, though he had more of the Small Pox than he designed. : . .

" He solemnly declares that, having when at school, as I formerly said, rubb'd the skin off his left hand, where the scar is now very visible, with the back edge of his penknife, till the blood began to appear, he apply'd the variolous matter to that part. . . .

"There are now living in this Town [Haverford West] and neighbourhood five or six persons, who undoubtedly had that distemper after taking the foresaid method to infect themselves: one of whom, a young woman aged twenty-three, told me (since I received your letter) that, about eight or nine years ago, in order to infect herself, she held twenty pocky scabs (taken from one toward the latter end of the distemper) in the hollow of her hand a considerable time; that about ten or twelve days afterwards she sicken'd, and had upwards of thirty large pustules in her Face and other parts; and that she has since freely conversed with such as have had the Small Pox on them."

Mr. Wright,[1] surgeon, of Haverford West, also gave a description of buying the Small Pox in a letter to Mr. Sylvanus Bevan, an apothecary in London :—

" I received yours the 9th instant, and in answer to it will readily give you all the satisfaction I can, in relation to a very antient custom in this country; commonly called *buying the Small Pox*, which, upon a strict inquiry, since I had your letter, I find to be a common practice, and of very long standing; being assured by persons of unquestionable veracity, and of advanced age, that they have had the Small Pox communicated to themselves this way,[1] when about sixteen or seventeen years of age, they then being very capable of distinguishing that distemper from any other.; and that **they have parted with the matter contained in the pustules to others, producing the same effects.** There are two large

---

[1] Wright, *Phil. Trans.*, 1722, p. 267.

villages in this county near the harbour of *Milford* more famous
for this custom than any other, namely, *St. Ishmaels* and *Marloes.*
The old inhabitants of those villages, with which they abound,
being in a healthful situation, say that it has been a common
practice with them time out of mind ; and what was more remarkable, one, *William Allen* of *St. Ishmaels*, ninety years of age (who
died about six months ago or thereabouts), declared to some
persons of good sense and integrity, that this practice was used
all his time ; that he very well remembered his mother's telling
him, that it was a common practice all her time, and that she got
the Small Pox that way. These, together with the many other
informations I have met with from almost all parts of the county,
confirm me in the belief of its being a very antient and frequent
practice among the common people ; and to prove that this
method is still continued among us, I will give you the relation of
an elderly woman, a midwife, who accidentally came into company when your letter was reading, whose name is *Joan Jones*,
aged seventy years, of good credit and perfect memory. She
solemnly declares that about fifty-four years ago, having then the
Small Pox, one *Margaret Brown*, to the best of her remembrance
then about twelve or thirteen years of age, bought the Small Pox
of her ; that the said *Margaret Brown* was seized with the Small
Pox a few days afterwards ; that the said *Margaret Brown* had
not had the Small Pox a second time a twelvemonth ago, and she
verily believes that she had not had them since. She farther says
that she has known this way of procuring the Small Pox practised
from time to time above fifty years ; that it has been lately used
in her neighbourhood, and she knows but of one dying of the
said distemper when communicated after the method aforesaid,
which accident happened within these two years last past ; the
person who miscarried (a young woman about twenty years of
age) having procured the distemper from a man then dying of a
very malignant Small Pox. The above relation I heard the old
woman declare two days ago, and she was willing to take her
oath of it before Dr. Williams, who is a magistrate. As to what
you mention concerning the manner of communicating the infectious matter to the blood, by scraping the skin thin with a
penknife and so rubbing in the matter, that was only the case of

one particular gentleman, Mr. Owen, a counsellor at Law, whom I heard several times positively affirm that he bought the Small Pox when at school, and of such a Lady, now living, and gave her threepence for the Matter contained in twelve pustules. That hundreds in this country have had the Small Pox this way is certain ; and it cannot produce one single instance of their ever having them a second time."

In Scotland.—In the Highlands of Scotland, where, according to Kennedy[1] and Munro,[2] Small Pox inoculation was early employed, the disease was induced by a method somewhat similar to that of holding variolous scabs in the hand ; worsted threads charged with variolous matter being tied round the wrists.

"When Small Pox appears favourable in one child of a family, the parents generally allow commerce of their other children with the one in the disease ; nay, I am assured that in some of the remote Highland parts of this country, it has been an old practice of parents whose children have not had the Small Pox to watch for an opportunity of any child of their neighbours being in **good mild Small Pox,** that they may communicate the disease to their own children by making them bedfellows to those in it, and by tying worsted threads wet with the pocky matter round their wrists."

In the island of St. Kilda, Small Pox was communicated by rubbing the variolous matter upon the skin of the elbow joint.

Inoculation was not practised by surgeons in Scotland until 1726, when Mr. Maitland performed this operation upon ten persons ; but as one of these cases

---

[1] Kennedy, *loc. cit.*, p. 157. 1715.
[2] Monro, *Observations on the Different Kinds of Small Pox*, p. 54. 1818.

proved fatal, such a prejudice was excited that
twenty years elapsed before an attempt was made to
revive the practice. At Dumfries, where they had
suffered very greatly from Small Pox, inoculation
was introduced in 1733, but in other parts of North
Britain it was not adopted until 1753.

In Ireland.—Inoculation was first performed at
Dublin in 1723. In this and in the three following
years, twenty-five subjects were inoculated, and as
three out of this number died, the results were not
very encouraging. Two of these deaths occurred in
one family, in which five children had been inoculated.

The history of these cases was published by Dr.
Bryan Robinson, and as they well illustrate a very
common result of inoculation at this period, it will not
be without interest to produce his account in full.

" Various Reports having been spread concerning five Children,
upon whom the *Small Pox* was *inoculated*, I have been desired
to publish the true Account of their Case; which is as
follows.*

" A Gentleman had six Children, five Sons and a Daughter;
who from their Infancy had been kept to a regular cooling Diet,
and had scarcely tasted Flesh-meat 'till about a Year ago, and
since that time, eat only such as was of easy Digestion, and
that sparingly once a Day. The fourth Son, aged between

---

* " I was a Stranger to the Children, and was not consulted about them
'till the eleventh Morning after their Inoculation; and therefore am
obliged to their Parents, and those who attended them, for what relates
to their Diet, their Conſtitutions, the Manner of their being prepared
for the Disease, and the Effects produced by the Inoculation before I
saw them.

nine and ten Years, of a healthy Constitution, took the *Small Pox* in the natural Way on the 18th of *August*, 1725. His *Pock* being *distinct* and good, the Parents resolved to have the rest of their Children *inoculated* from him ; which was accordingly done on the 26th of *August*, the ninth Day of their Brother's Illness. They were each of them prepared for the Distemper by two Doses of a purging Infusion, one of which was given on the 21st, and the other on the 23rd. From the time of *Inoculation*, they were kept from Flesh-meat, and were only allow'd Bread and Milk, Bread and Butter, light Pudding, Tea with Milk, and things of that Nature.

" I. The eldest Son aged thirteen Years was nursed in the Country, where he continued 'till he was a Year and a half old, and was then brought home to his Parents in a very poor and weak Condition. Soon after he grew *rickety*, but recovered from that Disease in less than a Year. In some Months after his Recovery, he got a swelling in his Foot which suppurated, broke, and ran for several Weeks. After this was healed, he continued well for about three Years, then he had an Abscess in his Belly below the Navel, which suppurated, broke and was healed in about two Months. Since that time he enjoyed a very good state of Health, and was a strong lusty Boy when he was *inoculated*.

" On the eighth Day after *Inoculation*, he began to be dis-ordered with a Head-ach and Vomiting. His Vomiting was frequent and violent 'till the third Day of his Illness, and then it abated but did not cease, for he vomited at times 'till the fourth Day at Noon. No *Pock* appeared, but on the third, at Night, purple Spots of different sizes were observed all over his Body, many of which were as large in Diameter as a midling Pea. About this time he fainted ; and died in the Evening of the fourth Day, about twenty-four Hours after the first Appear-ance of the Spots. He was extreamly thirsty during his Illness, and for the most part pale and cold.

" His Incision had a good Digestion at the second Dressing, which was on the third Day after it was made, and continued in this State till the Day on which he sickened ; then it grew pale, flaccid, and had little or no Discharge. It continued thus 'till the third Day of his Sickness ; then it turned blackish, and was perfectly dry on the fourth, the Day on which he died.

"II. The second Son aged eleven Years of a healthy Constitution, began to be disordered on the Seventh, at Night. He first complained of a Pain in his Bones and Back, and the next Morning of a Pain in his Head, and was very dozy all that Day. On the third, he was very restless, raved much, and had a very uneasy Night. He vomited a little on the third and fourth, and what he threw up was blackish and mixed with Clots of Blood. The *Pock* began to appear on the fourth towards Night, and upon the Eruption all the fore-mentioned Symptoms vanished. He then bled two or three Spoonfuls from his Nose. On the fifth, in the Morning he was very easy and without a Fever. On the sixth, he complained of a sore Throat, began to spit, and continued spitting three or four Days. His *Pock* was *distinct*, ripened well, and he recovered.

"His Incision had a good Digestion on the third Day after *Inoculation*, and continued to make a good Discharge 'till he sickened ; then it grew pale and flaccid, and continued so 'till the seventh Day of his Sickness : From the seventh to the ninth it was blackish, and somewhat dry, but after that it again came to a good Digestion.

"III. The third Son aged about ten Years, a fresh colour'd, strong, healthy Boy, who never had had any Sickness, began to be disordered on the eighth Day after *Inoculation;* in the Evening he complained of a Pain in his Head and Belly. He was very hot, thirsty and restless all that Night. The next Day which was the second of his Sickness, he vomited in the Morning and continued vomiting at Times 'till the third Day in the Evening. Then the Eruption began, and on the fourth, in the Morning, it appear'd in his Face like an *Erysipelas*. I could not at that time discover any *Pustules* either on his Body or Limbs, but he had many purple Spots all over him, especially in his Neck and Loins, many of which were as large in Diameter as a great Pin's Head. On the fifth, the *Pock* began to appear in his Body and Limbs, and came out thick on the sixth. He was extreamly restless, and raved much from the Beginning of the Eruption to the sixth Day, but was pretty quiet that Night, slept and began to spit. On the seventh, his Face was swell'd, his Spitting continued, and he had some Sleep. On the eighth, he continued much in the same state, only drank and slept more than he had done before. On the ninth, in the morning, the swelling of his Face abated. On the eleventh, his Breath grew short, his Spitting stopt, and he died in the Evening. His *Pock* was the worst sort of the *confluent* Kind, it never fill'd nor digested; but continued flat and watery 'till his Death. He had no Thirst, and wou'd drink but little during his Illness.

" His Incision discharged a well digested Matter from the third Day after *Inoculation* 'till the Day on which he sickened: Then it grew pale, flaccid, and had little or no Discharge. It continued thus to the eighth Day of his Sickness, then it turned black and was scarified: On the ninth, it discharged a little thin Sanies: It grew quite dry on the tenth, the Day before he died.

" IV. The fifth Son, strong and healthy, aged about eight Years, began to be disordered on the seventh at Night with a feverish Heat, and a Pain in his Head. These Symptoms continued much the same all the next Day; but towards Evening the Fever encreased, and he had a very uneasy Night; he grew easier the following Morning, and continued so 'till Evening, when the *Small Pox* appeared. He sweated much all that Day. His *Pock* was *distinct* and good; he had but few, and recovered without any ill or irregular Symptoms.

" His Incision suffered no Change at the time of his Sickening, but discharged plentifully throughout the Distemper.

" V. The Daughter aged six Years, of a pale Complexion, but always healthy, began to be disordered on the seventh Day after *Inoculation*: Towards Night she grew hot and complained of a Pain in her Head. On the Day following, she vomited in the Morning; towards Evening her Fever encreased, and she had a very restless Night. She was much easier the third Morning, and continued so 'till Evening, when the *Pock* began to appear. She dozed all the fourth Day, had a Looseness, and vomited once or twice; towards Evening were observed many purple Spots, especially on her Neck and Breasts, the largest of which were not greater in diameter than a midling Pin's Head. She

had a *distinct Pock*, but was very full, especially in her Face
and Limbs. On the tenth, she had some loose Stools, two or
three whereof were bloody. The *Pock* fill'd, digested well, and
she recover'd.

" Her incision in the beginning had but an ill digestion : from
the time of her sickening it was pale and flaccid 'till the eighth
Day, then it grew blackish and was scarified, the Slough separated
on the tenth, and after that it had a good Discharge."

Inoculation in England.—The profession in
England was persuaded to adopt variolous inoculation
by Lady Mary Wortley Montagu.[1]

Kennedy, in his account of inoculation as practised in
the East, had rather advised against its introduction
into England. The accounts by Timoni and Pylarini,
which appeared in the *Transactions of the Royal Society*,
merely described the method. But in 1717, Lady Mary
Wortley Montagu, whose husband was ambassador at
the Ottoman Court, wrote a letter from Adrianople to a
friend, Mrs. S. C. (Miss Sarah Chiswell), in which she
expressed her determination to persuade the physicians
in London to resort to inoculation.

" *Apropos* of distempers, I am going to tell you a thing that I
am sure will make you wish yourself here. The Small Pox, so
fatal and so general amongst us, is here entirely harmless by the
invention of *ingrafting*, which is the term they give it. There
is a set of old women, who make it their business to perform the
operation every autumn in the month of September, when the great
heat is abated. People send to one another to know if any of

---

[1] *Letters and Works of Lady Mary Wortley Montagu*, vol. i., p. 184
New Edition. 1887.

their family has a mind to have the Small Pox. They make parties for this purpose, and when they are met (commonly fifteen or sixteen together), the old woman comes with a nutshell full of the matter of the **best sort of Small Pox**, and asks what veins you please to have opened. She immediately rips open that you offer to her with a large needle (which gives you no more pain than a common scratch), and puts into the vein as much venom as can lie upon the head of her needle, and after binds up the little wound with a hollow bit of shell; and in this manner opens four or five veins. The Grecians have commonly the superstition of opening one in the middle of the forehead, in each arm, and on the breast, to mark the sign of the cross; but this has a very ill effect, all these wounds leaving little scars, and is not done by those that are not superstitious, who choose to have them in the legs, or that part of the arm that is concealed. The children or young patients play together all the rest of the day, and are in perfect health to the eighth. Then the fever begins to seize them, and they keep their beds two days, very seldom three. **They have very rarely above twenty or thirty in their faces, which never mark; and in eight days' time they are as well as before their illness.** Where they are wounded, there remain running sores during the distemper, which I don't doubt is a great relief to it. Every year thousands undergo this operation; and the French Ambassador says pleasantly that they take the Small Pox here by way of diversion, as they take the waters in other countries. There is no example of any one that has died in it, and you may believe I am very well satisfied of the safety of the experiment, since I intend to try it on my dear little son. I am patriot enough to take pains to bring this useful invention into fashion in England; and I should not fail to write to some of our doctors very particularly about it, if I knew any one of them that I thought had virtue enough to destroy such a considerable branch of their revenue for the good of mankind. But that distemper is too beneficial to them not to expose to all their resentment the hardy wight that should undertake to put an end to it. Perhaps if I live to return, I may, however, have courage to war with them. Upon this occasion admire the heroism in the heart of your friend."

Lady Mary Wortley Montagu accordingly desired Mr. Maitland, surgeon to the Embassy, to procure variolous matter from a suitable subject, and an old Greek woman, many years in the habit of inoculating, was employed to insert it. The woman inoculated one arm, and Maitland the other; the disease ensued in due course, with an eruption of about one hundred pustules. This took place in March 1717, and was the first time that the Byzantine method of inoculation was performed on an English subject; but this method was not employed in England until the year 1721, and in the same year the first essay was published in which inoculation was recommended.

Dr. de Castro[1] stated that it was employed by the Greeks, Turks, and Italians, and that it was probably introduced by ignorant peasants.

"That it first proceeded from some of the populace who were neither men of Fortune, Character, nor Learning, seems to me very probable, in that it appeared in the World without the least recommendation from any of the Learned, and met with very considerable opposition from the rich."

We learn from this essay that inoculation was at this date secretly employed in London.

"I have had it very well attested to me, that a Certain Gentleman of this City had the operation performed upon two of his Children this last winter; and that his expectations were fully answered in the event."

De Castro advocated arm to arm variolation.

[1] *A Dissertation on the Method of inoculating the Small Pox.* By J.C., M.D., 1721.

" There are few or none that make use of the Pus extracted from any who have this Disease by transplantation, but this being of a milder Disposition (I am very inclinable to believe), will be as proper as any other."

His pamphlet concludes by a recommendation to physicians to introduce the practice, as it was always attended with success.

" There, if I am not very much mistaken (being a real matter of fact), may be a sufficient encouragement to all, especially the *Fair Sex*, to endeavour to have this method introduced and practised in this Kingdom ; as also to the Physicians to direct their Friends and Acquaintances to admit of the operation."

Very shortly after the issue of this pamphlet, Dr. Harris delivered a lecture [1] before the College of Physicians of London, and described the Byzantine and Chinese methods. He was the first to mention inoculation by means of a *thread* imbued with the variolous pus, which method had been successfully practised upon four children of the French Consul at Aleppo, when secretary to the Marquis de Chateauneuf at Constantinople.

But it was not, as already stated, until April 1721 that, owing to the enthusiasm of Lady Mary Wortley Montagu, the Byzantine method was openly employed in England. After the successful result of the inoculation of her son in Turkey, Lady Mary determined to submit her daughter, an infant three months old, to the same operation. This was postponed for a while,

---

[1] *De Peste Dissertatio*, 1721 (quoted by Woodville).

but was eventually carried out in England by Maitland, in April 1721.

Maitland performed a second inoculation, in the following May, upon the son of Dr. Keith, with a favourable result. This was soon generally known in London, for the news spread rapidly, and excited the greatest interest among people of all ranks. Nevertheless, inoculation made very little progress, for it was regarded with so much fear and suspicion, that several months elapsed before a third trial took place in London. In fact, inoculation was regarded as of such a dangerous nature, that an attempt was not again made until there was an opportunity of inoculating some criminals in Newgate, who were promised a full pardon if they submitted to the experiment. They accepted the offer, and were accordingly inoculated by Maitland on the 9th of August, 1721. None of them had the disease severely; in fact, there were only sixty pustules on the one in whom the operation produced the most effect. A seventh criminal was experimented upon by the Chinese method. The disease followed in a mild form, but the patient suffered from severe pains in her head, from the commencement of the eruption to the maturation of the pustules. These cases, however, were not sufficient to convince the public of the safety and advantage of inoculation; and many contended that as the eruptions were so few, the true disease had not been communicated, and therefore the inoculated were liable to the disease contracted in the ordinary way. Consequently Maitland inoculated only eight persons in the following six months.

In the account given by Maitland[1] of these cases, we have the first intimation of a danger arising from this practice, which a century later was the strongest argument for not only abandoning it, but also for suppressive legislation. The first of these patients was Mary Batt, two years old, the daughter of a Quaker, inoculated October 2nd, 1721. This child, having only twenty pustules, soon recovered.

"But what happened afterwards was, I must own, not a little surprising to me, not having seen or observed anything like it before. The case was in short this: Six of Mr. Batt's domestic servants, who all in turn were wont to hug and caress this child whilst under the operation, and whilst the pustules were out upon her, never suspecting them to be catching (nor indeed did I), were all seized at once with the right natural Small Pox of several and very different kinds."

In spite of this disaster, the practice was adopted by Dr. Nettleton, of Halifax, Yorkshire, who in three months inoculated forty persons. Dr. Nettleton introduced a system of preparing his patients by means of purgatives, emetics, and occasionally by bleeding. Two incisions were made, one in the arm, and the other in the leg of the opposite side, and variolous matter dropped into the wounds. Later he employed a simpler method, cotton-wool being impregnated with variolous

[1] Maitland. *Account of inoculating the Small Pox.* 1722.

pus, and applied to the incisions for twenty-four hours, by means of a plaster.

In 1772, inoculation was more generally adopted. The Princess of Wales ordered it to be practised upon some charity children, and the successful result induced Her Royal Highness to have the two young princesses inoculated. They were both successfully infected, and the example of Her Royal Highness was followed by others, and thus much encouragement was given, for a time, to the new practice.

It was, however, soon destined to receive a great check, for the Hon. William Spencer and the butler of Lord Bathurst had both of them a copious eruption, and the disease in both cases terminated fatally. Another patient, Miss Rigby, died about eight weeks after inoculation, so that there were 3 deaths in 182 inoculations, or nearly 1 in 60.

The ill-success that had attended Maitland's inoculations in this country, caused him to be severely criticised, and it was generally considered that he had been imposed upon by the old women in Turkey. For he had described the treatment employed in Turkey, as very mild, and yet he had had deaths in consequence ; and further, he had committed himself to the opinion that the inoculated Small Pox was not infectious.

Woodville,[1] writing more than seventy years afterwards, refers to these failures in the following terms :—

---

[1] Woodville, *loc. cit.*, p 123.

" That inoculation did not constantly succeed in producing the distinct or favourable kind of Small Pox was at that time, and still continues to be, a melancholy truth; but the inoculators were at first unwilling to acknowledge it, and by attempting to attribute the death of persons inoculated to other accidental causes, exposed themselves to just censure."

A strong feeling of opposition to the practice arose, and both clergymen and physicians became ardent anti-inoculators. In 1722, an anonymous pamphlet[1] appeared, which described inoculation as the outcome of atheism, quackery, and avarice. The Rev. Mr. Massey preached a sermon, in which he condemned it as a dangerous and sinful practice; and Dr. Wagstaffe,[2] a physician of St. Bartholomew's Hospital, expressed a desire to have further evidence of the efficacy of inoculation, and considered that posterity would marvel that a practice employed by a few ignorant women amongst an illiterate and unthinking people, should have so suddenly been adopted by one of the politest nations in the world. In criticising the cases in the family of Mr. Batt, he said :—

"I am well informed by Persons of unquestionable reputation, that the Town of Hertford is a lamentable Evidence of the danger of this practice, where the Distemper was spread by it to that degree, as not only to make an havock of the Inhabitants, but to hinder the Commerce of the place. Thus the Operator has it in his power to convey the Small Pox to distant Places and Persons, who neither

[1] *The New Practice of Inoculation considered, and an Humble Application to the Approaching Parliament for the Regulation of that Dangerous Experiment.*

[2] Wagstaffe. A letter to Dr. Freind. 1722.

avow his practice or desire his experiment : And if 'tis possible
that the *ingrafted Pox* can be so poysonous as to communicate
certain death to all around by this method, they may ingraft as
violent a Plague as has been known among us.   How far the Legislature may think fit to interpose, in order to prevent such an
artificial way of depopulating a Country, is not my Province to
determine."

The anti-inoculators were in turn answered by Drs.
Crawford,[1] Brady,[2] Williams,[3] and Maitland.[4]   The subject gave rise to such an acute controversy, that these
publications were in turn replied to in the same year.

Mr. Tanner,[5] a surgeon at St. Thomas's Hospital,
declared that he had inoculated a person who had had
Small Pox several years previously, and that a discharge from the incisions, and irregular eruptions,
followed, " appearances which the inoculators in the
experiments at Newgate had deemed sufficient to
prevent the patient's having the Small Pox in future."

The opposition was counteracted by the letters of
Dr. Jurin,[6] who examined the question by means of
statistics.   He arrived at the conclusion that of all
children born, 1 in 14 dies some time or other of

---

[1] Crawford.   *The Case of Inoculating the Small Pox considered, and
its Advantages asserted.*

[2] Brady.   *Some Remarks on Dr.Wagstaffe's Letter and Mr. Massey's
Sermon.*

[3] Williams.   *Some Remarks on Dr. Wagstaffe's Letter, with an
Appendix.*

[4] Maitland.   *Mr. Maitland's Account of inoculating the Small Pox
vindicated.*

[5] Blackmore.   *Treatise on the Small Pox*, p. 92.

[6] Jurin.   *Letter to Dr. Cotesworth.*

Small Pox, while of all persons inoculated with choice of subjects, only 1 dies in 91. Jurin decided in favour of inoculation, and in consequence it continued to make steady progress.

In 1723, it was advocated by persons of rank, and by the heads of the Church. The number of persons inoculated during the years 1721-3 amounted to 474, 9 of whom died. There are several points of interest in the history of these cases. In the first place, in addition to the fact that 9 died as the result of inoculation, there were 29 in whom inoculation had no effect, and in 5 it had an imperfect effect. Of the 29 in which there was no effect, 9 occurred between the ages of twenty and fifty-two.

In 1724, there were only 40 persons inoculated; but Dr. Jurin considered that it was not unnatural that people should object to a practice in which there was risk, unless impelled to it by the dread of a greater danger; and in this year, natural Small Pox had somewhat abated. In 1725, natural Small Pox was very fatal, and people again resorted to inoculation. But in 1727-8, the practice began to decline, in spite of the fact that Small Pox generally prevailed. In these two years, only 124 were inoculated, 87 and 37 respectively, and 3 died from the effects of the operation. The first was a son of Mr. Wansey, of Warminster, aged one year and a half; the second was Enoch Trumble,

aged eight months.; and the third was a boy eleven
years old, the son of a person of rank in London,
whose name was concealed. Thus, during the first
eight years of inoculation in Great Britain, there were
897 persons inoculated ; 845 had true variolous pustules,
13 an imperfect eruption, in 39 no distemper was produced by the operation, and 17 died. With regard to
the 13 having an imperfect eruption, Dr. Scheuchzer [1]
says :—

"By having an *imperfect Small Pox* is meant the having
some slighter eruption of but a few days' continuance, but this
attended with an inflammation and running of the incisions
for the usual time, and generally preceded by some of the
common symptoms of the Small Pox ; this being esteemed by
the accounts from Turkey, and our own experience at home
as far as it goes, to be an effectual security against having the
Small Pox afterwards in the natural way."

In spite of the fatal cases, an advantage was claimed.
for inoculation, in that it had been calculated, that or
all those affected with Small Pox in the ordinary way,
about one in six died, whereas the deaths from inoculation contended for by the anti-inoculators amounted
to not more than one in fifty. In 1731, a pamphlet
was published exposing the fallacies in Dr. Jurin's
and Dr. Scheuchzer's statistics, and claiming that the
advantage of the inoculated Small Pox over the
natural disease was fictitious. The writer maintained

---

[1] Scheuchzer, *loc. cit.*

[2] *An Enquiry into the Advantages received by the First Eight Years'
Inoculation.* 1731.

that by inoculation the variolous infection was spread far and wide, and a considerable increase of mortality by Small Pox occasioned; thus the lives saved to the persons themselves inoculated fell short of the lives lost from the increased infection. To this pamphlet no direct reply was forthcoming, but papers both in favour of and against inoculation, continued to be issued from time to time. Dr. Warren regarded it as a " barbarous and dangerous invention imported from Turkey."

The successful and encouraging results reported from America, and the increase in the fatality of the natural Small Pox in Great Britain, led to a revival of the practice of inoculation, so that after 1738, it was very generally employed. In 5 towns, 2,000 were inoculated in 1742, of whom 2 women, both with child, died. In 1753, 422 inoculations were made, with 4 deaths. At Rye, in Sussex, 300 people were inoculated, with 1 death, and at Blandford, in Dorsetshire, 400, with only 1 death. In London, out of 1,500 cases, only 3 terminated unfavourably. At the Foundling Hospital, 186 were inoculated, and 1 died; and the same surgeon who had inoculated these cases lost, in private practice, only 1 case in 370. The progress made by inoculation at this period was in a great measure due to Dr. Mead's[1] publication in 1747, in which he devoted a chapter to inoculation, and

---

[1] Mead. *Small Pox and Measles.* 1747.

spoke in favour of it, and to Dr. Frewen's[1] work, which claimed a great success for this treatment. In the year 1746, the art of inoculation was still further encouraged by the establishment of an Inoculation Hospital. But the public were still very strongly prejudiced against it, and the patients on leaving the hospital were often abused and insulted in the street, so that they were not suffered to depart until the darkness of the night enabled them to do so without being observed.[2] These prejudices were gradually overcome in various ways. Dr. Maddox, Bishop of Worcester, President of the Small Pox Hospital, preached a powerful sermon, which was published, and passed through seven editions. This had a great effect upon the public mind, as well as the fact that out of 593 persons successfully treated, only 1 died. Inoculation now made uninterrupted progress. At the same time, the opposition of the anti-inoculators was not silenced. An anonymous discourse was published in 1751, and the Rev. Theodore De la Faye[3] preached a sermon as powerful as that of the Bishop of Worcester, and in opposition to his conclusions. The sermon was replied to by Mr. Bolaine[4] and Dr. Kirkpatrick.[5] These were answered by De

---

[1] Frewen. *The Practice and Theory of Inoculation, with an Account of its Success.*

[2] Woodville, *loc. cit.*, p. 238.

[3] De la Faye. *Inoculation an Indefensible Practice.* 1753.

[4] Bolaine. *Letter addressed to Mr. de la Faye.*

[5] Kirkpatrick. *The Analysis of Inoculation.*

la Faye,[1] which in turn called forth another pamphlet from Mr. Bolaine.[2] Mr. David Some and Dr. Dodd- ridge, " two respectable divines," were also in favour of the new practice.[3] Early in the year 1754, two works recommending inoculation were published, one by Mr. Burgess, and the other by Dr. Kirkpatrick.

In the same year, it was resolved to inoculate the three royal children who had not yet had Small Pox. In the meantime, the Prince of Wales took the disease casually, and Prince Edward and Princess Augusta were inoculated with variolous matter taken from him. This fact, and particularly the following declaration of the College of Physicians, still further tended to establish the practice.

" THE COLLEGE, HAVING BEEN INFORMED THAT FALSE REPORTS CONCERNING THE SUCCESS OF INOCULATION IN ENGLAND HAVE BEEN PUBLISHED IN FOREIGN COUNTRIES, THINK PROPER TO DECLARE THEIR SENTIMENTS IN THE FOLLOWING MANNER, VIZ. :—THAT THE ARGUMENTS WHICH AT THE COMMENCEMENT OF THIS PRACTICE WERE URGED AGAINST IT HAVE BEEN REFUTED BY EXPERIENCE ; THAT IT IS NOW HELD BY THE ENGLISH IN GREATER ESTEEM, AND PRACTISED AMONG THEM MORE EXTENSIVELY THAN EVER IT WAS BEFORE ; AND THAT THE COLLEGE THINKS IT TO BE HIGHLY . SALUTARY TO THE HUMAN RACE."

In 1758, an anonymous address was published, in which the writer wished to restrict the practice of

---

[1] De la Faye. *A Vindication of a Sermon, etc.*

[2] Bolaine. *Remarks on the Rev. Mr. de la Faye's Vindication of his Sermon.*

[3] Some and Doddridge. *The Case of receiving the Small Pox by Inoculation impartially considered.*

inoculation to the physicians. This was speedily answered by Mr. Cooper, a surgeon. In 1759, Dr. Franklin gave an account of the success of inoculation in England and America, and wrote to the effect "that it did not seem to make that progress among the common people of America which at first was expected." Dr. Heberden followed with *Plain Instructions for Inoculation,* and in 1761, a second edition of Dr. Kirkpatrick's work appeared. He was the first writer to give an account of inoculation by vesication or blister, a method which appears to have been made use of in Paris by Dr. Tronchin as early as 1756. In 1764, Dr. Alexander Munro gave an account of the inoculation of Small Pox in Scotland, and in 1765, the practice of inoculation was "impartially considered" by Dr. Andrews, of Exeter, and its "signal advantages fully approved."

A new epoch in the history of inoculation commenced with the introduction of the Suttonian method, which "in the year 1765, had extended so rapidly in the counties of Essex and Kent, as to much interest the public, who were not less surprised by the novel method in which it was conducted, than by the uninterrupted success with which it was attended, upon a prodigious number of persons."

Mr. Robert Sutton, who acquired great celebrity as an inoculator, lived at Debenham in Suffolk, where he practised surgery and pharmacy. He began the prac-

tice of inoculation in 1757, and in eleven years inoculated
2,514 persons. His sons, Robert and Daniel, following
the medical profession, assisted him during the first three
years of his practice. Robert established himself as
an inoculator at Bury St. Edmunds, while Daniel,
after being an assistant to a surgeon at Oxford, returned
to Debenham, and suggested to his father a new plan
of inoculation. It was said that he proposed to shorten
the time of preparation to a few days, and not to confine the inoculated patients to the house, but to
oblige them to be exposed as much as possible to
the open air. The father condemned the scheme;
but the treatment was so approved of by the patients,
that they desired to be inoculated by the son, rather
than by the father, which led to a quarrel and a
separation. Mr. D. Sutton then opened an Inoculation House near Ingatestone, in Essex. Here he
made known, by advertisements and handbills, his
intention of inoculating on an improved principle, and
hinted that by the use of certain medicines, he could
keep the disease entirely under his control. His
system was so appreciated, that at the end of the first
year, his practice produced him two thousand guineas,
and in the second year, his fees amounted to more
than three times that sum. He obtained such a
widespread reputation, and his patients were so
numerous, that it was difficult to accommodate them
in the village of Ingatestone. Mr. Sutton also

employed a clergyman, who preached sermons, and wrote exaggerated accounts of his results. The Rev. Robert Houlton, the advocating clergyman, attributed the success to Mr. Sutton's treatment. He said "that not one person out of a thousand inoculated by Mr. Sutton had more variolous pustules than he could wish, and that *if any patient had twenty or thirty pustules he was said to have the Small Pox very heavily.*" The reason that Mr. Houlton gave for this was, that Mr. Sutton, perceiving a symptom in the patients of great fever, or a probability of their having more pustules than they would choose, quickly prevented both by virtue of his medicines, for "the Sutton family is in possession of an inestimable medicine, by use of which too great a burden of pusules can infallibly be prevented." According to Mr. Houlton, the number of persons inoculated by Mr. Daniel Sutton, from 1764-6, amounted to 13,792 ; and, with the aid of his assistants, he had inoculated altogether 20,000 persons. He denied that a single patient had died *fairly* from the inoculation, the deaths which had occurred being attributed to other causes.

Woodville,[1] in referring to this new method, says :—

"Though this and other accounts of Mr. Sutton's practice magnified it beyond its real merit, yet not a doubt was entertained but that the Suttonian plan of inoculation was incomparably more successful than that of any other practitioner." . . .

_____

[1] Woodville, *loc. cit.*, p. 353.

It is not surprising that physicians were extremely anxious to find out the secret of Mr. Sutton's success. Dr. Baker[1] was one of the first to get detailed information of the new method, and he published an account of it. Dr. Rushlin, by means of an "ingenious gentleman who was conversant with Mr. Sutton's patients," obtained samples of the medicines, and subjected them to analysis. Dr. Langton described the method as a gross imposition, and argued that the matter communicated was not the Small Pox.

He pointed out that the practice was, to take the virus the fourth day after the incision was made.

"By this means you have a *contagious caustic water* instead of laudable pus, and a slight ferment in the lymph is raised, producing a few watery blotches in the place of a perfect extrusion of the variolous matter."

In 1767, the arguments of Dr. Langton and Mr. Bromfield were replied to by Dr. Giles Watts.[2] To explain why the effect of the new treatment was so slight, and to justify it, it was said that the aim was to get inoculation without pustules, because they were mindful of the observation of Dr. Boerhaave, that the Small Pox often happened without any pustules at all. That the result of the Suttonian inoculation was, as a rule, very slight indeed, was admitted.

---

[1] Baker. *An Inquiry into the Merits of a Method of Inoculating the Small Pox.* 1766.

[2] Giles Watts. *A Vindication of the New Method of Inoculating the Small Pox.* 1767.

"To say the truth, it is a fact well known to inoculators in this way, and I have sometimes known the same happen in the old, that the patients pretty often pass through the Small Pox so easily, as to have no more than five pustules. Nay, it happens every now and then in this way of inoculation, that even an adult patient shall pass through the distemper without having one, or even so much as a single complaint other than perhaps a slight shivering chill or some such trifling disorder, which he would hardly have taken the least notice of at any other time, so very powerful is the present method of preparation and management in lessening the violence of the distemper. When this happens, and especially if it happens without a considerable inflammation of the skin round the puncture, the patient can hardly be brought to believe he has had the Small Pox. In such cases, it is ever prudent in the operator for the satisfaction of the patients to inoculate them again."

Dr. Giles Watts also considered that Dr. Langton's criticism was wide of the mark.

"It was, without doubt, the practice of Mr. Sutton to inoculate from the punctures on the arms of his patients *while the matter in them was yet crude, and before the eruptive symptoms came on.* And it seems as if he looked on this as a necessary caution, in order to render the distemper, so inoculated, light on the patient."

But while admitting this, Dr. Giles Watts was of opinion that it did not matter whether the patient were inoculated with crude variolous lymph or yellow concocted variolous matter.

In spite of criticism, the Suttonian method of inoculation gained general approval; and even in 1815, Moore[1] spoke disapprovingly only of Sutton's unprofessional conduct.

---

[1] Moore, *The History of the Small Pox*, p. 270. 1815.

"It is much to be regretted that Daniel Sutton should have stooped to employ such unworthy devices, for his plan of treatment was greatly superior to that of any former practitioner, and had he followed the correct rules of open professional conduct, his name would have been recorded with honourable distinction."

It was impossible to entirely conceal the method. Physicians and chemists not only analysed his medicines, but endeavoured to find out the whole system. Information was obtained from his patients, and as he communicated his treatment to many distant practitioners on condition of half profits, the secret could not long be kept. The essential points were all discovered. Dr. Dimsdale[1] was one of the first to turn the Suttonian system to good account. He adopted the method in his own practice, and incorporated an account of all the essential part of the new method in a treatise on inoculation.

Dimsdale became so famous for his inoculations, that when the Empress of Russia desired to be submitted to the operation, he was appointed to perform it. His tracts on inoculation, which were written and published at St. Petersburg, will be referred to in detail in discussing the Suttonian method and its results.

In consequence of Dimsdale's works, inoculation became for a time very much more popular than before. It was rivalled by Cow Pox inoculation in 1798, and finally forbidden by Act of Parliament in 1840.

---

[1] Dimsdale. *The Present Method of Inoculating for the Small Pox.* 1779.

CHAPTER III.

THE OPERATION OF INOCULATION.

THE accounts of inoculation which have already been given, have included several different methods of performing the operation. But the writers who first described the custom which prevailed in different parts of the world, of " buying " or " ingrafting " the Small Pox, were unacquainted with the details which were essential for the performance of the operation with comparative safety ; and it is only by regarding their descriptions in the light of events which followed the introduction of the practice into this country, that we can fully appreciate the fact that inoculators in the East were taught many necessary precautions by long experience.

Practice of the Brahmins.—In Hindostan, the operation was performed only at certain seasons of the year, and a preparatory regimen was enforced. Probably, the Brahmins selected the subjects for inoculation, as well as the subjects from whom they took the variolous matter. They had certainly learnt by experience the varying intensity of the contents of the Small Pox pustule, for they were credited with being able to control the amount of eruption by the method of operation.

Practice of the Greeks.—The old Grecian women were still more cautious in their procedure, and, according to Gatti,[1] inoculated tens of thousands without an accident. They dispensed with a preparatory treatment, as they only operated upon those in perfect health.

"All that is considered is whether the breath is sweet, the skin soft, and whether a little wound in it heals easily. Whenever these conditions are found, they inoculate without the least apprehension of danger."

Having selected their subjects, they made punctures with *needles*, and were particularly careful "*in the choice of the Ferment;*" variolous matter being used in the *crude* state, freshly obtained from "*the kindly pustules of a young child.*"

Maitland's, or the English Practice.—When Lady Mary Wortley Montagu had her child inoculated at Pera, an old Greek woman was employed to insert the variolous matter. But Mr. Maitland, who was present, disapproved of the method, of which he gave the following account :—

"But the good woman went to work so awkwardly, and by the shaking of her hand put the child to so much torture with her blunt and rusty needle, that I pitied his cries, and therefore inoculated the other arm with my own instrument, and with so little pain to him that he did not in the least complain of it."

When the same surgeon operated on the Newgate

---

[1] Quoted by Baker, *loc. cit.*, p. 26.

criminals, *incisions* were made through the cutis, and pledgets applied which had been steeped in variolous pus from *ripe* pustules. This method, called the Improved or Reformed operation, was soon modified, for frequently very troublesome ulcers resulted. Kirkpatrick mentions the case of a young gentleman who, with a favourable eruption by inoculation, had nevertheless an arm so terribly ulcerated that amputation was apprehended.

Maitland performed the operation without selection 'of subjects or other precautions, and consequently with occasionally disastrous results similar to the examples which have already been given.[1]

Jurin's Practice.—In 1729, Dr. Jurin recommended—

" *Firstly.* Great care to be taken only to inoculate none but persons of a good habit of body, and free not only from any apparent, but, as far as could be judged, from any latent disease.

" *Secondly.* The body, especially if plethoric, ought to be prepared by proper evacuations, bleeding, purging, vomiting, etc.

" *Thirdly.* The utmost caution ought to be used in the choice of **proper matter** to communicate the infection. It should be taken from a young subject, otherwise perfectly sound and healthful, who has **the Small Pox in the most favourable manner.** When the pustules were **perfectly maturated,** and just upon the turn or soon after, two or three of them should be ripped with a glover's needle or small lancet, and a couple of small pledgets of lint or cotton are to be well moistened with the matter, and immediately put into a little vial or box, and carried in the warm hand or bosom of the operator to the house of the person to be inoculated.

[1] *Vide* pp. 20, 28, 37.

"*Fourthly*. The incisions are usually made with a small lancet in the brawny part of both arms, or in one arm and the opposite leg, cutting just into or at most through the cutis or true skin for the length of a quarter of an inch, half an inch, or at most an inch. This being done, one of the pledgets moistened with the infectious matter is to be laid upon each incision, and to be kept on, by means of a bit of sticking plaister laid over it, for about four and twenty hours; after which, all may be taken off, and the incision dressed with common diachylon, or with only warm cabbage and colewort leaves once a day at first; and afterwards, when the discharge is considerable, twice a day till they heal; or only with a linen roller to defend them from the air.

"*Fifthly*. The person inoculated sometimes receives the Small Pox without any previous sickness, as often happens in the most favourable sort in the natural way. But the greater part begin to be a little feverish, and have more or less of the usual symptoms preceding the natural Small Pox, most commonly upon the eighth day from inoculation, though pretty often upon the seventh, and very rarely a day or two sooner or later.

"*Sixthly*. The patients are sometimes taken with flushing heats, which disappear again in a little time, about the fourth or fifth day; but the eruption of the pustules happened generally within a day, or sometimes two or three after the sickening, viz., most commonly on the ninth day, less frequently on the tenth, and still less on the eighth or eleventh. In a few cases it appeared on the seventh or twelfth, in one case on the eighteenth, in one on the twenty fourth, and in one on the sixth, and in one on the third. The last patient but one had the confluent sort, and died. The last was very full of the distinct kind, and recovered.

"*Seventhly*. The incisions begin to grow sore and painful about the fourth or fifth day, and about the sixth, seventh, or eighth, they begin to digest and run with a thick purulent matter, which gradually increases till about the turn of the distemper, during which time the wounds grow wide and deep; afterwards, the running gradually abates, and they usually heal up in about a month, sometimes in three weeks; though, in some, they continue running five or six weeks, or sometimes longer. The greater the discharge is by the incisions, the more favourable the distemper is found in other respects. **When the inoculation does not take effect, the incisions heal up in a few days, like a common cut."**

Dr. Jurin says nothing about medicinal treatment; but, according to Dr. Whitaker, the patients were restricted to a vegetable diet, and were never exposed to the cold air, but were kept in a warm room, especially during the eruptive fever. · When the fever was considerable, bleeding, blistering, and diaphoretics were employed, with occasional recourse to anodynes. After the appearance of the eruption, the same treatment as was followed in the natural Small Pox.

Practice of Burgess.—In spite of the precautions which had been recommended by Jurin, inoculation still continued to be followed occasionally by bad results. It was by no means a safe operation, and in order to diminish the risks, Mr. James Burgess published, in 1766, an account of the necessary preparations and management, with additions and improvements.

Method of Preparation.—The patient was enjoined · to avoid all excesses, and to be regular and moderate in taking exercise; the latter was considered necessary in order to promote the natural secretions and diminish the disposition of the blood to inflammation. Diet was to be restricted both in quantity and quality. A gentle purgative was administered at the end of the second week of preparation, and this was repeated three times, at intervals of three days. For children a dose of manna or syrup of roses was sufficient. Adults were to be entirely free from business of all kinds during this period, to avoid all close application and sitting long at reading, being recommended to pass the time agreeably with a few friends. Exercise was to be taken only during the day and when the weather was fine; all fatigue of body and anxiety of mind carefully avoided. In fact, the course of preparation could be summed up in three words—"temperance, quiet, and cheerfulness." The patient, being in a proper state of body and mind, would then pass safely through the distemper, his system being "cleared from those obstructions that so often proved dangerous to those who have neglected the opportunity of being properly prepared for the reception of the infectious venom." Individual temperaments were also taken into account, as well as age and season. It was necessary to be informed of the exact state of the patient's health, both before and at the time of inoculation.

The Operation and its Accidents.—When the patient was considered in a fit state, the operation was performed in the following way :—An incision of about an inch long was made on each arm through the cuticle into the skin, but *not so deep as to wound the cellular membrane*. A thread, saturated with vario-lous matter, was laid along the whole length of the

wound, and covered with a pledget of digestive ointment, fastened on with a digestive plaster and secured
with a thin linen roller. This dressing was continued
for two days, and on examining the wound on the
third day, it was found slightly inflamed. Two or
three days after, the edges of the wound looked
whitish, a certain sign that the inoculation had taken.
On the seventh day after the operation, or soon after,
the patient experienced chilliness, with slight shiverings, pains in the back and limbs, weight and pain in
the head, and sickness.

Young children became drowsy and heavy, and
sometimes suffered from frequent convulsions ; they were
kept in bed, and supplied with warm liquids, and these
symptoms gradually abated, and sweating ensued. On
the second day after the first appearance of constitutional
symptoms a rash, resembling flea-bites, often made
its appearance, sometimes closely simulating the rash
of scarlet fever. About the fourth day, all other
symptoms decreasing, the variolous eruptions commenced as small red spots, which by the beginning
of the fifth day had risen apparently above the skin.
From this time the pimples daily rose higher, and
gradually changed from red to a whitish-yellow hue,
till, on the seventh day from the eruption on the face,
they became pustules charged with matter, and by
the ninth day the same alteration occurred upon the
limbs ; from this time all the outward marks of

inflammation ceased entirely, the skin of the pustules shrivelled, the matter contained in them thickened into a scab, and the patient was out of danger.

This was the regular course of inoculated Small Pox, but sometimes children suffered from diarrhœa, adults with bleeding at the nose; sometimes much more serious symptoms ensued.

Management after Inoculation. — The patient was confined to his apartment and carefully dieted. If there were depression or nervousness, a little wine was allowed. On the seventh day, when the constitutional symptoms showed themselves, the patient was put to bed, and any tendency to constipation was corrected by means of roasted apples, currants boiled in a bag and squeezed into water gruel, or fruit boiled in oatmeal. If these were insufficient, a clyster was administered, or a gentle purge given. When there were more severe symptoms, the patients were bled and blistered. When the eruption began to appear, the symptoms were relieved, but the patient was kept in bed until after the crisis, and then allowed to sit up, care being taken to avoid a chill. Abstinence from solid animal diet was enforced, unless the attack was very slight, in which case fish was allowed.

Accidents after Inoculation.—Sometimes open sores, with central sloughs, resulted. The slough often extended in breadth and depth, and the wound discharged an ichorous pus, which corroded the adjoining

parts, and the inflammation extended down to the
elbow; in others the wounds were very well condi-
tioned, and the discharge moderate. The wounds
often continued discharging about a fortnight or three
weeks after the turn of the Small Pox, or even
longer, and then healed up kindly under some simple
dressing; but poultices were sometimes necessary, and
bleeding and gentle purging resorted to, to encourage
the wound to heal.

Failure of the Operation.—Sometimes it happened
that the inoculation did not take, although it had been
correctly performed, and the matter good and properly
taken, the incision healing in a few days. In reference
to these results Burgess says :—

"When this is the case the patient is not secure from the
danger of contracting the disease afterwards ; but if the sores
keep open, and the feverish symptoms come on at the usual time,
though not a single pustule should appear, I am convinced that the
patient is as secure from ever having the Small Pox as if there had
been a plentiful eruption."

Practice of the Suttons and Dimsdale.—The
extraordinary popularity of the New Method, or Suttonian system, led to much curiosity among physicians,
and we are indebted to Dr. Baker for the earliest
account of the method employed by the Sutton
family. The details of the management and mode of
operation were obtained from informants who had
themselves been operated upon by Sutton.

" All persons are obliged to go through a strict preparatory regimen for a fortnight before the operation is performed ; during this course, every kind of animal food (milk only excepted), and all fermented liquors and spices, are forbidden ; fruit of all sorts is allowed, except only on those days when a purging medicine is taken. In this fortnight of preparation, a dose of a powder is ordered to be taken at bedtime, three several times ; and on the following mornings, a dose of purging salt. To children, only three doses of the powder are given, without any purging salt. The composition of this powder is industriously kept a secret. But that it consists partly of a mercurial preparation, is demonstrated by its having made the gums of several people sore, and even salivated others. The months of May, June, July, and August are preferred as the most seasonable for inoculation. But healthy people are inoculated at any season of the year, indifferently. The autumn is held to be the worst season ; and an aguish habit the least proper for this operation. No objection is made to any one on account of what is vulgarly called a scorbutic habit of body, or bad blood. . . . The person who is to be inoculated, on his arrival at the house used for this purpose is carried into a public room, where very probably he may meet a large company assembled, under the several stages of the Small Pox. The operator then opens a pustule of one of the company, chusing one where the matter is in a crude state, and then just raises up the cuticle on the outer part of the arm where it is thickest with his moist lancet. This done, he only presseth down the raised cuticle with his finger, and applieth neither plaster nor bandage. What is extremely remarkable, he frequently inoculates people with the **moisture taken from the arm before eruption of the Small Pox**, nay, within four days after the operation has been performed. And I am informed, at present, he gives the preference to this method. He has attempted to inoculate by means of the blood, but without success. If the operator happeneth not to be at home when the new patient arriveth, this is looked upon as a matter of no importance ; and so far is he from any apprehension of accumulating infection, that it is very common for persons just inoculated to lie in the same bed with a patient under any stage of the disease, as it may happen; nay, sometimes, in a room where four or five people are sick.

"On the night following the operation the patient takes a pill. This medicine is repeated every other night until the fever comes on. All this time, moderate exercise in the air is strongly recommended. In twenty four hours after the inoculation, the operator can often distinguish whether or no the patients be infected. He, every day, examines the incision, and from thence seems to prognosticate with some degree of certainty concerning the degree of the future disease. In three days after the operation (provided that it has succeeded), there appears on the incision a spot like a flea-bite, not as yet above the skin; this spot by degrees rises to a red pimple, and then becomes a bladder full of clear lymph. This advanceth to maturation like the variolous pustules, but is the last which falleth off. In proportion as the discoloration round the place of incision is greater, the less quantity of eruption is expected. And, therefore, whenever a small discoloured circle is observed, purging medicines stronger than ordinary, and more frequently repeated, are held to be necessary. There never is any sore in the arm, or discharge, but constantly and invariably a large pustule.

"The preparatory diet is still continued. If the fever remain some hours without any tendency to perspiration, some acid drops are administered, the effect of which is to bring on a profuse sweat; but, in some cases, where the fever is very high, a powder or pill, still more powerful, is given. . . . In general, during the burning heat of the fever, the inoculator gives cold water; but, the perspiration beginning, he orders warm Baum tea, or thin water gruel. As soon as the sweat abates, the eruption having made its first appearance, he obliges everybody to get up to walk about the house or into the garden. From this time to the turn of the disease he gives milk gruel *ad libitum.* On the day following the first appearance of the opaque spot on the pustules, to grown people he gives an ounce of Glauber's purging salt. To children he gives a dose of it proportioned to their age; then, if the eruption be small, he allows them to eat a little boiled mutton and toast and butter, and to drink small beer. But, in case of a large eruption, he gives them, on the third day after their having taken the first dose, another dose of the same salt, and confines them to the diet ordered during the preparation. . . .

"What is above written is to be considered as relating only to the practice of one gentleman. There are in different parts of the country several other inoculators, some of whom are said to have surpassed this person in the boldness of their practice. We have heard of patients who have been carried into the fields while shivering in a *rigor;* of their having been allowed no liquor except what they have been able to procure for themselves at the pump, while the fever has been upon them ; and of their having been indiscriminately exposed to the air, in all sorts of weather and in all seasons, during every period of the eruption. This and more has been related upon good authority ; and, indeed, it is certain that many thousands of all constitutions and ages, even to that of seventy years, have within these few years been inoculated according to the general method above described, and in general have gone through the disease almost without an unfavourable symptom. According to the best information which I can procure, about seventeen thousand have been thus inoculated, of which number no more than five or six have died."

Dr. Baker was of opinion that the value of the practice depended upon the free use of cold air. Dr. Glass, of Exeter, attributed it to the patient being sweated. Dr. Chandler, who made a minute examination of Dr. Sutton's system, concluded that the success of the celebrated inoculator did not depend upon his medicinal preparations, nor the free exposure of his patients to cold air ; Mr. Sutton never made a point of sweating his patients, and, therefore, but little efficacy could be attributed to the *punch* which was given ; the pills were useful merely as evacuants, and not as possessing specific power. But the grand

secret of the new system of inoculation, according
to Mr. Chandler,[1] was—

"The taking of the infected humour in a crude state before it has
been, if I may be allowed the expression, ultimately variolated by the
succeeding fever."

This was confirmed by the Rev. Mr. Houlton's
publication, in which it was asserted that Mr. Sutton
never brought into Chelmsford a patient who was
capable of infecting a bystander, though such patient
could convey infection by inoculation.

In spite of unfavourable criticisms which had been
passed upon the Suttonian method, Dr. Dimsdale[2]
appreciated the satisfaction which it gave to the
public, and was not slow to adopt the method in
his own practice. He published a work on the
subject, which was to a certain extent a *résumé* of
the methods of the Suttons, but it was not until
some years afterwards, that he openly adopted the
Suttonian plan in its entirety. Dimsdale laid considerable stress upon age, constitution, and season.
It was not considered desirable to inoculate children
under two years, from the tendency to convulsions,
and as they usually had a larger share of pustules
than those who are advanced in life, and many had
died. Those who laboured under acute or critical

---

[1] Chandler. *An Essay towards an investigation of the present successful and most general method of Inoculation*, p. 37. 1767.

[2] Dimsdale, *loc. cit.*, 1779.

diseases or their effects were "obviously unfit and improper subjects ;" and those who had marks of "corrosive, acrimonious humours," or were suffering from "a manifest debility of the whole frame from inanition or any other cause."

Dr. Heberden[1] had some time previously, in a communication to Dr. Kirkpatrick, insisted upon attention to the existence of any disease at the time of inoculation.

"It seems a reasonable practice to take some care that at the Time of his Receiving the Infection of the Small Pocks, the Person should be as free as may be from any other distemper, lest Nature should be hindered in producing, maturating, or rightly discharging them ; or lest he should sink under the oppression of two Distempers at the same Time."

All Dimsdale's patients had to undergo special treatment previous to the introduction of the disease. Persons inoculated in the spring generally had more pustules than at any other time of the year ; but it was considered safe to inoculate at all seasons, provided that care was taken to keep the patients as cool as possible during the heat of summer, and to prevent them from keeping themselves too warm or too much shut up in winter.

Preparation.—The general aims of preparation were to reduce the patient if in high health, to a low state ; to strengthen the constitution, if too low ; and to clear the stomach and bowels as much as possible

[1] Kirkpatrick, *loc cit.*, p. 271.

from "all crudities." The patients were enjoined to abstain from all animal food, fermented liquors, and spices; the diet to consist of pudding, gruel, sago, milk, fruit, and vegetables, and care was to be taken not to overload the stomach. This treatment was carried out nine or ten days before the operation, and during this period the patients were directed to take a powder composed of eight grains of calomel, the same quantity of compound powder of crabs' claws, and one-eighth part of a grain of tartar emetic. Three doses of this were given; one at the commencement of the course, the second in three or four days, and the third about the eighth or ninth day.

Mode of Inoculation.—Dimsdale had been in the habit of applying a piece of thread, which had been drawn through a *ripe* pustule and well moistened with the matter, to an incision in one or both arms. But this method he had now abandoned.

"The patient to be infected being in the same house, and, if no objection is made to it, in the same room, with one who has the disease, a little of the variolous matter is taken from the place of insertion, if the subject is under inoculation, or a pustule, if in the natural way, on the point of a lancet, so that both sides of the point are moistened. With this lancet an incision is made in that part of the arm where issues were usually placed, just deep enough to pass through the scarf skin, and just to touch the skin itself, and in length not more than one-eighth of an inch; the little wound being then stretched between the finger and thumb of the operator, the incision is moistened with the matter by gently touching it with the side of the infected lancet."

Dimsdale sometimes employed the following modification :—

> "A lancet being moistened with the variolous fluid in the same manner as the other, is gently introduced in an oblique manner between the scarf and true skin, and the finger of the operator is applied on the point, in order to wipe off the infection from the lancet when it is withdrawn."

It was said to be of no consequence whether infective matter were taken from the natural or the inoculated Small Pox. Dimsdale used both, and he did not consider it of consequence whether the matter were taken before or at the crisis of the disease.

> "It is, I believe, generally supposed that the Small Pox is not infectious till after the matter has acquired a certain degree of maturity; and in the common method of inoculation this is much attended to; and where the operation has failed it has commonly been ascribed to the unripeness of the matter. But it appears very clearly from the present practice of inoculation, that so soon as any moisture can be taken from the infected part of an inoculated patient, previous to the appearance of any pustules, and even previous to the eruptive fever, this moisture is capable of communicating the Small Pox with the utmost certainty. I have taken a little clear fluid, from the elevated pellicle on the incised part, even so early as the fourth day after the operation, and have, at other times, used matter, fully digested at the crisis, with equal success. I chuse, however, in general to take matter for infection during the fever of eruption, as I suppose it at that time to have its utmost activity."

No bandage, dressing, or application whatsoever was employed in this method.

" *Progress of Infection.*—The day after the operation is performed, though it takes effect, little alteration is discoverable. On the second, if the part is viewed with a lens, there generally appears a kind of orange coloured stain about the incision, and the surrounding skin seems to contract. A dose of the calomel pill was given at bedtime.

" On the fourth or fifth day, upon applying the finger, a hardness is to be felt by the touch. The patient perceives an itching on the part which appears slightly inflamed, and under a kind of vesication is seen a little clear fluid, the part resembling a superficial burn. About the sixth, most commonly some pain and stiffness is felt in the axilla, and this is a very pleasing symptom, as it not only foretells the near approach of the eruptive symptoms, but is a sign of a favorable progress of the disease. Sometimes on the seventh, oftener on the eighth day, symptoms of the eruptive fever appear, such as slight pains in the head and back, succeeded by transient shiverings, and alternate heats, which in a greater or less degree continue till the eruption is perfected. At this time, also, it is usual for the patient to complain of a very disagreeable taste in his mouth, the breath is always fetid, and the smell of it different from what I have ever observed in any case, except in the variolous eruptive fever.

" The inflammation in the arm, at this time, spreads fast, and upon viewing it with a good glass, the incision, for the most part, appears surrounded with an infinite number of small confluent pustules, which increase in size and extent as the disease advances. On the tenth or eleventh day, a circular or oval efflorescence is usually discovered surrounding the incision, and extending sometimes near half round the arm ; but, more frequently, to about the size of a shilling ; and being under the cuticle is smooth to the touch, and not painful. This appearance is also a very pleasing one ; it accompanies eruption, every disagreeable symptom ceases, and at the same time it certainly indicates the whole affair to be over, the pain and stiffness in the axilla also going off. The feverish symptoms are, for the most part, so mild as seldom to require any medicinal assistance, except a repetition of the same medicine that was directed on the second night after the operation, and in the morning, this laxative draught to procure three or four stools; infusion of senna two ounces, manna half an ounce, tincture of jalap two drams. . . .

"Being now arrived at the most interesting period of this distemper, the eruption, a period in which the present practice I am about to recommend differs essentially from the method heretofore in use, and on the right management of which much depends, it will be requisite to give clear and explicit directions on this head, and to advise their being pursued with firmness and moderation. Instead of confining the patient to his bed or his room when the symptoms of the eruptive fever come on, he is directed, as soon as the purging medicine has operated, to keep abroad in the open air—be it ever so cold, as much as he can bear—and to drink cold water if thirsty; always taking care not to stand still, but to walk about moderately while abroad. . . .

"In general the complaints in this state are very moderate, and attended with so little illness that the patient eats and sleeps well the whole time; a few pustules appear, sometimes, equally dispersed; sometimes the inflammations on the arms spread and are surrounded with a few pustules, which gradually advance to maturity, during which time, for the most part, the eruption proceeds kindly, and there is much more difficulty to restrain the patients within due bounds, and to prevent their mixing with the public and spreading the infection (which I always endeavour to prevent), than there was at first to prevail upon them to go abroad.

"The system of purging and the free use of cold air were credited with preventing either alarming symptoms, or a large crop of pustules. Those who had the disease in the slightest manner—that is to say, without any appearance of eruption except on the inoculated part—were soon allowed to go about their usual affairs. Those who had it in a greater degree were confined a little longer. Occasionally there were dangerous symptoms, and accidents of various kinds. Sometimes the inoculated part showed certain marks of infection a day or two after inoculation, the incision appearing considerably inflamed and elevated.

"The patient about this time frequently makes some of the following complaints: viz., chilliness; itchings and small pricking pains in the part, and sometimes in the shoulder; giddiness, drowsiness, and a slight headach, sometimes attended with a feverish heat, but often without any. . . . These complaints seldom last twenty-four hours, often not so long. . . . The inflammation on the arm, at the time of the complaint, advances apace, and feels hard to the touch; but, upon their wearing off, the inflamed appearances gradually lessen, and the part dries to a common small scab; the skin that was before red turns livid, and the party is quite well, and nothing more is heard of the distemper. . . .

"In some instances, these symptoms attack much later; even on the seventh or eighth day, when an eruption might be expected in consequence of them, yet none appears; but the arm gets well very soon, and the disease is at an end."

Similar appearances resulted in other cases, though there were only a few pustules which, moreover, did not look like true pocks. When such cases first occurred in Dimsdale's practice, he was in doubt whether the patients would be quite secure in future from an attack of the disease; and, in order to test whether they were so, he inoculated them a second time, and caused them to associate with persons in every stage of the disease, and exposed them to all other means of catching the infection; but there was no instance of its producing any disorder, so that they were pronounced to be perfectly safe.

Dimsdale explained how it was that he was led to try the new method of inoculation in 1765. He had heard that inoculation of the patients with fluid matter, and exposure to the open air, produced results that were appreciated, and therefore he borrowed the practice. He concluded by saying :—

"Should it be asked, then, to what particular circumstance the success is owing, I can only answer that, although the whole process may have some share in it, in my opinion it consists chiefly in the method of inoculating with *recent fluid matter*, and in the management of the patients at the time of eruption. If these conjectures should be true, perhaps we should be found to have improved but little upon the judicious Sydenham's cool method of treating the disease, and the old Greek woman's method of inoculating with fluid matter carried warm in her servant's bosom."

Dimsdale now became recognised as a specialist in the art of inoculation. He was summoned to Russia, in 1768, to inoculate the Empress, and his procedure may be followed in some detail, as the results led to the revival of inoculation in England. Dimsdale, on arrival at St. Petersburg, resolved to commence operations by experimenting on two young gentlemen of the Cadets Corps.[1] These boys, Basoff and Swieten, were about fourteen years old. The matter for their inoculation was taken from a child of a poor man in the suburbs of St. Petersburg, who was "pretty full of a distinct kind of Small Pox." Every one was anxious for the success of this first attempt, and the experiment caused Dimsdale considerable anxiety. On the second day after inoculation, Basoff was seized "with great sickness and vomiting," attended with other symptoms of fever; but it was subsequently "discovered that he had improperly overcharged his stomach with a quantity of dried fruits, which it was

---

[1] Dimsdale. *Tracts on Inoculation written and published at St. Petersburg in the year* 1768, *with additional observations.* 1781.

hoped might be the sole occasion of that disorder."
Dimsdale's anxiety was relieved, for the symptoms of
the eruptive fever were moderate, and only two or
three pustules followed on the arm. Swieten's arm,
which had never seemed likely to produce any eruption,
remained well. Four more youths of the Cadets Corps
and a young maid-servant were selected for further
trials, and a case of natural Small Pox, with the eruption
in a suitable stage for the purpose, was chosen.

" The child from whom we were to take matter for inoculation
was rather full of Small Pox, the kind was favourable and distinct, and near the time of maturation. . . .

"As we were extremely anxious for the event of this inoculation, our observations were carefully and frequently made on the
progress of it in the five patients ; . . . on the punctured part
almost immediately arose a pimple, which soon became one large
pustule filled with yellow matter, very much resembling the Small
Pox completely maturated. This continued to the seventh and
eighth days, when the eruptive symptoms might, in the common
course, be expected. Not one of them, however, had any illness,
nor did I then expect they would, and in short the experiment
turned out wholly ineffectual. The wounds upon the arms dried
up, and the patients continued in perfect health."

Dimsdale was strongly disposed to believe that
these patients had passed through Small Pox at some
early period of their lives, but no evidence whatever
existed in support of this theory. He proposed that
the same persons should be inoculated a second time
in the old and original manner. The patients were
also recommended to frequent the rooms of those

who were under the natural Small Pox, even of the
worst sort ; that they should handle those labouring
under Small Pox, and expose themselves in every
way to infection. This proposal was carried into
execution, but the result was that not the least
symptom of infection was produced.

The Empress was now determined to undergo inoculation. A child " on whom the Small Pox *had
just commenced to appear,*" was selected and taken to
the palace. The operation was secretly performed.

"The Empress, during this interval, took part in every amusement with her usual affability, without showing the least token of
uneasiness or concern, constantly dined at the same table with
the nobility, and enlivened the whole Court with those peculiar
graces of conversation for which she is not less distinguished than
for her rank and station."

Dimsdale also recommended inoculation of the Grand
Duke, if it were performed by *a very slight puncture
of a lancet wet with recent and fluid variolous matter,*
as some anxiety was felt about the state of his health.
After relating these facts and occurrences, Dimsdale
remarks :—

"But I must not omit mentioning that both the Empress and
the Grand Duke were pleased to permit several persons to be
inoculated from them, and, by this condescension, the prejudice
which had reigned among the inferior ranks of people, that the
party would suffer from whom the infection was taken, was most
effectually destroyed."

For these services, Dimsdale was made a Baron of

the Russian Empire, appointed Councillor of State, Physician to Her Imperial Majesty, and awarded a sum of £10,000 in addition to an annuity of £500.

The following is a short account of the progress of inoculation of the Empress :—

Previous to inoculation she abstained " from animal food at supper, and at dinner ate such only as was easy of digestion." The day before inoculation " she took 5 grains of mercurial powder." Sunday, 12th, late in the evening, she was inoculated with *fluid matter* by one puncture in each arm, and "on the succeeding night was very restless, and complained of pains in different parts of her body." . . . On the 14th, "she passed a tolerable night, certain signs of infection appeared on the places of incision; a little pain was felt under the arm." . . . On October 15th, "the giddiness and the pain under her arm ceased. The places of incision became more red." On the 16th, she "complained of heaviness in her head at intervals; . . . four grains of the mercurial powder were given;" on the 17th, "she took half an ounce of Glauber's salt dissolved in warm water, but in the evening she complained of a pain in her head, and that her hands and shoulders seemed benumbed, and she was inclined to sleep. . . . The places of incision advanced properly, and with the assistance of a magnifying glass I could plainly discover small pimples around the part." On the 18th, "the incisions in the arm became more red and inflamed." On the 19th, "the incisions looked more red, and in the evening many of the pimples mentioned before appeared to unite in a general inflammation." About the 20th, "more pustules appeared around the incision, and the circumference of the wound itself looked more red than before. One pustule was also discovered in the face and two upon the wrist." October 21st, "some pustules appeared on the face and arms, and the fever was entirely gone." 22nd, "more pustules appeared, and advanced according to our wishes." On October 24th, there was "a large pustule on the upper part of the right tonsil." 25th, "the pain and swelling of the throat were abated ; . . . some of the pustules began to change their colour to a darker

hue." October 27th, "all the pustules had now become brown."
On October 28th, "she returned to St. Petersburg in perfect
health, to the great joy of the whole city."

The case of His Imperial Highness the Grand
Duke was still milder.

"The inoculation was performed on him with fresh fluid matter,
by one puncture in the right arm only; the matter was taken
from the youngest son of Mr. Briscorn, apothecary to the Court.
. . . November 4th, symptoms of infection appeared on the arm.
. . . November 5th, on examining the incision, the mark of the
infection very evidently appeared, and he complained of the part
around the wound being somewhat painful. . . . November 6th,
he had shivering, succeeded by a feverish heat; the quickness of
the pulse increased. . . . November 7th, he had slept the preceding night . . . a considerable shivering. November 9th, one
pustule appeared upon the chin, and three were discovered upon
the back. November 10th, more pustules appeared on different
parts; and he was quite free from complaints. . . . November
12th, his throat was sore and painful. November 14th, his throat
much better. From this time he was quite free from pain; the
pustules, which together did not exceed forty, matured kindly, soon
dried up, and the illness terminated very happily."

At the request of the Empress, Dr. Dimsdale proceeded to Moscow, where the citizens were desirous
of receiving the inoculation.

"I was informed that at Mosco, as well as at St. Petersburg,
every possible precaution was used to prevent the spreading of
the Small Pox, and it was very probable that much time might be
lost before the disease could be discovered there in a proper state
for inoculation. I therefore thought it advisable to make use of
an expedient that was thought pretty extraordinary: it was to
inoculate one or two children at St. Petersburg to take with us, to
answer the purpose of infection when we should arrive at Mosco.

It was with some difficulty that two children were procured, for
though the idea of arbitrary power conveys with it a presumption that nothing more would be wanting than an Imperial order
for us to fix on the persons we thought most eligible, yet such
mildness and benevolence;prevails under the Government of the
Empress, that no such compulsion is ever practised. After a few
days, two children were obtained, the one a boy about six years
old, the son of a sailor's widow, the other a girl about ten, the
daughter of a deceased subaltern German officer. . . . The
children were inoculated at St. Petersburg two days before the
time fixed for our setting out, and as it was expected that the
journey would be performed in four days, we hoped to arrive at
Mosco on the 6th after inoculation. . . .

"Many of the nobility instantly applied to have their families
inoculated, and as the patient that we brought with us was at that
time in a very proper state to take matter from, we began to
inoculate on the day after our arrival, so that in a few days we
had inoculated more than fifty patients from that girl only. After
the first were recovered, several others, encouraged by their
success, were desirous of being inoculated also."

Dimsdale published his experiences in Russia, in
1781, and appended a description of the points in
which, as the result of further experience, he had
modified his early practice. With regard to the
method of preparation, he had• come to the conclusion
that such was hardly necessary ; and he stated that
for some years past he had not been in the habit
of enjoining any restriction from diet, or prescribing
any special medicine before the operation, and more
caution was exercised in repeatedly giving mercurials
or other purgatives. With regard to the mode of
infection, he now restricted himself to inoculating by
means of a lancet, the point of which was slightly

dipped in recent variolous matter taken during the eruptive fever. The lancet was introduced obliquely beneath the superficial skin, making the smallest puncture possible, If there were no patients in a proper state to yield the variolous fluid, dried lymph was employed. A lancet, or a plate of glass or gold, was charged with matter in a fluid state, which was then allowed to dry. When required for use it was held over the steam of boiling water, or a small quantity of water, barely sufficient for dilution, was added to it, and the matter thus moistened was used for the purpose of inoculation. The practice of going out in the fresh cool air, and the use of aperients were still recommended ; but, when the complaint was moderate, a result which he always endeavoured to obtain, these injunctions were dispensed with.

Sometimes patients under inoculation passed through the illness in a manner that differed materially from natural Small Pox.

"Yet, where the infection appeared to have succeeded satisfactorily on a punctured part of the arm, although no eruption should be discovered in consequence of it, the party will never receive the disease in future."

In speaking of the different methods of communicating the infection employed by inoculation, Dimsdale states :—

"That if inoculation be performed by a slight puncture, and with fluid matter, the progress is usually this :—After two, three, or four days a small redness of a particular colour may be distinguished, which gradually rises to a pimple, resembling the Small Pox in its first appearance; this fills with a pellucid fluid. About the time of the commencement of the eruptive symptoms, the inflammation increases, very often during the fever.

"Now, when this gradual progress is observed to take place, I maintain that, although it be unattended with fever or derangement of health, and not followed by any eruption, the person will during the remainder of his life be secure from receiving the disease. I am emboldened to speak in this positive manner from having made repeated trials to infect such patients again, and in every instance ineffectually."

Finally, after discussing the old method of treatment, Dimsdale proceeded to give the credit of this more successful system to the family of the Suttons; the essential difference between them consisting in the return to the original method of slight puncture, and the use of recent fluid matter. The accounts of the wonderful effects of medicines, which were also alleged to cure the most malignant kind of Small Pox after the eruption had appeared, served to disguise the true secret of the new method.

Many years afterwards, Sutton[1] published an account of the practice which he had introduced. His method had been carried out in 100,000 cases. He acknowledged that he had relied upon the use of *crude fresh matter;* for in his experience with *concocted matter,* "the infection was not so rapid; the indications on the arm not so favourable; the conglobate glands in the axilla were more liable to suppurate;

---

[1] Sutton. *The Inoculator, or the Suttonian system of inoculation fully set forth.* 1763.

and the eruptive symptoms were more irregular and
ungovernable." In fact, the patient in all likelihood
encountered "a very copious Small Pox, which he
would not have had from the use of fresh matter."

Sutton describes the method which he employed
in the following words :—

"The lancet being charged with the **smallest perceivable
quantity** (and the smaller the better) of **unripe, crude, or watery
matter,** immediately introduce it by puncture, obliquely, between
the scarf and true skin, barely sufficient to draw blood, and
not deeper than the sixteenth part of an inch. Neither
patting, nor daubing of the matter, in or over the punctured
part, is at all necessary to its efficacy. This practice indeed is
rather prejudicial than otherwise, as it may affect the form of the
incision, and thus be apt to confound our judgment upon it.

"*Indications of the Incision.*—In the incipient state of variolous
increase in the incision, a small florid spot appears on the part of
access, resembling a flea-bite in size ; and on passing the finger
lightly over it, a hardness is felt not larger than a small pin's
head. This florid appearance and hardness denote that the
variolous principle is effectually imbibed, and their indications
point no farther, unless the progress to vesication be very slow,
in which case an uncomfortable number of pustules may be
expected to follow. The florid spot in most instances of inoculation is somewhat larger, or more extended, on the second than
on the third day after the insertion.

"About the fourth day from inoculation, should the incision
begin to vesicate, an itching sensation will be complained of on
the place of insertion ; the occurrence of which symptom is the first
indication of a favourable event, yet not of sufficient importance to
justify any present relaxation in the preparatory proceedings.

The vesication of the incision in most instances will begin to be
visible on the fourth or fifth day after the insertion of the matter ;
the sooner it becomes so, the more favourable may be expected to
be the event. The extent or diameter of the vesication at this

stage does not usually exceed that of a large pin's head, and it has invariably a dint or small depression."

It is interesting to note that Sutton frequently met with cases of insusceptibility. There were one, two, or three persons every day who could not be infected. In such cases the result of inoculation is thus described :—

" In a few hours after the insertion of the Small Pox matter, the part became considerably inflamed and hardened to the extent of a shilling, or wider, resembling the effects produced by the stings or bites of small venomous insects, and attended with an itching sensation. These effects increasing, continued for two, three, four, or more days, and then disappeared. In some instances of this sort, which have since happened to me, the part thus irritated has suppurated, and a small sloughing ensued ; but this matter will not give the Small Pox."

However, instances sometimes occurred of accidents and even death; but these were attributed to other causes, in order to save the new method from reproach, a fact which was many years afterwards commented upon by Moore [1] in the following words :—

" An empiric never hesitates at making positive declarations, and is never at a loss for pretexts to cover failures. Should an infant at the accession of the variolous fever be carried off by convulsion, he denies with effrontery that the Small Pox was the cause, and invents another upon the spot. Should the confluent Small Pox and death ensue, he soon detects that his instructions were not strictly complied with, but some important error was committed in regimen ; or, that the patient was too much or too little exposed to the air. In fine, the fault may be in the parents, in the nurse, or in the inoculated, but is never allowed fairly to fall upon the inoculator."

[1] Moore. *The History of the Small Pox*, p. 269. 1815.

CHAPTER IV.

HAYGARTH'S SYSTEM FOR PREVENTING SMALL POX.

THE history of Small Pox inoculation has been given in the preceding pages, from its first employment in England to the time of the general adoption of the Suttonian method. This practice, though so long continued, had not only failed to exterminate Small Pox, but, on the contrary, there can be little doubt that it actually assisted in spreading the disease. Instances occurred in which Small Pox was introduced by inoculation into towns which were and had been for many years perfectly free from the natural disease, and an epidemic followed.

The futility of inoculation led Dr. Haygarth in 1777 to suggest a new plan for exterminating Small Pox. In the year 1784, he published a work on this subject,[1] explaining his reasons and the means by which he proposed to carry out his scheme. It will be of interest to follow his argument and conclusions, which resulted in his anticipating, by nearly a century, the

---

Haygarth. *An Inquiry how to prevent the Small Pox.* 1784.

modern method of stamping out infectious diseases.
Haygarth pointed out, first, that Small Pox is an
infectious distemper ; secondly, that Small Pox was
never known since its original commencement to be
produced by any other cause than infection.

"That at present it is occasioned by neither climate, soil, nor
season, but by infection only. The world had existed about
four or five thousand years before history takes any notice of
this distemper. It is universally allowed to have been originally
endemic in or near Arabia. All Europe was infected from this
place, and all other parts of the world that were then known, or
have since been discovered. It did not appear in Greenland till
1733. The infection was carried thither by a native returning
home, in the distemper, from Copenhagen. In Minorca, it entirely
disappeared from 1725 to 1742—that is, for seventeen years. In
1745, it was again brought to Minorca by one of His Majesty's
ships ; and there can be no doubt that the former infection was
imparted by some ship, though unnoticed by the author. At
Boston, in New England, the Small Pox had been epidemical
only eight times from the first settlement of the province of
Massachusetts till 1752, as appears from the following table,
composed out of Dr. Douglas's *Historical and Political Summary
of North America.*

EPIDEMICAL SMALL POX AT BOSTON.							YEARS ABSENT.
1649	.	.	.	.	.	.	—
1666	.	.	.	.	.	.	17
1678	.	.	.	.	.	.	12
1689	.	.	.	.	.	.	11
1702	.	.	.	.	.	.	13
1721	.	.	.	.	.	.	19
1730	.	.	.	.	.	.	9
1752	.	.	.	.	.	.	22

"Before the epidemic of 1721, the Small Pox was imported
from Barbadoes, before that of 1730, from Ireland, and before
that of 1752, from London. At Rhode Island, in America, this

distemper was *never* epidemical, according to authentic intelligence which I have received from Dr. Moffat, who practised physic at Newport, their capital, from 1740 to 1765, and from Dr. Waterhouse, a native of the island. The former gentleman acquainted me with this fact in these words :—'The Small Pox was never epidemical during my residence in Rhode Island, nor before, that I ever heard of. As far as I can recollect, there never was, at the same time, more than five or six ill of the distemper. Such a happy exemption is accomplished by regulations established there for the purpose.'"

Haygarth was unable to obtain a sufficient number of facts to ascertain with certainty on which day of the disease a patient becomes infectious ; but the following evidence, he considered, would warrant a probable conjecture that the patient is seldom or never liable to communicate the disease before the eruption appears.

" 1st *and* 2nd *Cases.*—I attended a little boy, in the Small Pox, whose eruptions, of the distinct kind, appeared on the fourth day of the fever. His two sisters, on their appearance, were removed out of the house. One of them became feverish on the eleventh day after her removal, the other was not attacked till seven weeks after, on being exposed to another infection. As the former sister was only removed to a neighbouring house, there may be some doubt whether she might not be infected by some future communication. The other was sent to a much greater distance.

" 3rd *and* 4th *Cases.*—A gentleman's child became feverish on the Sunday ; two others of his children were daily in the same room, and one of them lay every night with the patient till Friday, the sixth day, and were then removed ; yet neither were infected, though the pustules had appeared a day or two before. One of them was inoculated soon after and had the distemper.

" 5th *Case.*—In a family where there were four children who had never been exposed to the infection, when the eruption appeared on the first patient, which was on the fourth day of the disease, the other three were separated from it and escaped infection."

As these observations were not sufficiently numerous to establish the truth, Haygarth quoted the testimony of Dr. Heberden, in confirmation of the theory he had advanced. This authority made the following statement in a letter to Haygarth :—

"Many instances have occurred to me which show that one who never had Small Pox might safely associate, and even lie in the same bed, with a variolous patient for the two or three first days of eruption without receiving the infection."

From this and other experience, Haygarth was of opinion that it was quite established—

"That when one person is accidentally seized with the Small Pox in a family where others are liable to it, the rest may generally avoid the natural infection either by separation or immediate inoculation."

Haygarth continued thus :—

"In an enquiry how to prevent the Small Pox, it is a point of consequence to determine *how long the variolous poison remains on the patient's body.* I have collected some authentic facts on this subject, chiefly from the register of the Small Pox Society. Out of 90 *single* patients the shortest continuance of the poison was to the tenth and the longest to the fortieth day from the commencement of the variolous eruption till the last scab dropt off, and of these only 16 were later than the thirty-eighth day.

Haygarth then pointed out that—

"All the discharges of a Small Pox patient, either of themselves, or the probable mixture of serum, pus, or scab may be infectious, and ought to be destroyed by cleanliness in order to prevent the propagation of the distemper. . . . That 'persons liable to the Small Pox are infected by breathing the air very near the variolous poison in a recent state,' is a medical opinion so well established as to require no proof. Let us reflect how widely and fatally this poison is dispersed among all ranks of people. It may be conveyed into any house unobserved from a great variety of families, adhering to clothes, food, furniture, etc., as—

"*Clothes:* 1, Linen ; 2, Cotton ; 3, Woollen (particularly flannel) ; 4, Silk ; 5, Millinery goods ; 6, Stockings ; 7, Stays ; 8, Gloves ; 9, Shoes.

"*Food:* 10, Bread ; 11, Cakes ; 12, Huxtery ; 13, Fruit ; 14, Butter ; 15, Milk ; 16, Sugar and other groceries ; 17, Salt ; 18, Tea ; 19, Nuts. N.B.—Food boiled or roasted at home is probably not infectious.

"*Furniture:* 20, Earthenware ; 21, Hardware ; 22, Dolls and other toys ; 23, Pens ; 24, Paper ; 25, Books ; 26, Letters ; 27, Money ; 28, Medicines. Tenfold more articles might be enumerated ; besides several of these I have mentioned, as linen, etc., includes four families each, who by this means may communicate the distemper, namely the seller, maker, washer, and wearer. . . .

"The clothes of a patient generally contain the largest quantity of variolous poison. However, all the enumerated articles and many more that come out of an infectious house or from an infectious person find their way unsuspected into all families of a certain rank. The poison is quickly and universally dispersed among the lowest class of people whose poverty renders them dirty."

As an instance of the long time that the variolous poison retains its infectious quality in clothes, the following example was quoted :—

"'About 1718, a ship from the East Indies arrived at the Cape of Good Hope. In the voyage, three children had been sick of the Small Pox ; the *foul linen* about them was *put into a trunk and locked up.* At the ship's landing, this was taken out and given to some natives to be washed. Upon handling the linen, they were seized with the Small Pox, which spread into the country for many miles, and made such a desolation that it was almost depopulated.[1]'"

Haygarth added :—

"From a variety of considerations I am inclined to believe, that the most usual method of transferring the Small Pox to a distant place is, by sending to relations and acquaintances clothes, etc., bedaubed with the variolous poison ; either shut up in boxes, or what has a similar effect, folded up in clothes, paper, etc., so as to exclude all access of fresh air. It has been remarked that relations at a distance are infected by this distemper nearly about the same time. This event, I believe, happens from a communication of dirty clothes, etc., and sometimes possibly from a letter. Whoever reflects that a piece of paper on which a letter is written may have lain on the bed where there is, or has been, a Small Pox patient, or on a table, chair, etc., where the foul handkerchiefs, clothes, etc., are thrown, or may be smeared with variolous matter by the unwashed hands of a servant, correspondent, or a patient ; that the letter is folded up carefully so as to exclude the air, that when opened it is held near the mouth and nose to be read, and afterwards a child puts it into the mouth, will not be surprised that it may sometimes communicate an infection."

Haygarth argued that the variolous poison, in the form of serum, pus, and scab, by impregnating the surrounding air, was the sole means of infection, and that if this were granted, the difficulty of prevention would be much diminished. A number of cases and arguments were produced, to show that the air is only rendered infectious to a slight distance by the variolous poison.

---

[1] Mead, *On the Plague.*

There was only one cause that would be likely to disperse the infection to a distance from the patient's room, viz., a strong wind; provided that the wind blew directly through the room, an uncommon circumstance.

"To diminish the force of this argument, it may be suggested that the variolous infection is a ferment which by an admixture of a few of its particles with blood occasions the generation of a large quantity of poison. It cannot be denied that by inoculation a very small portion of matter—and we may even allow that by natural infection, perhaps a much smaller quantity of miasms, dissolved in the air of a Small Pox chamber—can produce in some subjects so much variolous poison as would communicate the distemper to thousands; but when the infectious air is again diluted several hundred times with fresh air, we cannot suppose it to retain any mischievous energy. A fact respecting another kind of ferment sets this point in a true light. A pint of yest is sufficient to excite a fermentation in a barrel of ale; but 100th, much less 1000th part of this quantity of yest, would not have the effect."

In further support of his doctrine, Haygarth pointed out—

"That Small Pox was epidemical in Chester, from May, 1777 to January 1778. . . .

"(1) At the beginning, two or three families were seized, not immediate neighbours, but in the same quarter of the town.

"(2) Then the children of a neighbourhood comprehending an entry had the distemper, but it did not spread from them as a centre.

"(3) In no part of the town it has spread uniformly from a centre farther than thro' an entry or narrow lane, where all the children of a neighbourhood play together.

"(4) Afterwards the poor children in several parts of the town were attacked, at a considerable distance, in some places half a mile off each other.

"(5) Yet many portions of all the large streets were not

infected in November; but so late as December and January the
distemper returned to attack many who had escaped when it
was in their neighbourhood some months before.

" (6) In Handbridge, a part of Chester, only separated from
the rest of the town by the river Dee, not more than 7 had
been infected during the epidemic, tho' great numbers of
children in this quarter are liable to the distemper.

" (7) In the middle of the city, in one street (King's) of 24
who never had passed thro' the distemper, only 2, both in
the same house, were attacked.

" (8) During the summer and autumn of 1777, while this
epidemic was general in Chester, many of the surrounding villages
(as Christleton, Barrow, Tarven, etc.), and some larger towns (as
Nantwich, Neston, etc.) were visited by the Small Pox in one
or more families. Yet the distemper did not spread generally
thro' any of these towns. As both the state of the air and
the variolous poison were the same in these places as in Chester,
why did it not equally *infect* their *air* as well as ours?

" (9) At Frodsham the Small Pox began in May, and gradually
became more frequent, so as to be remarkably epidemical in one
part for several months; yet, nearly one half of the town,
Nov. 18, 1777, still remained quite uninfected. On the contrary, at Upton, a small village 2 miles from Chester, of
24 children, who had never been attacked by the distemper,
all, except one (who was also certainly exposed to the infection), had it in less than two months. The reason of its
speedy propagation I shall give in the words of Mr. Edwards,
surgeon, a very intelligent inhabitant of the place:

" 'The distemper has not been propagated by the air or contiguity
of houses, but has increased in proportion to the communication which
families have with each other. No care was taken to prevent the
spreading; but, on the contrary, there seemed to be a general wish
that all the children might have it.'

" (10) It is universally allowed that the variolous infection
attacks the children of the poor people first, and by far the most
generally; but the air is equally breathed both by rich and poor,
and, if infectious, would equally communicate the distemper to both

in proportion to their respective numbers. Many instances daily occur of a favourite child, living in large towns where the Small Pox almost constantly rages, who, by anxious care to avoid the distemper, has escaped it till arrived at maturity, and received the infection by inoculation or by mixing with society in a less cautious manner. Of many gentlemen's children liable to the distemper in Chester, not one was seized by the natural Small Pox, whose infection could not be accounted for, during the whole time of this epidemic." . . .

(11) A gentleman's family, of whom eight were children all liable to the Small Pox, became inhabitants of Chester, and on the occasion of their first walk in the town they met a child a year old with the Small Pox. The breadth of the path was a yard and a quarter. One of the children, a young girl, passed within half a yard of the child, and her brothers, she believes, were all as near. Both parties walked uniformly forward in opposite directions, except one of the brothers, who out of curiosity stopped to look at this Small Pox patient; he did not touch the child, but he approached nearer than any of the others of the party. This brother was the only one who was infected. At the same time all the other three were susceptible of Small Pox, for they were attacked on the 24th, 25th, and 26th day after they met the child, being infected from the brother; while another brother was seized on the 29th November, and another sister on December the second, who had not accompanied the others.

These facts afforded an opportunity of judging how small a distance in the open air a Small Pox patient exerts a pestilential influence. The following account indicated that the variolous poison in a house is not infectious to any persons out of it. Small Pox occurred in a family in a quarter of the town where there were numbers of children liable to infection. The new method of prevention was explained to a lady in order to prevent any of her neighbours catching the disease. "Tho' two of her children were attacked by the Small Pox, and one of them died, yet, except a boy who had been in the sick chamber before the directions were given, not a single child caught the disease, altho' two were liable to it, even at the next door, and not fewer than twenty six in the near neighbourhood."

These observations convinced Haygarth that Small Pox did not render the surrounding air infectious to such a distance, as to frustrate all human attempts to stop its progress, and he therefore formulated the following conclusions :—

"If the Small Pox be communicated by infection and by infection only ; if it be only caught by approaching very near to the variolous poison in a recent state, or that has been close shut up from the air ever since it was recent; and the variolous miasms do not render clothes, etc., infectious, *it follows that the Small Pox may be prevented by keeping persons liable to the distemper from approaching within the infectious distance of the variolous poison till it can be destroyed.* The variolous poison, if exposed to the air for sufficient time, is probably deprived of its infectious quality, being dissolved in the atmosphere. I have known several instances where Small Pox was communicated in the open air by two persons meeting and walking in opposite directions. These facts proved that an infectious quality is quickly given to the air, and consequently that it may soon be exhausted. . . . The epidemical Small Pox, which has been attributed to a peculiar constitution of the atmosphere by the sagacious Sydenham, and by most other physicians who have since written on the subject, may be supposed incompatible with this conclusion; but I think it can be explained in a satisfactory manner on the principles of this inquiry." . . .

I request the reader to consider the following table :—

DEATHS BY THE SMALL POX IN 1781.

	Manchester.	Warrington.	Chester.
January	3	7	1
February	5	8	0
March	10	5	0
April	17	5	1
May	31	5	0
June	44	6	0
July	55	3	0
August	46	4	1
September	53	3	0
October	36	0	2
November	31	2	1
December	13	2	1
	344	50	7

" Hence we see, on surveying several large neighbouring towns, as Manchester, Warrington, and Chester, that the distemper is very seldom absent from any of them, but that it becomes generally epidemical at uncertain periods in each, and at times which hold no correspondence with one another. In like manner, on comparing several neighbouring villages, we observe some entirely free from the distemper, others have a few only infected, others suffer a general seizure. . . . Whoever considers the numerous facts here faithfully related will perhaps be convinced that the distemper becomes epidemical neither thro' any peculiar state of the air, nor of the human constitution. No such difference can reasonably be supposed to exist in large towns within twenty miles of each other, much less in neighbouring villages, and least of all in different parts of the same town or village. If what is above advanced be true, the seeming mystery may be explained in a few words. **The Small Pox continues spreading as long as persons liable to the infection approach patients in the distemper, or infectious matter, either in the same chamber, or very nearly in the open air, and then ceases.** The next point was to inquire in what way this theory was capable of practical application, 'either by civil regulations, or by a private society founded on principles of charity and benevolence to mankind.' With this end in view Haygarth drew up the following instructions :—

" MANKIND ARE NOT NECESSARILY SUBJECT TO THE SMALL POX ; IT IS ALWAYS CAUGHT BY INFECTION FROM A PATIENT IN THE DISTEMPER, OR THE POISONOUS MATTER, OR SCABS THAT COME FROM A PATIENT, AND MAY ; BE AVOIDED BY OBSERVING THESE

"RULES OF PREVENTION.

"I. Suffer no person who has not had the Small Pox to come into the infectious house. No visitor who has had any communication with persons liable to the distemper, should touch or sit down on anything infectious.

"II. No patient, after the pocks have appeared, must be suffered to go into the street, or other frequented place.

"III. The utmost attention to *cleanliness* is absolutely necessary *during* and *after* the distemper. No person, clothes, food, furniture, dog, cat, money, medicines, or any other thing that is known or suspected to be daubed with matter, spittle, or other infectious discharges of the patient, should go out of the house till they be washed, and till they have been sufficiently exposed to the fresh air. No foul linen or anything else that can retain the poison should be folded up and put into drawers, boxes, or be otherwise shut up from the air, but immediately thrown into water and kept there till washed. No attendants should touch what is to go into another family till their hands are washed. When a patient dies of the Small Pox, particular care should be taken that nothing infectious should be taken out of the house, so as to do mischief.

"IV. The patient must not be allowed to approach any person liable to the distemper till every scab is dropt off, till all the clothes, furniture, food, and all other things touched by the patient during the distemper, till the floor of the sick chamber, and till his hair, face, and hands have been carefully washed. After everything has been made perfectly clean, the doors, windows, drawers, boxes, and all other places that can retain infectious air should be kept open till it be cleared out of the house."

As every restriction is attended with inconvenience, Haygarth proposed that a reward should be given for attention to the rules, and this was to be secured by annexing to them a

"PROMISSORY NOTE

"DATED . . . . . .

" *The* SOCIETY *for Promoting General Inoculation at stated periods, and for Preventing the Natural* SMALL POX *in Chester,* promises to pay . . . . . . the sum of [half-a-crown or a crown, or . . . . .] as soon as all the scabs have dropt off the patients in . . . . family, on condition that the said . . . . . . and . . . . . . family exactly observe the foregoing rules, and allow any member of the society, or their inspector, to inquire whether they are exactly observed : and as a farther encouragement to follow these directions attentively and faithfully, the society promise [double or . . . .] the reward if no neighbour or acquaintance be attacked by the Small Pox during the time it is in the family of the said . . . . , nor within 16 days after all the scabs have entirely fallen off the family.

"By order of the Society,

. . . . Inspector."

As there were inhabitants to whom it would be improper to offer pecuniary reward, it was thought desirable to affix the following request in such cases to the rules:—

" The independent citizens to whom the rewards of the Society will not be worth acceptance, are earnestly requested to observe these regulations through motives of humanity, in order to preserve their fellow creatures from so fatal a pestilence as the natural Small Pox; and to permit the inspector, if they have no other medical visitor, to see that they are observed, lest their servants inadvertently spread the contagion."

An inspector was to be appointed, to see that these rules were observed, and to keep a register containing full information of families attacked with the Small Pox. The name, address, and occupation of each patient were to be entered, with the following particulars : date when the Small Pox fever began, date of information, date of receiving the rules of prevention, whence infected, date of death or last scab, date of being washed and aired, whether infection was communicated or not, whether the rules were observed or transgressed.

It was also considered desirable that, where it was possible, the inspector should write down in the register the proofs of infection. Thus, in one family it was necessary to move into another house while they were suffering from Small Pox. One of the children, with the eruption upon her, ran against a child belonging to another family who probably carried home some of the poison upon her clothes. Some children had been allowed, contrary to the promise of the parents, to play in the street, and they communicated the Small Pox to another family. In another instance, a child with the eruption upon him was playing in a street window; he gave a teetotum through the sash to a boy, and communicated the Small Pox to a family. Again, bed-clothes that had been made foul by children who had died from the Small Pox were sent to a distant part of the town nearly a mile off, to be washed, and communicated the distemper to another family. Haygarth anticipated that experience would discover defects in the regulations, but it was reasonably hoped that such defects would admit of a practical correction. Haygarth also stated that he could deduce many facts from other infectious distempers in favour of the doctrine maintained in the inquiry; but he considered that argument from analogy would be superfluous after so many direct proofs had been produced.

As the result of these sanitary measures, we find that in a report by the inspector, it was certified that the Small Pox had been stopped in ten different parts of the city, and that so far as could be learned from minute inquiries, there were only three Small Pox patients in Chester, results which were principally produced by the rules and the rewards of the Society for preventing the Small Pox.

When in 1778, Haygarth submitted the preceding inquiry to the consideration of his friends, including Dr. Waterhouse, he ascertained that this practice had actually been carried out for a long series of years in Rhode Island. In Boston and Rhode Island, inoculation was discouraged, and the following method was employed for preventing the Small Pox :—

If any who resided in those parts had gone to the Southern Provinces to be inoculated they were enjoined

"never to bring back any of their clothes worn during their stay at the inoculating place. Never to quit it till a certain space of time—fixed by the inoculators—be the disease ever so slight. And if they have any sores about them when they arrive in the harbour, not to come on shore till they are examined by the inspector appointed for that purpose."

If a case of Small Pox occurred in the town the inspector was sent for; if, in his opinion, the person were infected, he took with him some *overseers of the Small Pox*, and if they—in conjunction with a practitioner—pronounced it to be a case of the Small Pox, the family had little more to do with the patient, who was, from that time to the conclusion of the disease, wholly under the direction of these officers, who removed him to an island where everything convenient was already provided.

If the disease were so far advanced before it was known to be the Small Pox, that the patient could not be removed without danger, the street was boarded up, the fact was advertised in the newspaper, and guards were placed to prevent any person coming to within a certain distance of the house. If a vessel arrived in the harbour with Small Pox on board, the sick were taken to the island before referred to, the ship was obliged to undergo quarantine and to hoist a jack in her shrouds, in which case no boats could board her. Dr. Waterhouse adds :—

"I acknowledge some of these rules are unnecessary and inconvenient, but the dread of this disorder induces the people to adhere to them with cheerfulness. A stranger would be ready to conclude that they could not be so scrupulously complied with, without exerting an authority disagreeable to the people ; but it is not the case, for the united voice of the people coinciding with the magistrate, gives every regulation its wished for effect ; so that it rather appears like a popular custom than the restraints of the law."

Haygarth proposed to have general inoculation at stated intervals, but it was only at such time as would be most agreeable to the inhabitants in general. The object of having a general inoculation was, of course, to avoid the danger of propagating the infection ; because, if the inoculation were general, no subject liable to infection would remain. It was only proposed to perform this at a fixed time once in about two years, or less frequently, and this was to be publicly made known, so that those who never had the disease might easily avoid all intercourse with the infectious. The practice of inoculation was to be altogether subsidiary to the plan of stamping out the disease by isolation, the latter system however was regarded by many as visionary, it was not generally adopted, and when the promise of perfect and ever-lasting security was made by the promoters of Cow Pox inoculation, Haygarth's system was ignored and lost sight of.

CHAPTER V.

THE TRADITIONS OF THE DAIRYMAIDS.

ADAMS in his work on Morbid Poisons writes:
" Shall we forget that to the barbers we owe the
bold use of mercury, to the Jesuits, of the Peruvian
bark, which they learned of the Indians, that an
African showed us the value of quassia, that a Greek
slave taught a woman the art of inoculation, the
blessings of which were for a time almost lost by our
fancied improvements and ill-directed cautions? Lastly,
shall we contrast all this with the manner in which a
Jenner has availed himself of the neglected traditions
of cowherds and dairymaids ? "

In some parts of the country, a belief existed among
those who had the care of cattle, that a disease of
cows, which they called Cow Pox, when communicated to the milkers, afforded them protection from
Small Pox.

It is not without importance to consider when, and
how, this belief arose. Pearson and Jenner were both
of opinion that it originated simultaneously with the

introduction of Small Pox inoculation. It remains to be seen how far their conclusion will enable us to explain the origin of this tradition of the dairymaids.

Had a belief in the protective power of Cow Pox existed prior to the practice of inoculation, the early writers on Small Pox would doubtless have mentioned it, and possibly explained it as the outcome of the experience of persons who had contracted Cow Pox and had not subsequently caught Small Pox. But, although Cow Pox and natural Small Pox have been known from time immemorial, there is no evidence to show that this belief originated simultaneously with the early experience of these diseases. How was it, we may ask, .that the tradition arose as a result of Small Pox *inoculation?* It was evidently failure in attempting to inoculate Small Pox on the arms of those who had recently contracted Cow Pox, which gave rise to gossip among the dairymaids, and laid the foundation of the popular tradition. The dairy-folk could not be expected to distinguish between inoculated Small Pox and Small Pox caught in the natural way, and the fact that some Cow Poxed milkers were proof against inoculation was so interpreted, as to afford a foundation for the popular belief that they were for ever after secured from the danger of catching the Small Pox. In many parts of the country, the tradition was unknown amongst those who were quite familiar with Cow Pox; and this may be explained by the fact that inoculation of Small Pox was much more commonly practised in some counties than in others. Another circumstance which points to the relation between this tradition and the inoculation of Small Pox, is, that the resistance in some cases of those who had had Cow Pox was known to those who practised inoculation in the country, long before it was brought to the notice of the profession generally. Thus, it was alleged that the following statements were found among the papers of Mr. Nash[1] after his death :—

"It is rather remarkable that no writer should have taken notice of the Cow Pox.

"I never heard of one having the Small Pox who ever had the Cow Pox. The Cow Pox certainly prevents a person from having the Small Pox. I have now inoculated about sixty persons who have been reported to have had the Cow Pox, and I believe at least forty of them I could not infect with the variolous virus ; the other twenty, or nearly that number, I think it very reasonable to presume (as they were no judges), had not the real Cow Pox. It is not my own opinion only, but that of several other medical gentlemen, that convinces me the Cow Pox is a prophylactick for the Small Pox.

"I have not been able to discover that the human species get it from the cows in any other manner than by contact with the parts immediately infected, such as in milking ; neither do I apprehend that one of the human species can communicate it to another but by the same means, as I have known some of the inhabitants of a house where it was escaped, but none of those who lay in the same bed with the diseased person.

[1] Pearson. *An Examination of the Report of the Committee of the House of Commons*, 1802, p. 24.

"*In Mrs. Scammell and Mrs. Bracher*, inoculation produced no eruption, no sickness, and little or no suppuration of the arm, the place punctured not being bigger when inflamed and suppurated than a large pin's head. It frequently leaves considerable marks, which are much larger than those of the Small Pox, as large (I have measured some) as a silver threepence.

"My principal intention in publishing being to recommend to the world *a method of inoculation* that is far superior, in my opinion (and I judge it from experience), to any yet made known, therefore I hope and trust, although I have no medical friend to enforce it upon the world, that they will give me so far credit for my assertions as to make the experiment, and then it will sufficiently introduce itself. But if, from my being so little known, they should disregard it, I cannot but remind them that we had the art of inoculation first from Grecian women, who were both ignorant and illiterate, and put them in remembrance of the saying of Hippocrates, *Mη οκνεειν*, etc. Upon looking into the systematic writers, as Sauvages and Machide, or those who have made catalogues of definitions of disease, as Linnæus, Vogel, and Cullen, I do not find any disease mentioned by them at all like the Cow Pox.

" Although some people cannot, from the peculiar nature of their constitutions, take the Small Pox ; but that cannot be the reason of so many persons in one part of the country, and no other, being incapable of taking the Small Pox.

"That it is not more surprizing that no one has written on the Cow Pox, since Dr. Heberden was the first who described the Chicken Pox, which had been in the country one hundred years.

"When those who have had the Cow Pox are inoculated, the arms inflame, but never, or at least seldom, form an abscess, but some hard tumour in the muscular flesh.

" On cows, the Cow Pox usually appears at first in round pustules, afterwards in ulcers upon the teats and udders, but principally upon the teats. They do not appear to have any sickness before it comes out. Their teats are so far injured by the inflammation it produces, that people are frequently obliged to open the tubes through which the milk passes with a knitting needle or some such instrument. One cow having it will communicate it to a whole dairy. It continues after a long time upon them unless proper 'means' be employed to cure them, which means are the unguents to the sore parts. The best, I am told, is soot and butter. This disease is not very frequent in this country.

"Cows have the disease but once.

"I have not yet been able to determine whether a person who has had the Small Pox can receive this disease.

"In those who have had the Cow Pox, the arm on inoculation for Small Pox is inflamed to a greater extent than in those who have not had it; but then there is little or no matter in the middle, where the puncture was made, nor does it fill as in those who have not had this disease, but soon heals and dries."

Mr. Nash's observations were written in the year 1781, and he died in 1785. The papers, on his death, were sent by his mother to her brother, Mr. Battiscombe. They passed, about 1795, to Mr. Thomas Nash, and from him, in 1799, to Mr. Robert Keate. It was rumoured that Jenner was acquainted with Nash.

Similar testimony was afforded by Mr. Rolph,[1] who had practised for nine years in Gloucestershire, and was well acquainted with Cow Pox, and had experienced many failures to inoculate milkers who had contracted this disease. Mr. Rolph for two years was a partner of Mr. Grove, who had been a medical practitioner at Thornbury for nearly forty years, and the following facts related by Mr. Rolph were rom his own observations and the experience of Mr. Grove:—

---

[1] Pearson, *loc. cit.*, p. 13.

" Cow Pox is very frequently epizootic in the dairy-farms in the spring season. It especially breaks out in Cows newly introduced into the herds. When a number of Cows on a farm are at the same time affected, the infection seems generally to have originated in the constitution of some one Cow, and before the milker is aware of the existence of the disease, the infectious matter is probably conveyed by the hands to the teats and udders of other Cows. Hence they are infected. For if the disease in the Cow first affected be perceived in a certain state, and obvious precautions be taken, the infection does not spread, but is confined to a single beast. Whether the morbific poison is generated in the Cow first diseased in a farm, *de novo*, from time to time, and disseminated among the rest of the herd, or, like the Small Pox poison, is only communicated from animals of the same species to one another, is not ascertained. No cow has been known to die, or to be in danger from this disorder."

Numbers of cases of milkers suffering from Cow Pox had fallen under Mr. Rolph's observation, and many hundreds more under that of his late partner, Mr. Grove; but not a single fatal or even dangerous case had occurred. The patients ordinarily were ill of a slight fever for two or three days, and the local affection seldom called for the assistance of a medical practitioner.

Mr. Rolph added :—

" There is not a medical practitioner of even little experience in Gloucestershire, or scarce a dairy farmer, who does not know, from his own experience or that of others, that persons who have suffered the Cow Pox are exempted from the agency of the variolous poison.

" The late Mr. Grove was a very extensive Small Pox inoculator, frequently having two hundred to three hundred patients at one time, and the fact of exemption, now asserted, had been long before his death abundantly established, by his experience of many scores of subjects, who had previously laboured under the Cow Pox, being found unsusceptible of the Small Pox either by inoculation or by effluvia."

Mr. Rolph estimated that while he practised at Thornbury, not less than threescore instances of failure in attempting to produce the Small Pox by inoculation occurred in his own practice, and all these were cases of persons who had been previously affected with the Cow Pox; almost all freely associated with those who took Small Pox, and many were repeatedly inoculated, without being infected. Mr. Rolph was not able to recollect any instances of persons taking the Small Pox after the Cow Pox, but he was of opinion that cases may have, and indeed had, occurred to others.

Mr. Dolling, a practitioner at Blandford, had inoculated a number of persons who said they had had Cow Pox, and very few of them took the infection.

Mr. Fewster, who in his early days was associated with Sutton in the practice of inoculation for Small Pox, had repeatedly heard the tradition that Cow Pox afforded security against Small Pox, and had met with cases in his own practice which seemed to support the tradition.

About seventeen years before the publication of Jenner's *Inquiry*, a woman who had had Cow Pox went to an Inoculation Hospital to ascertain whether there was any truth in the common belief, in order to satisfy her brother's curiosity. This circumstance is thus related by Dr. Lettsom in his *Observations on the Cow Pock*, published in 1801, just three years after the publication of Jenner's *Inquiry*.

"Although the Cow Pock has long since been found by incidental experience a security against the Small Pox, it had never been applied to any beneficial purpose till the genius of Jenner discriminated its powers, and introduced it into practice as a permanent security against the variolous infection. This preventive quality of the vaccine fluid was certainly known even to scientific professional men many years ago; but, strange as it may now appear, no one, till Jenner promulgated his discovery, had ever improved that knowledge by applying it to the process of inoculation. About *twenty years* ago, when Dr. Archer was the physician of the hospital for inoculation, Catherine Wilkins, now Titchenor, from Cricklade in Wiltshire, who had had the Cow Pock in consequence of milking cows, came to her brother in London (where she is now resident), who, being desirous of ascertaining whether this circumstance could be depended upon as preventive of the Small Pox, sent her to the hospital for inoculation, when she received the variolous matter from Dr. Archer, against which, however, she was proof, and the Small Pox, of course, could not be communicated ; but no advantage was derived from the fact."

Not only was the tradition well known to inoculators, but we are also informed that there were many who did not believe it ; for it was equally well known that many who had contracted Cow Pox had subsequently suffered from Small Pox. It was owing to this that when Jenner mentioned to his professional neighbours the subject of the prophylactic power of Cow Pox, their reply was not very encouraging.[1]

---

[1] Baron. *Life of Edward Jenner*, vol. i., p. 125.

"We have all heard" (they would observe) "of what you mention, and we have even seen examples which certainly do give some sort of countenance to the notion to which you allude ; but we have also known cases of a perfectly different nature,— many who were reported to have had the Cow Pox having subsequently caught the Small Pox. The supposed prophylactic powers probably, therefore, depend upon some peculiarity in the constitution of the individual who has escaped the Small Pox, and not on any efficacy of that disorder which they may have received from the cow. In short, the evidence is altogether so inconclusive and unsatisfactory that we put no value on it, and cannot think that it will lead to anything but uncertainty and disappointment."

In ·Dorsetshire, according to Mr. Downe,[1] a similar disbelief prevailed among the public as well as among some of the practitioners in those parts.

"The lower class of people still refuse the vaccine inoculation, from an opinion that the resistance to the Small Pox after it, will wear out in a few years, which opinion some medical practitioners encourage."

The tradition was founded on the fact that an attack of Cow Pox interfered with inoculated Small Pox, and it is not therefore surprising that it should have been generally accepted by the country people as worthy of credit, and that attempts should have been made to communicate the disease by different methods, with a view to afford the benefits that were alleged to result, when the disease was contracted by the milkers. Two methods would naturally suggest themselves to the peasant mind : either, to handle the teats of the cows,

[1] Letter from Mr. N. S. Downe, Surgeon, dated Bridport, June 7, 1802, to Dr. Pearson.

or to inoculate themselves in the arm with a needle, according to the method commonly employed in some parts of the country in the practice of buying the Small Pox.

Dr. Pulteney [1] had heard of an instance in which Cow Pox had been contracted intentionally by contact.

"A very respectable practitioner informed me that of seven children whom he had inoculated for the Small Pox, **five had been previously infected with the Cow Pox purposely, by being made to handle the teats and udders** of infected Cows ; in consequence of which they suffered the distemper. **These five,** after inoculation for the Small Pox, did not sicken ; the other **two** took the distemper."

Mr. Downe gave the following history of intentional inoculation in the year 1771 :—

"Robert Fooks, a butcher near Bridport, 31 years ago, when about 20 years of age was at a farmhouse when the dairy was infected with the Cow Pox. It being suggested to him that it would be the means of preserving him from the Small Pox, which he had never taken, if he would submit to be inoculated with the Cow Pox matter, he gave his consent : he was infected by a needle in two or three places in his hand. In about a week, the parts began to inflame and his hand to swell, his head to ach, and many other symptoms of fever came on. The parts inoculated left permanent scars. He was afterwards inoculated twice by my grandfather, and a considerable time after, twice by my father, but without any effect than a slight irritation of the part, such as is occasioned in the arms of persons who have already had the Small Pox. The Small Pox has been repeatedly since in his own

---

[1] Letter from Dr. Pulteney to Dr. Pearson, dated Blandford, July 14, 1798.

family, and he never avoided it, being confident that it was not possible to infect him with this disease."

Mr. Nicholas Bragge,[1] an apothecary, reported in a letter written in 1802, that a farmer's wife had performed a similar operation.

" It is now, I believe, twenty years ago that Mrs. Rendall, the wife of a respectable farmer in the parish of Whitechurch, near Lyme, in Dorsetshire (who is at this time a tenant to Lady Caroline Damer, in the same parish for which I have been concerned as an apothecary for the poor ever since I have been in business), inoculated herself and three or four children for it ; **and those children, who have long arrived at manhood, have since inoculated their friends and neighbours whenever an opportunity has offered.**"

But these inoculations were not only performed by farmers' wives. Mr. Nicholas Bragge appears himself to have inoculated Cow Pox, and to have advocated its prophylactic efficacy.

" It is now more than thirty years ago that I first made experiments, and proved that the Vaccine Distemper was a preservative against the Small Pox ; and it is, I believe, more than twenty years ago, that, through the Rev. Herman Drew, I acquainted Sir George Baker with the observations and experiments I had then made, which I am certain Sir George will readily acknowledge."

This statement was supported by Mr. Tucker,[2] in a letter in 1802, in which he wrote that Mr. Bragge,

---

[1] Mr. Nicholas Bragge's Letter, dated Axminster, April 12, 1802, to Sir William Elford, Bart.

[2] Letter from William Tucker, Esq., of Coryton, in Devonshire, to Sir William Elford, Bart., April 12, 1802.

twenty years ago, with great assiduity recommended the practice of vaccine inoculation, and had furnished Sir George Baker, through the Rev. Herman Drew, with a variety of papers in proof of its being a sure guard against Small Pox.

The Rev. Herman Drew[1] was not only interested in Mr. Bragge's researches, but in a letter conveys the impression that he too had performed some experiments about 1782.

"Nearly twenty years ago, I wrote sheets of paper to Sir George Baker on this disorder, and I know not what occasioned his laying aside his intention of publishing his investigations. He had had a previous correspondence with Dr. Pulteney of Blandford on the subject. . . .

"No one can have an higher opinion of the good effects of the vaccine inoculation than I have. It has occupied my thoughts for years, and nothing but Horace's advice, 'Ne sutor ultra crepidam,' has checked me from the use of the infected lancet or saturated cotton. *Entre nous, I have had a little successful practice.*"

According to Dr. Barry, the casual Cow Pox (or Shinach) had been known in Ireland, perhaps, as long as the Small Pox. Instances had occurred of persons having had the Cow Pox about 1750, and one woman, eighty years of age, asserted that as long as she could remember, the opinion prevailed that *people who had the Cow Pox cannot take the Small*

---

[1] Letter from the Rev. Herman Drew to Sir William Elford, Bart., dated Abbots, near Honiton, April 1, 1802.

Pox; and that people purposely exposed themselves to it to protect themselves from the Small Pox.

Two cases of intentional inoculation in Ireland were related by Dr. Barry.[1]

"A woman ill of the casual Cow Pox, by handling her infant then at her breast, produced Cow Pox. Two years after this child slept with another child with Small Pox, and was also inoculated for Small Pox, but without exciting the disease."

"A gardener gave himself the Cow Pox purposely by rubbing himself against some person who was affected with it, from a conviction that it would prevent the Small Pox. This happened several years ago ; and though he has often put himself in the way of Small Pox infection, and even lain in the same bed with his children when they were covered with it, he has not taken the disease. If I had time to make the necessary inquiries I am sure I could multiply instances of this kind."

Mr. Jesty.—It may perhaps be said, that there is very little interest in the accounts which have just been related, owing to the absence of sufficiently reliable evidence, to entitle them to be regarded as authentic. But this cannot be said of the inoculations performed by Mr. Jesty. I shall give in full all the evidence which I have been able to collect from different sources, with a view of establishing Jesty's experiment as an historical fact, for Jenner regarded the account of it as an invention to deprive him of the merit of discovering Cow Pox inoculation. Baron, the biographer of Jenner, turned a deaf ear to anything

---

[1] Letter to Dr. Pearson, Oct. 16, 1800, and *Medical and Physical Journal*, p. 503. 1800.

which he considered might detract from Jenner's credit, and only referred in his biography to Jesty's *alleged* vaccinations; and in more recent times in Simon's history of vaccination there is no mention of Jesty whatever.

Benjamin Jesty held, at one time, a large farm at Yetminster in Dorset, and carried on an extensive business by sending cattle to the London market. From Yetminster, he removed to the farm of Down-shay, belonging to Mr. Calcraft, not very far from Swanage. There, many years afterwards, he formed the acquaintance of the Rev. Dr. Bell,[1] who had introduced the practice of vaccination into Swanage. Jesty, having inoculated his wife and two children with Cow Pox in 1774, became anxious that his claims to the original discovery should be known; and he accordingly gave Dr. Bell an account of his proceedings, and suggested that he was entitled to some reward as well as Jenner. Dr. Bell was much struck with Jesty's narrative, and drew up the following paper on the subject, though he was afraid that Jesty was too late in making his claim, as he had not made his discovery known at the time, and had only practised inoculation on members of his own family.

"*Of the Vaccine Inoculation as performed thirty years ago.* 1st August, 1803.

"The inoculation with vaccine matter, as taught by Dr. Jenner and diffused over the globe by the ability, industry, and well

---

[1] Southey. *The Life of the Rev. Andrew Bell*, vol. ii., p. 98.

directed exertions of that great benefactor of the human race, now rests on such universal experience as might seem to require no further support or illustration. Sir Isaac Newton, Dr. Franklin, Monsieur Lavoisier (or, if you chose, rather Dr. Black), and Harvey, could not, in the same short period, boast of equal success in the spread of their respective discoveries; still, however, there are some who question the efficacy of vaccination as a preventive of the Small Pox.

"After I had last spring, by way of introducing (for that was all I proposed in the first instance) the practice into this peninsula, inoculated, with vaccine matter which I brought from a distance of five hundred miles, upwards of three hundred persons—men, women, and children—in my insulated parish and neighbourhood (Isle of Purbeck), where the visitation of Small Pox is a stranger, having only occurred twice in forty years, once by infection, and once by inoculation, I have the mortification to find that the efficacy of this disorder is still disputed, and that parents still decline to submit their children to this simple operation. Even learned and able physicians have argued that Dr. Jenner's discovery is not of sufficient standing to establish that the vaccine inoculation is a security against the variolous infection for a longer period than his practice extends.

"It may not therefore be altogether useless to bring forward a fact which, in an earlier stage of Dr. Jenner's practice, would (had it been known to him) have given weight to his doctrines, and which still perhaps may be thought not unworthy of a place in the history of the Cow Pox. If it should have any influence with those parents who decline the offer made to them of having their children vaccinated, my object is attained; and let Mr. Jesty have that share of credit (whatever it may be) which attaches to his bold and successful experiment.

"In the spring of the year 1774, Farmer Benjamin Jesty, then of Yetminster in Dorset, now of Downshay, Isle of Purbeck, inoculated with vaccine matter, his wife[1] and two sons, Robert

---

[1] He is said to have had the infection himself by casually taking it from the cows before this.—BELL.

and Benjamin, of three and two years of age, and all three now alive. Mrs. Jesty was inoculated in the arm under the elbow, her sons above the elbow. The incision was made with a needle, and the virus taken on the spot from the cows of Farmer Elford of Chittenhall, whither Mr. Jesty carried his family for that purpose. The sons had the disorder in a favourable way, but Mrs. Jesty's arm was much inflamed; and the boldness and novelty of the attempt produced no small alarm in the family, and no small sensation in the neighbourhood. Fifteen years afterwards (1789), the sons were inoculated for the Small Pox by Mr. Trowbridge, surgeon, of Cerne Abbas, along with others who had not had the Cow Pox. The arms of the former inflamed, but the inflammation soon subsided, and no fever or other variolous symptom was observable; the latter went through the fever eruption and usual course of the inoculated Small Pox. Mrs. Jesty and the two sons have often since been exposed to the variolous contagion.

" It may be inquired by the future historian of the Cow Pox what led to this early essay of introducing the vaccine virus into the human frame ? and how it happened that this successful attempt fell still-born from the cow ? Mr. Jesty's relation is to this effect :—

" When the Small Pox raged in the vicinity and inoculation was introduced into the village (Yetminster), alarmed for the safety of his family, he bethought himself of this expedient. There had been, in his family, two maid servants, Ann Notley and Mary Read, who, after having the disorder from the cows, and knowing this to be a preventive of the Small Pox, had attended, the one her brother, the other her nephew, in the natural Small Pox without taking the infection. This circumstance led Mr. Jesty to communicate by inoculation the disorder of the cows to his family. For this purpose he carried them to the field of a neighbouring farm, and, as has been related, performed the operation on the spot.

" To the other question, how did it happen that this discovery expired at its birth, a ready solution will be found in the character of the ingenious farmer, whose pursuits were widely different from those of medicine, or literature, or science, and in the natural prejudice of mankind strengthened by the alarm which the inflammation of Mrs. Jesty's arm had excited. To such a height was this prejudice carried that a neighbouring surgeon, whose name I have not been able to learn, had almost lost his practice from the bare proposal of following up Mr. Jesty's bold and successful experiment.

"With those who objected to introducing the bestial disorder into the human frame, already liable to so many diseases, the farmer has been heard to say that he argued after this manner :—

"For his part he preferred taking infection from an innocuous animal like a cow, subject to so few disorders, to taking it from the human body, liable to so many and such diseases ; and that he had experience on his side, as the casual Cow Pox was not attended with danger like the variolous infection ; and that beside, there appeared to him little risk in introducing into the human constitution matter from the cow, as we already without danger eat the flesh and blood, drink the milk, and cover ourselves with the skin of this innocuous animal."

This statement was forwarded some time afterwards to the Jennerian Society, and a copy was also sent to the Right Hon. George Rose. In a note accompanying the latter, Dr. Bell said :—

"If you think it worth the previous notice of your friends, Mr. Pitt, Sir H. Mildmay, etc., or of being otherwise disposed of, you have my leave. I have many apologies to offer for obtruding upon you at this time, but as this affair has long lain dormant, and is now to be forwarded to the R.J.S., I am exceedingly desirous of presenting to you this simultaneous communication."

An answer was returned by the secretary of the Jennerian Society, stating "that he had received Dr. Bell's very interesting paper of the vaccine inoculation, and that he should have an opportunity of laying it before the two boards at their meeting on the following evening." At the time that Dr. Bell drew up this statement, he was not aware of Dr. Pearson's pamphlet, in which Mr. Jesty's name had already been mentioned.

Indeed, Dr. Bell had obtained his information directly from Mr. Jesty, and quite independently of Dr. Pearson; and this is sufficient to show how utterly unjustifiable was Jenner's view that the whole story was a "trick" invented by Pearson. Dr. Pearson's publication fell into Dr. Bell's hands shortly afterwards, and he wrote immediately to the Secretary of the Jennerian Society :—

> " CENTRAL HOUSE, SALISBURY SQUARE,
> " *July 7th*, 1804.

"SIR,—In Dr. Pearson's pamphlet which has just been put into my hands, I read as follows :—'Mr. Justins' (a mistake for Jesty), 'a farmer of Yetminster in Dorset, inoculated his wife and family with matter taken from the teat of a cow that had the Cow Pox. In about a week from the time of inoculation, their arms were very much inflamed, the patients were very ill, and the man was so much alarmed as to call in medical assistance (Mr. Read, of Cerne). The patients soon got well, and they have since been inoculated for the Small Pox by Mr. Trowbridge, of Cerne, but without effect.'

"'I cannot inform you at what period Mr. Justins inoculated his family, but I have no doubt it was previous to Dr. Jenner's practice.

"'The farmer alluded to in Mr. Pulteney's letter to you, who inoculated his wife and children with matter taken from a cow, and the person mentioned in Mr. Drew's letter, viz., Mr. Justins, is the same person. Both Mr. Pulteney's and Mr. Drew's intelligence came from me, I am not certain at this time as to the year, but I believe it was on or before the year 1786. The farmer is still living, of whom I can have the particulars.

"'In a subsequent letter to Dr. Pearson, dated Chattle June 15th, 1802, Mr. Dolling informed him that Mr. Benjamin Jesty (not Justins) performed the inoculation above mentioned as early as 1774,[1] and he is still living.

"'I know a medical man in this country who was greatly injured in his practice by a prejudice raised against him long ago for his intention of substituting the Cow Pox for the Small Pox.'

"These extracts, had I seen Dr. Pearson's pamphlet, should have preceded the statement which I forwarded to you in my late letter, and you will perhaps agree with me in opinion that they should still be subjoined in a note. The facts which I have detailed were communicated to me by the parties themselves, and their accuracy may be depended on."

Mr. Banks, the member for Corfe Castle, wrote to Dr. Bell on the same subject :—

"*October 16th*, 1804.

"SIR,—A fact relating to a farmer in Dorsetshire, which I take to be the same that is mentioned in the enclosed papers,[2] given in evidence before the committee of the House of Commons, to whom Dr. Jenner's petition was referred, and if I am not mistaken was printed in their report. There was, I am sure, abundant proof of the disorder being known, and of its preventive power, long before Dr. Jenner's name was heard ; nor, at this moment, do those who continue to doubt the complete efficacy of the Cow Pock deny its success in innumerable instances."

The Jennerian Society now became desirous of seeing Mr. Jesty, and an endeavour was made to induce him to go up to London ; but, fearing an

---

[1] "Dr. Jenner is said first to have considered the subject in 1775, but it was not until 1796 that he made his first experiment."—BELL.

[2] Dr. Bell's statement.

attack of gout, to which he was subject, he declined to undertake the journey. In the course of the next year, the following letter was addressed to him by the secretary of the society :—

"LONDON, *July 25th*, 1805.

"SIR,—I am desired by the medical establishment of this institution to propose to you that, provided you will come to town at your own convenience, but as soon as possible, to stay not longer than five days, unless you desire it, for the purpose of taking your portrait as the earliest inoculator for Cow Pock, at the expense of the institution, you will receive 15 guineas for your expenses, and the members of the establishment will be happy to show you any civility during your stay in London, on which account it is hoped you will be put to little or no expense.

"I have the honour to remain, Sir,

"Your Obedient, Humble Servant,

"WILL SANCHO."

Mr. Jesty accepted this invitation, taking with him his son Robert, whom he had inoculated in 1774.

"They met with great attention from the members of the society, who were much amused with Jesty's manners and appearance. Before he left home, his family tried to induce him to attire himself somewhat more fashionably, but without effect. 'He did not see,' he said, 'why he should dress better in London than in the country;' and accordingly wore his usual dress, which was peculiarly old-fashioned. In order to prove their statement, Mr. Robert Jesty willingly consented to be inoculated for the Small Pox, and his father for the Cow Pock, but neither took effect.

"Mr. Jesty was presented with a pair of very handsome gold-mounted lancets, and his portrait was also taken by Mr. Sharpe; but he proved an impatient sitter, and could only be kept quiet by Mrs. Sharpe's playing to him on the piano."

The portrait, from which an engraving was made, was exhibited at Somerset House, and afterwards placed in the Vaccine Institution; it then fell into Dr. Pearson's hands, and on his death, passed to his son-in-law, who, finding that Jesty's family were anxious to possess it, presented it to Robert Jesty. After Robert Jesty's death, the portrait remained with his widow for a time at Wraxall House, near Maiden Newton.

During my inquiries in Dorsetshire, early in 1888, I was fortunate enough to obtain one of the original engravings, made from this portrait, of which the frontispiece is a reduced fac-simile. I also ascertained that the portrait was in the possession of Jesty's great-grandson, Mr. Frank Pope, of Chilfrome, near Dorchester; I thus had an opportunity of seeing the portrait, and of acquiring much interesting information.

The following statement was also drawn up and signed by the members of the Jennerian Society, and presented with the portrait :—

"Mr. Benjamin Jesty, farmer, of Downshay, in the Isle of Purbeck, having, agreeable to an invitation from the Medical establishment of the Original Vaccine Pock Institution, Broad Street, Golden Square, visited London in August, 1805, to communicate certain facts relating to the Cow Pock Inoculation, we think it a matter of justice to himself and beneficial to the Public, to attest that, among other facts, he has afforded decisive evidence of his having vaccinated his wife and two sons, Robert and Benamin, in the year 1774, who were thereby rendered unsusceptible of the Small Pox, as appears from the exposure of all the parties to that disease frequently during the course of thirty-one years, and from the inoculation of the two sons for the Small Pox fifteen years ago. That he was led to undertake this novel practice in 1774, to counteract the Small Pox at that time prevalent where he then resided, from knowing the common opinion of the country ever since he was a boy, now about sixty years ago, that persons who had gone through the Cow Pox naturally (*i.e.*) by taking it from the cows, were unsusceptible of the Small Pox; by himself being incapable of taking the Small Pox, by having gone through the Cow Pox many years before; from having personally known many individuals who, after the Cow Pox, could not have the Small Pox excited; from believing that the Cow Pox was an affection free from danger; and from his opinion that by the Cow Pock inoculation he should avoid engrafting various diseases of the human constitution—such as the evil, madness, lues, and many bad humours, as he called them.

"The remarkably vigorous health of Mr. Jesty's wife and two sons, now thirty-one years subsequent to the Cow Pox, and his own healthy appearance, at this time seventy years of age, afford a singular proof of the harmlessness of that affection. But the public must, with particular interest, hear that during their late visit to town, Mr. Robert Jesty very willingly submitted publicly to inoculation for the Small Pox in the most rigorous manner, and that Mr. Jesty also was subjected to the trial of inoculation for the Cow Pock after the most efficacious mode, without either of them being infected.

"The circumstances in which Mr. Jesty purposely instituted the vaccine pock inoculation in his own family—viz., without any precedent, but merely from reasoning upon the nature of the affection among cows, and from knowing its effects in the casual way among men, his exemption from the prevailing popular prejudices, and his disregard of the clamorous reproaches of his neighbours, in our opinion will entitle him to the respect of the public for his superior strength of mind; but, further, his conduct in again furnishing such decisive proofs of the permanent anti-variolous efficacy of the Cow Pock, in the present discontented state of many families, by submitting to inoculation, justly claims at least the gratitude of the country. As a testimony of our personal regards, and to commemorate so extraordinary a fact as that of preventing the Small Pox by inoculation for the Cow Pock thirty-one years ago, at our request a three-quarter length picture of Mr. Jesty is painted by that excellent artist Mr. Sharpe, to be preserved at the original Vaccine Pock Institution.

Physicians.	*Consulting Surgeons.*	*Surgeons.*
George Pearson,	—— Wheate,	Joseph Constantine,
L. Nitell,	F. Foster.	Carpue,
Thos. Nelson.		J. Doratt.

Visiting Apothecaries.	*Treasurers.*
Fra. Rivers,	J. Heaviside,
Everard A. Brande,	T. Payne."
Philip de Bruyn.	

Jesty's visit to London had satisfactorily established his claim as the first inoculator of Cow Pox, but there the matter ended ; and while he was in London he does not seem to have pressed for any pecuniary reward. The following year, however, he wrote to Dr. Pearson on the subject, and his letter was communicated to the members of the Institution. The secretary wrote to Jesty in answer, stating that they would endeavour to promote his views, but they were afraid it was very improbable that any such reward would be obtained. After this, Jesty gave up all expectations ; and his circumstances were such as to render it a matter of little importance.

But the interest of his family in the subject did not on that account cease. His son Benjamin became an enthusiast in the cause of Cow Pox inoculation. In the year 1809, he is said to have performed the operation on great numbers, and to have kept a regular register of the names of the individuals, and of the progress of the disorder in each.

There is also additional local evidence, proving the accuracy of Dr. Bell's account, in a letter written by the Rev. J. M. Colson, of Swanage, to the Rev. F. F. Tracy.

"*February* 16*th*, 1860.

"My Dear Sir,—"I have a perfect recollection of old Jesty coming to our house at Corfe, the one now inhabited by Mr. Bradley, to borrow of my father a pair of saddle-bags to contain his clean shirts when he was going to London to give evidence on his discovery of vaccination, and being *vice* the saddle-bags (a thing of bygone ages, now quite an *extinctum genus*), supplied with a portmanteau as a more convenient vehicle. On his return, he gave a very unfavourable report of the metropolis.; but, *per contra*, said there was one great comfort there indeed—viz., that he could be shaved *every day*, instead of wearing his beard from Saturday to Saturday, on which day alone—when he rode into Wareham market—was he relieved of that encumbrance (as it was then thought, *now, tempora mutantur*). I cannot precisely date this event. We lived at Corfe from May 1800 till October 1810, and my belief is that it must have been about 1805, 6, or 7. Some years before this, he had lived at a farm in the neighbourhood of Cerne, of this county (Dorset), and there he first practised vaccination on his own children. Fever ran high with his patients, and he called in Mr. Trowbridge, the medical man of Cerne (whom I full well remember in later years when we lived near that place), and told him what he had done. Trowbridge said, ' You have done a bold thing, but I will get you through it if I can ; ' treated it as fever, and was

---

¹ Papers read before the Purbeck Society, p. 244. .1860.

successful. I should have said that old Jesty, not being equipped with a lancet, performed the operation with a stocking needle! ! . . .

" Believe me,

" Truly yours,

" J. M. COLSON."

Jesty died in 1816, and was buried in the church-yard of Worth Matravers, near Swanage. On the tombstone is the following inscription :—

Sacred
To the Memory
of
BENJ^N. JESTY (OF DOWNSHAY),
Who departed this life
April 16th, 1816,
AGED 79 YEARS.

He was born at Yetminster in this County, and was an upright honest man ; particularly noted for having been the first Person (known) that introduced the Cow Pox by inoculation, and who, from his great strength of mind, made the experiment from the Cow on his wife and two sons in the year 1774.

The anxiety which Jesty must have felt when his inoculations were in progress, can be well understood in the light of later experiences. Those severe symptoms occurred, which have so commonly followed the use of lymph direct from the cow. Fever ran high with his patients, and he was obliged to call in medical aid ; in fact, he met with similar occurrences to those which many years afterwards alarmed Jenner, Bousquet, Estlin, and others to whose lot it has fallen to observe the full effects of the Cow Pox virus.

Mrs. Jesty, who was thus the first person known to have been intentionally Cow Poxed, not only recovered from the operation, but lived to the age of eighty-four, a result which if it was not actually credited to the beneficial effects on the constitution alleged to follow the operation, was certainly testimony that it had produced no permanent ill effects.

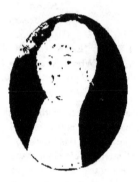

ELIZABETH JESTY.   Inoculated with Cow Pox in 1774.

Mrs. Jesty was buried by the side of her husband in the churchyard of Worth Matravers, and her tombstone bears the following inscription :—

Sacred to the
Memory of
ELIZABETH JESTY,
Relict of the late
BENJAMIN JESTY,
of Downshay, who departed
this life, Jan. 8, 1824,
AGED 84 YEARS.

To the descendants of Jesty, still living in Dorsetshire, I am indebted for the copy of the portrait of
Mrs. Jesty, which is here reproduced. It affords additional evidence of the fact that the above accounts
are records of persons whose existence was not merely
imaginary.

CHAPTER VI.

EDWARD JENNER was a native of Berkeley, in Gloucestershire. He was born in 1749, and was the third
son of the Rev. Stephen Jenner, M.A., Vicar of
Berkeley. Jenner's father had been tutor to a former
Earl of Berkeley, who had a great regard for all the
family.

In the Berkeley manuscripts, published by Thomas
Dudley Fosbrooke in 1821, it is remarked that the
foundations for Jenner's subsequent investigations on
the subject of protection from Small Pox, were probably
laid in an early period of his life. He was eight
years of age when he was put under the preparatory
regimen for inoculation. This lasted for six weeks,
during which time he was bled, purged, kept on
very low diet, and dosed with "a diet drink to
sweeten the blood." After this "he was removed
to one of the then usual inoculation stables, and
haltered up with others in a terrible state of disease,
although none died." By good fortune, Jenner escaped

with a mild attack. Such is the incident on which Fosbrooke felt justified in making the following comment :—

"It is, without superstition, a noticeable incident in a biographical account that the misery endured in the Small Pox process should have laid the foundation for the extermination of the disease, and it is strongly indicative of a philosophical bias in the character. It exhibits impression accompanied with reflection, and a view to the removal of the evil. Whereas common man takes such incidents as usual inevitable occurrences, feels irritable, swears stoutly, and then forgets."

Shortly afterwards, Jenner was sent to school at Cirencester, where he stayed half a year ; but his health not being reinstated, he was placed with a private tutor. The effect of the preparation and inoculation was said to be this : "As a child he could never enjoy sleep, and was constantly tormented by imaginary noises and a sensibility too acutely alive to these, and sudden jars subsisted through many years." As a schoolboy, Jenner is said to have been "enamoured of natural history," as evidenced by his possessing a dormouse, and making a collection of birds' nests. At thirteen years of age, Jenner was placed under the care of the Messrs. Ludlow, then eminent practitioners at Sodbury, near Bristol, and remained with them six years. It was during his apprenticeship there, that, according to Baron, an incident happened which laid the foundation of Jenner's future observations.

"It has been stated that his attention was drawn forcibly to the nature of Cow Pox while he was yet a youth. The event was brought about in the following manner :—He was pursuing his professional education in the house of his master at Sodbury ; a young countrywoman came to seek advice; the subject of Small Pox was mentioned in her presence ; she immediately observed, ' I cannot take that disease, for I have had Cow Pox.' This incident rivetted the attention of Jenner."

That such an event occurred is extremely probable, for the famous tradition was part of the stock gossip of the dairymaids, and was well known to many practitioners in dairy districts. But if it "rivetted the attention of Jenner" at this period, it is somewhat extraordinary that Fosbrooke should have made no allusion to such an interesting incident, especially as the first biography was written during Jenner's life, and the anecdotes it contained were written on authority. Baron nevertheless attributes the greatest importance to this incident.

"Newton had unfolded his doctrine of light and colours before he was twenty; Bacon wrote his *Temporis Partus Maximus* before he attained that age ; Montesquieu had sketched his *Spirit of Laws* at an equally early period of life; and Jenner, when he was still younger, contemplated the possibility of removing from among the list of human diseases one of the most mortal that ever scourged our race."

Jenner's hypochondriacal habit, attributed to the Small Pox inoculation, still existed at this period, though it is said to have gradually diminished. After the usual course of instruction in materia medica and surgery, Jenner became, at the age of twenty-one, house pupil to John Hunter, and is said to have mentioned the subject of Cow Pox to him. He assisted him in forming his valuable museum, and on his return to Berkeley, undertook anatomical and physiological researches (suggested by Hunter), while he at the same time commenced practice. It was at this stage, we are told, that the first great event of his professional career occurred. During the indisposition of the senior surgeon of the Gloucester Infirmary, he operated with success on a case of strangulated hernia.

Jenner was also interested in pharmaceutical chemistry, and as, in his experience, some of the preparations were by no means perfect, he was led to investigate them. This was particularly the case with tartar emetic. He wrote a small pamphlet on the subject, apparently his earliest publication, and he also communicated the results of his inquiries to Hunter, which were acknowledged in the following letter [1] :—

MR. HUNTER TO E. JENNER.

"DEAR JENNER,—

"I am puffing off your tartar, as the tartar of all tartars, and have given it to several physicians to make trial, but have had no account yet of the success. Had you not better let a bookseller have it to sell, as Glass of Oxford did his magnesia? Let it be called Jenner's Tartar Emetic, or any body's else you please. If that mode would do, I will speak to some, viz. Newbery, etc. You are very sly, although you think I cannot see it: you very modestly ask for a thermometer; I will send one, but take care

[1] The original letter is in the library of the Royal College of Surgeons.

that those d——d clumsy fingers do not break it also. I should be glad to have a true and particular account of the cuckoo, and as far as possible under your own eye. To put all matters out of dispute, if the cuckoo's eggs were taken out of the hedge-sparrow's nest in which they were laid, and put into another by human hands, there could be no supposition that the parent cuckoos would feed, or take any care of them. I also want some young ones. I had a series from you, but a moth got in among them, and plucked them.

"Let me hear from you when you can.

> "Yours,
> "J. HUNTER."

Jenner made some original observations on the natural history of the cuckoo, which he made the subject of a paper for the Royal Society. It was returned with a letter from Sir Joseph Banks, who wrote :—

"In consequence of you having discovered that the young cuckoo, and not the parent bird, removes the eggs and young from the nest in which it is deposited, the council thought it best to give you a full scope for altering it, as you shall choose. Another year we shall be glad to receive it again and print it. Your other papers I hope you will proceed with, when your leisure allows you opportunity."

The paper was finally read on March 13th, 1788, and published in the *Philosophical Transactions* for that year. According to Fosbrooke

"It proved the very singular fact that the infant cuckoo reared from the egg in the sparrow's nest expelled the young of that bird by placing them upon its shoulder, on a depression, which Nature gives for the purpose, on the back of the unfledged cuckoo, and throwing them out of the nest. There are also other phenomena never before noticed. These curious incidents were affirmed by Pennant to have eluded research from the time of Aristotle."

On the continent, the paper appears to have been read with interest, and to have received the highest praise from at least one person. In a postscript, Blümenbach wrote to Jenner :—

"Give me leave, Sir, to tell you also that I, as a very warm friend and even teacher of Natural History, long very eagerly to see at once your paper on the migration of birds, mentioned in your **masterly observations on the cuckoo.**"

After the publication of this paper, Jenner was elected a Fellow of the Royal Society. Soon afterwards he was married to Miss Kathleen Kingscote, and he was assisted in his practice by his nephew, Henry, whom he had taken as his apprentice. From the proceeds of his practice, and a patrimonial inheritance, Jenner in 1792 took out a diploma. He then settled down in Chauntry Cottage, Berkeley, where he devoted a good deal of his spare time to landscape gardening. In 1794, he had a severe attack of typhus, and was confined to his house by debility till the spring of 1795. He removed to Cheltenham during the season, and was occasionally called in consultation by local practitioners. From Fosbrooke we learn that

"it was chiefly during these periods of residence in Berkeley and Cheltenham (because he was not then burdened with the labours which vaccine has generated) that Dr. Jenner used to

.amuse · himself with extemporaneous effusions in poetry, not intended for the press. In this way his taste generally took an epigrammatical turn, but was strictly confined to harmless gentlemanly facetiousness."

The statement of Fosbrooke, that up to the year 1795, Jenner was not burdened with the labours which vaccine had generated, is important, and leads one to ask how it is that the *Inquiry*, published in 1798, has been described by Simon[1] as the outcome of thirty years of incessant thought, watching, and experiment.

" Thirty years elapsed before the fruit was borne to the public ; but incessantly he thought, and watched, and experimented on the subject."

Baron is responsible for this illusion. The incident at Sodbury, in 1770,[2] was credited with riveting the attention of Jenner. When Jenner returned from London and settled in practice, his attention was again drawn to the subject of Cow Pox, and it is stated that in 1780, he conversed on the subject with his friend Gardner. Baron[3] gave the following account of this conversation:

"It was not till 1780 that he was enabled, after much study and inquiry, to unravel many of the perplexing obscurities and contradictions with which the question was enveloped, and which had impressed those who knew the traditions of the country with the opinion that it defied all accurate and satisfactory elucidation. In the month of May of the year just mentioned, he first disclosed his hopes and his fears respecting the great object of his pursuit,

---

[1] Simon. *Papers relating to the History of Vaccination*, 1857.

[2] *Vide*, p. 127.

[3] Baron, *loc. cit.*

to his friend Edward Gardner. By this time Jenner's mind had caught a glimpse of the reputation which awaited him, but it was still clouded by doubts and difficulties. He then seemed to feel that it might, in God's good providence, be his lot to stand between the living and the dead, and that through him a plague might be stayed. On the other side, the dread of disappointment, and the probability of failing to accomplish his purpose, restrained that eagerness which otherwise would have prompted him prematurely to publish the result of his inquiries, and thereby, probably, by conveying insufficient knowledge, blight for ever his favourite hope.

" He was riding with Gardner, on the road between Gloucester and Bristol, near Newport, when the conversation passed of which I have made mention. He went over the natural history of Cow Pox ; stated his opinion as to the origin of this affection from the heel of the horse ; specified the different sorts of disease which attacked the milkers when they handled infected cows ; dwelt upon that variety which afforded protection against Small Pox ; and with deep and anxious emotion mentioned his hope of being able to propagate that variety from one human being to another, till he had disseminated the practice all over the globe, to the total extinction of Small Pox. The conversation was concluded by Jenner in words to the following effect :—' Gardner, I have entrusted a most important matter to you, which I firmly believe will prove of essential benefit to the human race. I know you, and should not wish what I have stated to be brought into conversation ; for should anything untoward turn up in my experiments, I should be made, particularly by my medical brethren, the subject of ridicule, for I am the mark they all shoot at."

Jenner was evidently much interested in the natural history of Cow Pox, and, in 1787, it is related that his nephew, George Jenner, accompanied him into the stable to look at a horse with diseased heels. " There," said Jenner, pointing to his horse's heels, " is the source of Small Pox. I have much to say on that subject, which I hope in due time to give to the world."

In 1788, Jenner took a drawing of the hand of a milker with Cow Pox, to London, and showed it to Sir Everard Home and others. The subject of Cow Pox now became a topic of conversation in the profession, and was mentioned to students by more than one lecturer. Seven years after the incident of 1787 he wrote :—

"Our friend ————, at our last meeting, treated my discovery as Chimerical. Farther investigation has convinced me of the truth of my assertion, beyond the possibility of a denial. Domestication of animals has certainly proved a prolific source of disease among men. But I must not anticipate ; you shall have a paper."

Jenner had always freely conversed with others on this subject, and in the same year his intimate friend Dr. Worthington gave an account of his work (without mentioning his name) to Dr. Haygarth, who in replying made the following criticisms :—

"Your account of the Cow Pox is indeed very marvellous : being so strange a history, and so contradictory to all past observations on this subject, very clear and full evidence will be required to render it credible.

"You say that this whole rare phenomenon is soon to be published ; but do not mention whether by yourself or some other medical friend. In either case, I trust that no reliance will be placed upon vulgar stories.

"The author should admit nothing but what he has proved by his own personal observation, both in the brute and human species. It would be useless to specify the doubts which must be satisfied upon this subject, before rational belief can be obtained.

"If a physician should adopt such a doctrine, and, much more, if he should publish it upon inadequate evidence, his character would materially suffer in the public opinion of his knowledge and discernment."

The subject of Cow Pox was not only mentioned in conversation and lectures in London, but was referred to in medical works.

Dr. Adams, in his work on Morbid Poisons, published in 1795, says :—

"The Cow Pox is a disease well-known to the dairy-farmers in Gloucestershire. The only appearance on the animal is a phagedænic ulcer on the teat, without any apparent inflammation. When communicated to the human, it produces, besides ulceration in the hand, a considerable tumour of the arm, with symptomatic fever, both which gradually subside. What is still more extraordinary, as far as facts have hitherto been ascertained, the person who has been infected is rendered insensible to the variolous poison."

In the second edition of this work, published in 1807, in a footnote he adds :—

"Though this description of Cow Pox is incorrect, excepting in· its consequence on the human, I have preserved it as an historical register of my imperfect knowledge of this disease when the first edition was published. There was then no printed account of the Cow Pox. Mr. Cline, knowing the object of my enquiries, acquainted me with what he had heard from Dr. Jenner, and by his correspondence procured me further information."

From this it would appear that Adams had independently commenced inquiries, though, in a letter to

Jenner, Cline thought that he was entirely responsible for Dr. Adams' information on the subject.

"I am very glad to learn that you are prosecuting your inquiries on the Cow Pox, for it is a most interesting and curious subject. All that Adams had heard of the disease was from me."

The same year as Adams' first publication, Dr. Beddoes[1] wrote as follows :—

"I have learned from my own observation, and the testimony of some old practitioners, that susceptibility to the Small Pox is destroyed by the Cow Pox, a disease from cows, which is a malady more unpleasant than dangerous."

And the year following, 1796, Dr. Woodville referred to the same subject, in a footnote in his *History of Small Pox Inoculation.*

"It has been conjectured that the Small Pox might have been derived from some disease of brute animals ; and if it be true that the mange affecting dogs can communicate a species of itch to man, or that a person having received a certain disorder from handling the teats of cows, is thereby rendered insensible to variolous infection ever afterwards, as some have asserted, then indeed this conjecture is not improbable."

Jenner had not only heard of cases of immunity from Small Pox after Cow Pox, but he had made notes of a few which had been brought to his notice. In 1778, he inoculated a Mrs. H. unsuccessfully, which result he attributed to her having had Cow Pox

---

[1] Dr. Beddoes, *Queries concerning Inoculation*, 8vo. 1795.

when very young. Simon Nichols had Cow Pox in
1782, and "some years afterwards" inoculation failed,
and in 1795, Jenner failed to inoculate Joseph Merret,
who had had Cow Pox in 1770.

In 1796, an opportunity occurred for an experiment
of a different kind. Cow Pox occurred at a farm near
Berkeley, in May, and a dairymaid, Sarah Nelmes,
caught the disease. On May 14th, matter was taken
from a sore on her hand and inserted by means of two
superficial incisions (as in the method of performing
Small Pox inoculation) into the arm of James Phipps,
a healthy boy about eight years old. The inoculation succeeded, the result being described as much
the same as after inoculation in the same way with
variolous matter, except that the usual efflorescence
had more " of an erysipelatous look." The whole
died away, leaving " scabs and subsequent eschars."
Jenner was so impatient to try the effect of variolous
inoculation, that on July 1st, only six weeks after
the insertion of the Cow Pox matter, variolous lymph
was applied, by means of punctures and slight incisions.
Jenner communicated his experiments on Phipps to
his friend Gardner.

" DEAR GARDNER,

    " As I promised to let you know how I proceeded in my
inquiry into the nature of that singular disease the Cow Pox,
and being fully satisfied how much you feel interested in its
success, you will be gratified in hearing that I have at length
accomplished what I have been so long waiting for, the passing of

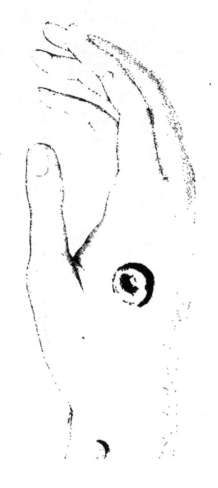

CASUAL COW POX (JENNER).
Case of Sarah Nelmes.

the Vaccine Virus from one human being to another by the ordinary mode of inoculation.

"A boy of the name of Phipps was inoculated in the arm from a pustule on the hand of a young woman who was infected by her master's cows. Having never seen the disease but in its casual way before, that is, when communicated from the cow to the hand of the milker, I was astonished at the close resemblance of the pustules, in some of their stages, to the variolous pustules. But now listen to the most delightful part of my story. The boy has since been inoculated for the Small Pox which, as I ventured to predict, produced no effect. I shall now pursue my experiments with redoubled ardour.

"Believe me yours, very sincerely,

"EDWARD JENNER.

"BERKELEY, *July* 19, 1796."

Jenner had now materials for another paper for the Royal Society, but he waited a year in order to add two or three more cases, of failure to inoculate after casual Cow Pox. In February 1797, William Rodway's case was added, and a month later the cases of Sarah and Elizabeth' Wynne.

Jenner lost no time in finishing his paper, but he little anticipated the reception it was destined to meet with. Baron says:—

"It was his intention that it should first have appeared before the public in the *Transactions of the Royal Society*, but this design was abandoned, and the work appeared as a separate publication."

Baron does not say here, why the idea was abandoned, and James Moore was the first to publish what actually took place. In 1796 or 1797, Jenner

transmitted his manuscript to a correspondent, who
was in the confidence of Sir Joseph Banks, President
of the Royal Society, not doubting that it would
be printed in the *Transactions of the Royal Society.*
The perusal of his cases and experiments produced
no conviction whatever, and he received a friendly
admonition in reply, that as he had gained some reputation by his former papers to the Royal Society,
it was advisable not to present this one, which would
injure his established credit.   In the second volume
of the Biography, published in 1837, Baron, no
longer, suppressed the details in connection with
this incident, but published a letter of Jenner's, in
which a reference is made to the rejection of the
paper :—

"I explained in conversation, as I said before, all that passed
respecting my first paper on the Cow Pox intended for the Royal
Society. It was not with Sir Joseph, but with Home ; he took
the paper. It was shewn to the Council, and returned to me.
This, I think, was in the year 1797, after the vaccination of one
patient only ; but even this was strong evidence, as it followed
that of the numbers I had put to the test of the Small Pox
after casual vaccination."

After making a few additional experiments, Jenner
resolved to publish the paper himself.   In June, 1797,
he wrote :—

"I have shown a copy of my intended paper on the Cow
Pox to our friend, Worthington, who has been pleased to express
his approbation of it, and to recommend my publishing it as a
pamphlet, instead of sending it to the Royal Society."

His friends, Gardner and Hicks, were often consulted about it, and it was shown to and scrutinised
by a number of his particular associates. It was
also submitted to Woodville, who endeavoured to
persuade Jenner to leave out his speculations with
regard to the origin of Cow Pox from " the grease ; "
but Jenner would not hear of it. The *Inquiry* was
published about the end of June, 1798, Jenner having
left Berkeley for London to see the printers on the
24th of April, and returned home on the 14th of July.
While in London, Jenner had another opportunity of
speaking about this subject to his professional brethren,
but he was unable, during the whole time that he was
in the metropolis, to procure a single person on whom
he could exhibit the results of inoculation. Some of
the virus, however, which he carried with him was
presented to Mr. Cline, who, at the end of July,
inserted it into the hip of a patient by two punctures.
This patient had some affection of the hip joint, and
it was thought that the counter-irritation, excited by
the Cow Pox, might prove beneficial, and it was
intended to convert the ulcer, which was anticipated,
into an issue. This operation is referred to in the
following extract from Jenner's Journal :—

EXTRACTS FROM JOURNAL OF 1798.

"That the matter of Cow Pox, like the Small Pox matter, may
be preserved without any diminution in its active qualities is
evinced by the following experiment.

"Mr. Cline inoculated a child with matter that had been taken from the pustule on the arm of Hannah Excell (see page 39 pamphlet) when in a limpid ichorous state, and dried by exposure to the air, after being preserved three months on a quill in a seal. The following is the result:—

"Copy of Mr. Cline's Letter.

"Lincoln's-Inn Fields, 2d Aug. 1798.

"The Cow Pox experiment has succeeded admirably. The child sickened on the seventh day; and the fever, which was moderate, subsided on the eleventh day. The inflammation extended to about four inches diameter, and then gradually subsided without having been attended with pain, or other inconvenience. The ulcer was not large enough to contain a pea, therefore, I have not converted it into an issue as I intended.[1] I have since inoculated him with Small Pox matter in three places, which were slightly inflamed on the third day, and then subsided.

"Dr. Lister, who was formerly physician to the Small Pox Hospital, attended the child with me, and he is convinced that it is not possible to give him the Small Pox.

"I think the substituting of Cow Pox poison for the Small Pox promises to be one of the greatest improvements that has ever been made in medicine: for it is not only so safe in itself, but also does not endanger others by contagion, in which way the Small Pox has done infinite mischief. The more I think on the subject, the more I am impressed with its importance.

"With great esteem I am, dear Sir,

"Your faithful servant,

"Henry Cline."

"With the intention of proceeding with the experiments, Mr. Cline took matter from the pustule, and with it inoculated three other children; but on none of these did it take any effect."

---

[1] This boy was brought to town on account of some disease in the joint of the hip. Mr. C. therefore inoculated near the part, with the view of exciting inflammation, and subsequently of forming an issue.—E. J. [See vol. ii., p. 184.]

"I have observed that the matter of Cow Pox appears to lose its powers of infection after it ceases to be limpid. Probably it might have passed the bounds of perfection when Mr. Cline made his second experiment."

"HENRY CLINE, ESQ., TO DR. JENNER.

"LINCOLN'S-INN FIELDS, *18th August*, 1798.

"MY DEAR SIR,—Seven days since, I inoculated three children with Cow Pox matter, and I have the mortification of finding that the infection has not taken, and I fear I shall be entirely disappointed unless you can contrive to send me some fresh matter. I think it might come in a quill in a letter, or inclosed in a bit of tin-foil, by the same conveyance,.or in any other way that may be more convenient.

"With much esteem, I am, dear Sir,

"Your faithful servant,

"HENRY CLINE."

Mr. Cline having failed to carry on the disease from the first case of vaccination in London, and Jenner also having failed in the country, the stock of lymph was lost, and the latter was therefore unable to supply those who were anxious to try the new inoculation, and to test its alleged prophylactic powers.

According to Baron, Mr. Cline was more than satisfied with the result of his experiment.

"Mr. Cline, perceiving at once from the success of his first trial what incalculable blessings were connected with the diffusion of the practice, with just a becoming regard for the welfare of Jenner, wished his personal advantage to keep pace in some degree with the benefits which he had it in his power to impart to mankind. He, therefore, immediately advised him to quit the country, and to take a house in Grosvenor Square, and promised him £10,000 per annum as the result of his practice."

Another friend endeavoured to persuade him to seize this as an opportunity of acquiring fame and fortune. But Jenner declined, and in a letter in answer to his friend the reason is made apparent. Jenner preferred retirement in the country, because he knew that his theory would be rigidly tested in London, and he was not prepared to face failures. At this early stage, he was evidently conscious of the fact that the variolous test would break down, as he was already prepared with an answer to meet the results he anticipated.

"CHELTENHAM, *September 29th.*

"It is very clear from your representation that there is now an opening in town for any physician whose reputation stood fair in the public eye. But here, my dear friend, here is the rub. . . .

"How very few are capable of conducting physiological experiments! I am fearful that before we thoroughly understand what is Cow Pox matter, and what is not, some confusion may arise, for which I shall unjustly be made answerable. In the first place, instances will occur where those who have truly had the disease shall be subjected to the common process of inoculation, inflammation, vesication, and even pus will appear on the wounded part. The axilla will show that the lymphatics have been active, and the system may even, in a very limited degree, feel the consequence. What would the enemies to the improvement of science say to this? I leave you to answer this question. But the very same thing has happened again and again to those who have had the Small Pox; and do not those (nurses for example) who are much exposed to the contagion of Small Pox?" . . .

[The rest of this letter is unfortunately lost.]

But in the seclusion of his country home, Jenner

was able to ponder over unfavourable criticisms, and exercise his ingenuity in finding explanations. It was not long before the anticipated opposition had to be encountered.

Dr. Ingenhousz, a distinguished physician and man of science, was on a visit to the Marquis of Lansdowne, at his seat in Wiltshire.

Ingenhousz had made a special study of Small Pox, and having read Jenner's publication, at once instituted inquiries among the dairies in Wiltshire.

His experience was communicated to Jenner in a letter written from Bowood Park, October 12th, 1798 :—

DR. INGENHOUSZ TO DR. JENNER.

"SIR,—Having read with attention your performance on the Variolæ Vaccinæ, and being informed by everyone who knows you that you enjoy a high and well-deserved reputation as a man of great learning in your profession, you cannot take it amiss if I take the liberty to communicate to you a fact well deserving your attention, and with which you ought to be made acquainted. I prefer this private method of conveying my information to any other which might expose you to the disagreeable necessity of entering into a public controversy, always disagreeable to a man so liberal-minded and well-intentioned as your treatise indicates you to be.

" As soon as I arrived at the seat of the Marquess of Lansdowne, Bowood, near Calne, I thought it my duty to inquire concerning the extraordinary doctrine contained in your publication, as I knew the Cow Pox was well known in this country. The first gentleman to whom I addressed myself was Mr. Alsop, an eminent practitioner at Calne. This gentleman made me acquainted with Mr. Henry Stiles, a respectable farmer at Whitley, near Calne,

who, thirty years ago, bought a cow at a fair, which he found to
be infected with what he called the Cow Pox. This cow soon
infected the whole dairy ; and he himself, by milking the infected
cow, caught the disease which you describe, and that in a very
severe way, accompanied with pain, stiffness, and swelling in the
axillary glands. Being recovered from the disease, and all the
sores dried, he was inoculated for the Small Pox by Mr. Alsop.
The disease took place : a great many Small Pocks came out ,and
he communicated the infection to his father, who died of it. This
being an incontrovertible fact, of which I obtained the knowledge
from the very first man to whom I addressed myself, cannot fail
to make some impression on your mind, and excite you to inquire
farther on the subject, before ·you venture finally to decide in
favour of a doctrine, which may do great mischief should it
prove erroneous." . . .

Dr. Jenner to Dr. Ingenhousz.

" Dear Sir,—I shall ever consider myself as under great
obligations to you, for the very liberal manner in which you have
communicated a fact to me on a subject in which at present I feel
myself deeply interested ; a subject of so momentous a nature
that I am happy to find it has attracted the attention of some of
the first medical philosophers of the present age, among whom it
is no compliment in me to say that I have long classed you.

" It will doubtless, in the course of time, meet with a full investigation ; but as that moves on (and from the nature of the inquiry
it must move slowly) I plainly foresee that many doubts will arise
respecting the validity of my assertion, from causes which ought
to be examined with the nicest inspection before their convictive
force be fully admitted.

" Truth, believe me, Sir, in this and every other physiological
investigation which has occupied my attention, has ever been the
object which I have endeavoured to hold in view. In the publication on the Variolæ Vaccinæ, I have given little more than a
simple detail of facts which came under my own inspection, and to
the public I stand pledged for its veracity. In the course of the
inquiry, which occupied no inconsiderable portion of my time and
attention, not a single instance occurred of a person's having the

disease, either casually or from inoculation, who on subsequent exposure to variolous contagion received the infection of the Small Pox, unless that inserted in page 71[1] may be admitted as an exception. And from the information you have given me, and from what I have obtained from others who have perused the pamphlet, I am induced to suppose that my conjecture respecting the cause of that patient's insecurity, namely, her having had the disease without any apparent affection of the system, might have been erroneous; and that the consequences might be more fairly attributable to a cause on which I shall, in my present address to you, feel it my duty to speak explicitly. Should it appear in the present instance that I have been led into error, fond as I may appear of the offspring of my labours, I had rather strangle it at once than suffer it to exist, and do a public injury. At present, I have not the most distant doubt that any person, who has once felt the influence of perfect Cow Pox matter, would ever be susceptible of that of the Small Pox. But on the contrary, I perceive that after a disease has been excited by the matter of Cow Pox in an imperfect state, the specific change of the con-stitution necessary to render the contagion of the Small Pox inert is not produced, and in this point of view, as in most others, there is a close analogy between the propagation of the Cow Pox and the Small Pox. Therefore, I conceive it would be prudent, until further inquiry has thrown every light on the subject which it is capable of receiving, that (like those who were the objects of my experiments) all should be subjected to the test of variolous matter who have been inoculated for the Cow Pox."

When discussing the subject of Cow Pox with neighbouring practitioners, Jenner had previously been confronted with the statement that there were un-doubted instances of Small Pox occurring after Cow Pox, and he had met this argument by the assertion that there were two kinds of Cow Pox; and those cases which had been subsequently variolated must have

---

[1] Vol. ii., p. 32.

had "false" Cow Pox, while those which had not
been variolated had had "true" Cow Pox. Ingenhousz
had independently brought forward the argument of the
neighbouring practitioners, and this led Jenner to realise
still more the weak point of his case. He keenly felt
the necessity for disseminating, far and wide, the
doctrine of spurious Cow Pox, which would cut away
the ground from under the feet of a host of objectors.
In this cause, he enlisted the assistance of his friend
Gardner.

DR. JENNER TO MR. EDWARD GARDNER.

"DEAR GARDNER,—I fully depend upon meeting you at Eastington to-morrow to sit in council on several subjects of high import.
My friends must not desert me now. Brickbats and hostile wea-
pons of every sort are flying thick around me; but with a very
little aid, a few friendly opiates seasonably administered, they
will do me no injury.

"Ingenhousz has declined my offer of receiving my letter in
print—so that must be modelled anew. We must set off by
impressing the idea that there will be no end to cavil and controversy until it be defined with precision what is, and what is not
Cow Pox.

"The *true* has many imitations by the *false* on the cow's udder
and nipples; and all is called *Cow Pox*, whether on the cow or
communicated to the human animal.

"My experiments move on—but I have all to do single-handed.
Not the least assistance from a quarter where I had the most right
to expect it ! !

"Bodily labour I disregard, but pressures of the mind grow too
heavy for me. Added to all my other cares, I am touched hard
with the reigning epidemic—Impecuniosity.—Any supplies from
the paper-maker ?　　　　"Adieu !

　　　　　　　　　　　　　　"Your faithful friend,

"*Wednesday morning.*"　　　　　　　　　　"E. J.

Jenner recognised a formidable antagonist in Ingenhousz, whose opposition bid fair to wreck his theory. He therefore deputed Mr. Paytherus, who was well trained in the cause of Cow Pox inoculation, to endeavour to gain over the enemy by personal explanations. Mr. Paytherus, however, entirely failed in his mission.

T. PAYTHERUS, ESQ., TO DR. JENNER.

" *December* 14*th*, 1798.

" DEAR JENNER,—The moment I received your letter I called on Ingenhousz ; he was in the country, but expected in town the next day. Yesterday I called a second time, and made an appointment for this morning, in consequence of which I have had an interview with this very interesting character.

" A more determined or a more formidable opponent you need not covet or desire. Unfortunately for your hypothesis, he made his first inquiry of a Mr. Alsop, of Calne, who immediately named a person who had had the Small Pox after the Cow Pox. This person he was afterwards introduced to, and satisfied himself of the *fact.* The second application was to Major-General Hastings : he also pointed out an instance of the Small Pox subsequent to the Cow Pox at Adlestrop.

" Dr. Garthshore has also at Dr. Ingenhousz's request written to Dr. Pulteney, of Blandford, who in reply has assured him that the inoculators of his neighbourhood have known many instances of the Small Pox happening after the Cow Pox. He believes that it does in many instances produce that change in the human constitution as to render it unsusceptible of the Small Pox, but not with certainty in *all* cases. He would not hear a word in defence of your opinion respecting its origin.

" He is confident that a spurious Small Pox cannot be produced by what you call putrescent variolous matter, and that whether the matter be kept in a wet sponge, or on cotton, either in a moist or a dry state, it will uniformly produce the Small Pox. Yet he confessed in his own practice that the dried matter more generally produced a confluent Small Pox. In your last letter to him you speak of the putrescent state of the Cow Pox matter, and that the milk might likewise undergo a similar change. To this he objects, and says that milk will become acescent, not putrescent.

" That it should render the habit unsusceptible of Small Pox, and not of its own specific action, is to him incredible. You tell him in one of your letters that you have heard from Adlestrop, and that the father of the boy or girl now thinks that the Small Pox preceded the Cow Pox. To *think*, it seems, is to *doubt*, and he says the ambiguity on the part of the father confirms the first statement instead of weakening it. His respect for your character has kept him from publishing, and he declines entering into controversy with you. Had you been a less formidable antagonist he would have flogged you long since. He spoke very handsomely of you, and desired me to assure you that nothing would have kept him from answering your letters but the desire of satisfying his mind on the subject. He desires that you will not be in haste to publish a second time on the Cow Pox, but wait till you have collected a sufficient number of facts, and to secure your ground as you advance. He remarked that you would not be permitted to be judge in your own cause ; that you were now before the tribunal of the public, and so long as *sub judice lis est*, you ought not to risk an opinion."

* * * * * * *

Jenner keenly felt the antagonism of Ingenhousz, and was at a loss to know what to do. Again he writes to Gardner for sympathy and advice.

DR. JENNER TO MR. EDWARD GARDNER.

" BERKELEY.

" DEAR GARDNER,—We wondered at Ingenhousz's delay in answering my letters, particularly the long one that you inspected. A tempest is generally preceded by a calm. He has in some measure exemplified the remark. I know not what to do with him, and wish for your advice, after you have seen his letter. It is a matter of real moment—a matter on which, perhaps, much of my future peace may rest—indeed, my existence. I sometimes think that it would be most prudent to desire him to make public all he knows of the Cow Pox ; but would there not in this measure be a sort of defiance that might irritate ? The grand question to be determined at present is this : Shall I immediately publish an appendix, or say nothing till every bolt is flung, and then attack my adversaries ?

"This very man Ingenhousz knows no more of the real nature of the Cow Pox than Master Selwyn does of Greek. Yet he is among philosophers what Johnson was among the *literati*, and, by the way, not unlike him in figure; 'tis no use to shoot straws at an eagle. When shall I see you ?

"Yours sincerely,

"E. J."

After his return from London, in July 1798, Jenner spent most of his time until the following February at Cheltenham and Berkeley.

He had lost his stock of lymph, and now had encountered an antagonist on whose opposition depended not only his future peace, but his very existence. Such was the state of the Cow Pox question at that period, and Jenner might well have felt in despair ; but the fate of the new inoculation was not destined to be consigned to oblivion, for the much-needed help came from a very unexpected quarter.

The subject had been receiving increased attention from men of science in London. Some were anxious to obtain further information, others questioned the accuracy of Jenner's statements, and treated his doctrines as "conjectural and ridiculous." Among the former were Dr. George Pearson and Dr. Woodville, physicians to the Small Pox Hospital.

Dr. Pearson set to work with extraordinary zeal, making inquiries by means of correspondence with practitioners in all parts of the country, and in less than six months after the publication of Jenner's *Inquiry*, produced a volume in which he incorporated all the information which he had received as to the prevalence of Cow Pox and its alleged protective power, together with his own comments on the proposed substitute for Small Pox inoculation.

Dr. Pearson had not been able to make any experiments, as during the few months in which he had been making inquiries, he had not succeeded in meeting with an outbreak of Cow Pox; but having sent his book to press, his next wish was to inoculate. Thus he wrote to Jenner, on November 8th, 1798 :—

"Your name will live in the memory of mankind as long as men possess gratitude for services and respect for benefactors ; and if I can but get *matter*, I am much mistaken if I do not make you live for ever."

Dr. Pearson's book was issued by the publishers about the middle of November, a fact which he announced to Jenner in the following letter.

DR. PEARSON TO DR. JENNER.

"MY DEAR SIR,—Unexpectedly my pamphlet made its public appearance a day or two ago. I am sorry to trouble you to say by what conveyance I can send you a copy, and to what place. If you have any commissions to execute in London, you may as well have a parcel made up, and I will see it forwarded.

"I observe several errors since printing, partly mine and partly those of the printer; but I know other authors discover similar errors, and that readers do not perceive them.

"You cannot imagine how fastidious the people are with regard to this business of the Cow Pox. One says it is very filthy and nasty to derive it from the sore heels of horses! Another, 'O my God, we shall introduce the diseases of animals among us, and we have too many already of our own!' A third sapient set say it is a strange odd kind of business, and they know not what to think of it! All this I hear very quietly, and recollect that a still more unfavourable reception was experienced by the inoculation for the Small Pox.

"I wish you could secure for me matter for inoculation, because, depend upon it, a thousand inaccurate but imposing cases will be published against the specific nature of the disease by persons who want to send their names abroad about anything, and who will think yourself and me fair game. By way of *se defendendo* we must inoculate. I have thought it right to publish the evidence as sent to me, and also my own reasoning, because I know you are too good a philosopher to be offended at the investigation of truth, although the conclusions may be different from your own. I think, too, your principal facts will be the better established than if it had happened that I had uniformly acceded to all your doctrine.

"I am, with Mrs. P.'s best compliments to Mrs. Jenner and yourself,

"Your faithful Servant,

"G. PEARSON.

"LEICESTER SQUARE, *Nov.* 13*th*, 1798."

According to Baron, a few days afterwards (November 26th), Jenner succeeded in obtaining Cow Pox virus from a farm at Stonehouse, and on the following day, he inoculated two of the children of his friend, Mr. Hicks of Eastington. Baron relates this to disprove an assertion, subsequently made, that the first vaccinations performed by Jenner after the publication of the *Inquiry* were with lymph received from Pearson. This subject will be referred to again ; in the meantime the history of what occurred in London will be continued.

Dr. Woodville, as well as Dr. Pearson, were very curious to try the new inoculation ; and after patiently waiting, their wish was gratified, for the welcome news was received that Cow Pox existed in London dairies.

In January 1799, Mr. Wachsel obtained intelligence that Cow Pox had broken out among the cows in Gray's Inn Lane, and reported it to Woodville ; and at the same time, Pearson heard that the disease was raging among a large herd of cows in the New Road, near Paddington. With vaccine matter from these sources, Woodville experimented at the Small Pox Hospital, and Pearson also induced persons to be inoculated.

Jenner received information of the discovery, a few days afterwards, from Woodville.

DR. WOODVILLE TO DR. JENNER.

" ELY PLACE, *Jan.* 25, 1799.

" DEAR SIR,

    *   *   *   *   *   *   *

" On Sunday last, I was informed that the Cow Pox had broke out among Mr. Harrison's cows in Gray's Inn Lane   The next day I took Mr. Tanner with me to examine them ; and as he declared it to be the genuine disease, I that day inoculated six persons with the matter that he procured from a cow

¹ *Vide* p. 162.

which appeared to be the most severely affected with this pustular complaint. On Wednesday, I called again at the cow-house to make farther inquiries, when I was very much pleased to find two or three of the milkers were infected with the disease, one of whom exhibited a more beautiful specimen of the disease than that which you have represented in the first plate. From this person I charged a lancet with the matter, which appeared different from that taken from the cow, as that of the former was purely lymphatic, and the latter of a purulent form. With this lymphatic matter I immediately inoculated two men at the hospital.

"Finding now there could be no doubt of the disease, I the same day called upon Sir Joseph Banks, Dr. Pearson, Dr. Willan, etc., to inform them of the circumstance; and these gentlemen, together with Lord Somerville, Sir William Watson, and Mr. Coleman, met me the following day at the cow-keeper's, where your book was produced; and upon comparing *your figure* with the disease it was allowed by all to be a very faithful representation, and every gentleman seemed highly gratified at seeing so good an example of the Cow Pox. From this place we proceeded to the hospital, where I inoculated six patients, so that the whole number inoculated by me with the Cow Pox matter amounts to fourteen."

* * * * * * *

Jenner was quite satisfied from this description that Woodville had discovered "true" Cow Pox, and wished himself in London.

Dr. Jenner to Dr. Woodville.

"My Dear Sir,—I am extremely obliged to you for your letter, and most sincerely wish circumstances would admit of my being at your elbow while you conduct your experiments on the interesting subject before you.

"I answer your letter by return of post, to suggest (what perhaps is needless) the immediate propriety of inoculating those who may resist the action of the Cow Pox matter, and may have been exposed to variolous contagion at the hospital.

After the description you have given, there can be no doubt, I think, that the disease among the cows in Gray's Inn Lane is the true, and not a species of the spurious Cow Pox. In the account of the appearance on the milker's hand, the report of my friend Tanner merits great confidence. Whether to the cold season of the year or to what other cause it can be ascribed I know not, but out of six patients that I lately inoculated two of them only were infected. An inflammation was excited in the arms of all, and in some of those, whose constitutions would not feel it, it did not die away for more than a week, and even went on so as to leave a little scab behind.

"It has not happened so, generally. However, once in the course of the last summer, I was foiled in a similar way. Three or four servants at a farm were carefully inoculated with matter fresh from a cow:—they all resisted it, but in the course of the season, all of them were infected by milking the cows. As every case of Cow Pox is to be considered as a case of inoculation, I mention these facts to you, that it may be considered whether some mode more certain of infecting the subject than that at present in use with variolous matter may not be thought of.

" It would imitate the casual mode more closely were we first by scratch or puncture to create a little scab, and then, removing it, apply the virus on the abraded part.

"I am shortly going to publish an appendix to my late pamphlet (which, by the way, I hope you received, as I directed it to be sent to you before I left London) to mention the precaution of destroying the pustule, and the general sources of spurious Cow Pox, etc., etc.

" I shall also point out the result of one of the cases where caustic was used soon after the symptoms of infection appeared (see page 41[1]). This I shall concisely relate to you now. About six weeks ago, I inoculated M. James (see page 40[1]) with fresh Small Pox matter, and at the same time exposed her to the effluvia of a patient. The appearances of the arm were just the same as if she never had had either Small Pox or Cow Pox ; and on the eighth day, I expected, from the appearances, she

---

[1] *Vide* vol. ii., p. 174.

would be ill. She was a little hotter than usual during the
night, but slept well, and it was supposed that a rash appeared
for the space of a few hours about the wrists. I inserted matter
from her arm into two other subjects, a boy, and a woman of
fifty. The boy had about half a dozen pustules, two or three
of which were fairly characterised. Their appearance was
preceded by a pretty general rash. The woman, though she
felt an indisposition, had not a single pustule. A person near
sixty years of age, who had in the early period of her life been
exposed to the contagion of the Small Pox and resisted it,
fully exposed herself now to this infection. She sickened in
consequence, and had three pustules, one of which became a
perfect Small Pox pustule. It would be unfair to draw positive
conclusions from such scanty precedents, but yet they lead one
to hope that a mild variety of the Small Pox might thus be
actually created."

* * * * * * *

Jenner had recommended that caustic should be
employed to destroy the pustule, but this was
strongly objected to by both Pearson and Woodville. Pearson alluded to this in a letter, February
15th, and at the same time mentioned the prospect of
increasing opposition to the new practice.

"On telling Dr. Woodville that I had been anxious about
your publishing the use of the caustic, he replied 'that would
have damned the whole business.'

"Be assured that if the practice cannot be introduced without
the caustic, or call it by any other name, it will never succeed
with the public. I cannot yet tell whether all my patients have
had sufficient affection of the constitution. There has not been
time for a second inoculation and with variolous matter. Some
of the patients had undergone the Small Pox.

"Dr. Parr's letter you shall see in town, merely to satisfy
you, but it contains nothing that is relative beside what I
extracted from it. I must tell you that Dr. Parr has written

to me to say that although he 'is not yet convinced, he is staggered, and begins to doubt.' We shall have to experience soon a number of *gnat bites.* If the practice is likely to go forward, it will excite opposition. What obligation society owes to those worthy and liberal men who favour the public with their *a priori* opinions, having never seen the disease, and not even understanding the arguments ! ! Tantæne animis cœles- tibus iræ !

"I trust we shall establish facts enough to prove whether Cow Pox inoculation extinguishes that of the *variola* or not. We have got able, candid, and worthy men on our side, and proceeding, as we have all done, circumspectly, I do not feel any dread from the opponents who have yet taken the field."

In the same letter, Pearson enclosed a bit of thread infected with the virus, and Jenner made a number of inoculations, and reported the results.

DR. JENNER TO DR. PEARSON.

" BERKELEY, *March 13th,* 1799.

"MY DEAR SIR,—I received your letter while I was writing to Dr. Woodville, and requested him to transmit to you the result of the inoculation with the London virus. I hope he did not fail to execute my wishes. Twelve patients have since been inoculated with matter produced by this virus. They all took the infection. This is the ninth day, and they appear a little ill— no eruptions yet. The character of the arm is just that of Cow Pox, except that I do not see the disposition in the pustule to ulcerate as in some of the former cases. I am the more induced to believe this to be the *genuine* Cow Pox from the following circumstance :—

"One of the boys inoculated sickened the preceding day with the measles, which went through its course. Yet the pustule advanced with the same regularity as if the measles had not been present. Now this would not have been the case, I presume, had variolous matter been inserted into the skin under similar circumstances. No Cow Pox yet in the country !

Should it appear within a particular district I shall undoubtedly know it. It cannot now be long before I shall see you in town ; at least I can speak with as great a certainty of being soon there as a medical man can.

" I hear of a child covered over with pustules at the Small Pox Hospital. What are they ?

" I am glad to find that the disposition for forming eruptions among your patients does not increase, as you tell me that none of your last inoculated patients had any, and that Mr. Rolph's children went through the disease without them. Tanner, I find, could not succeed in giving the Cow Pox to the veterinary cow in a direct way, that is, by inserting the virus into a sound part of the nipple, in the same way as all experiments have hitherto been conducted to confute my notions with the matter of grease ; but when he found a part of the nipple that was previously affected with a sore, and applied the matter there, it took effect immediately. With best respects to Mrs. Pearson,

" I remain, dear sir,
" Yours very truly,
" E. JENNER."

In about two months, Pearson and Woodville had inoculated upwards of one hundred and sixty persons, and above sixty were afterwards inoculated with Small Pox, but none took the infection.[1]

On March 12th, 1799, Pearson sent a letter enclosing an infected thread to two hundred practitioners, requesting them to try its effects and report the results.

Pearson also sent virus to Paris, Berlin, Vienna, Geneva, and to Hanover, Portugal, America, and also supplied the army.

In May, 1799, Woodville published his report.

Vide, p. 163.

Between the 21st of January and the 18th of March, he had inoculated two hundred persons, and within a short time, four hundred more. In fact, Pearson and Woodville had so succeeded in promoting Cow Pox inoculation, by their energy and zeal, and by distributing lymph and disseminating information about the new inoculation, that the whole medical world was in a state of agitation.

It was obvious that Jenner's limited efforts, when compared with the work of Pearson and Woodville, were in danger of sinking into insignificance. Jenner without delay, issued a counterblast in the form of a pamphlet,[1] the data of which had been hurriedly put together. Criticisms also, were overwhelming him, and, according to Baron, he began to feel deeply the weight of the responsibility which rested on him from the publication of the *Inquiry*. Hence we find him again appealing to his friend Gardner for help.

DR. JENNER TO MR. EDWARD GARDNER.

" DEAR GARDNER,—There never was a period in my existence when my situation called so loudly for the assistance of my literary friends as the present. Though my bark will, with flying colours, reach the shore at last, yet it is now in a storm.

" I am beset on all sides with snarling fellows, and so ignorant withal that they know no more of the disease they write about than the animals which generate it. The last philippic that has appeared comes from Bristol, and is communicated by Dr. Sims of London. Sims gives comments on it in harsh and unjustifiable language. It is impossible for me, single-handed, to combat all my adversaries.

---

[1] *Vide* vol. ii., p. 155.

"Standing, as I do, before so awful a tribunal, my friends will volunteer their counsel and IMMEDIATELY appear in court.

" My intended pamphlet has only been looked over in a cursory way. Every sentence must be again revised and weighed in the nicest balance that human intellect can invent. The eyes of the philosophic and medical critic, prejudiced most bitterly against the hypothesis, will penetrate its inmost recesses, and discover the minutest flaw were it suffered to be present. Language I put out of the question : the matter is what I allude to.

" Give me as much of your company as you can, and as speedily.

" Yours, very faithfully,

" E. JENNER.

" *Thursday, March 7th*, 1799."

But more trouble was in store for him. George Jenner happened to be in London, and became greatly alarmed at the part played by Pearson and Woodville, particularly the former. He wrote off post-haste to his uncle, warning him that Pearson would become the chief person known in the business, and that, if he did not go at once to London, his chance of obtaining fame and fortune would be lost for ever.

G. C. JENNER TO DR. JENNER.

"NORFOLK STREET, *March* 11*th*, 1799.

" MY DEAR SIR,—After what Mr. Paytherus has written to you, it will be needless for me to say anything to urge the necessity of your coming to town to wear the laurels you have gained, or to prevent their being placed on the brows of another.

" I shall only state a few facts I have got possession of since I wrote to you last. Dr. Pearson is going to send circular letters to the medical gentlemen to let them know that he will supply them with Cow Pox matter upon their application to him, by which means *he* will be the chief person known in the business, and consequently deprive you of that merit, or at least a great share of it, which is so justly your due. Doctor P. gave a public lecture on the Cow Pox on Saturday last. Farmer Tanner was there. Doctor Pearson adopted your opinions, except with regard to the probability of the disease originating in horses' heels. He spoke of some unsatisfactory experiments having been made by inoculating from the greasy heels; but when we consider how difficult it was to communicate the disease from one cow to another by inoculation, we are not to wonder at the still greater difficulty in communicating it from the horse to the cow. The farmer says Dr. Pearson was wrong in some part of his lecture, which he *took the liberty to tell him.*

"Mr. Paytherus is much disappointed not to receive any letter from you by this day's post, but hopes you may be coming up to-day, and therefore did not write. All your friends agree that *now* is your time to establish your fame and fortune; but if you delay taking a personal active part any longer, the opportunity will be lost for ever. If Dr. Pearson does not intend to endeavour to give the merit to himself, why should he quibble about the name you gave the disease? The eruption he calls the *vaccinous* eruption.

"Your affectionate nephew,
"G. C. JENNER.

"Mr. Paytherus has just told me that a copy of Doctor Pearson's lecture was exhibited yesterday at Sir Joseph Banks's. When I get a sight of it I will send you an account of it."

Jenner promptly wrote to his counsellor and guide, proposing counter-action.

DR. JENNER TO MR. EDWARD GARDNER.

"BERKELEY, *Wednesday,* 1799.

"DEAR GARDNER,—A letter I have just received from G. Jenner informs me that Dr. Pearson on Saturday last gave a public lecture on the Cow Pox, and that it was publicly exhibited at Sir J Banks's on Sunday evening. He has also given out that he wil furnish any gentlemen at a distance with the virus.

" As this is probably done with the view of showing himself as the first man in the concern, should not some neatly-drawn paragraphs appear from time to time in the public prints, by no means reflecting on the conduct of P., but just to keep the idea publicly alive that P. was not the author of the discovery—I mean Cow Pox inoculation ?

" Yours truly,

"E. J."

On the 21st of March, Jenner acted on the advice of his friends, and left Berkeley for London. On the 23rd, he saw Woodville, who informed him that in one of his cases the Cow Pox was communicated by effluvia, and the patient had had it *in the confluent way.*[1] In the same month, Woodville published his *Reports*, in which he concluded that Cow Pox manifested itself sometimes as an eruptive disease of great severity, for three or four cases out of five hundred had been in considerable danger, and one case died. Baron says that these results proved well-nigh fatal to the cause of vaccination. However, in other localities where Woodville's lymph had been employed, much happier results were met with. One explanation was, that as Woodville had vaccinated in a variolous atmosphere, Cow Pox and Small Pox occurred simultaneously. Jenner had employed the Woodville lymph, and inoculated his grand-nephew, Stephen Jenner, and a boy of the name of Hill, who was about four years old. With

---

[1] Baron, *loc. cit.*, vol. i., p. 322.

lymph from the arm of the boy Hill, Jenner inoculated
two of the children of his friend, Mr. Hicks, and at
the same time, 16 others, and with matter taken from
this source, his nephew, Henry Jenner, successfully
vaccinated a child twenty hours old, and no eruptions
resulted in any. The same stock supplied Mr. Marshall
with virus for inoculations on 107 persons, and in only
one or two cases were there any eruptions.

Jenner had left London in June; but in order to
study the effects of lymph from the London dairies,
he procured before his departure some virus from
Mr. Clark's farm at Kentish Town, and sent it to Mr.
Marshall by his friend Mr. Tanner, who used it on 127
cases without any eruptions resulting. Jenner therefore concluded that, in Woodville's cases, the eruptions
resulted from " the action of variolous matter which
crept into the constitution with the vaccine."[1]

Both Woodville[2] and Pearson[3] acknowledged afterwards that the eruptions arose from variolation.

"It is true that many of these vaccine cases were conjoined
with the Small Pox from the influence probably of the variolous infection, but as the eruptive cases exhibited the genuine Cow Pock
on the part inoculated, and the matter of it very generally propagated the Vaccina without eruptions, in private practice and in the
country, it is fair to admit them into the class of Cow Pock cases."

[1] *Vide* vol. ii., p. 252; vol. i., p. 244 and p. 184; and Moore. *History
and Practice of Vaccination.* p. 26.

[2] Woodville. *Observations on the Cow Pox.* 1800. p. 21.

[3] Pearson. *An Examination of the Report of the Committee of the
House of Commons.* 1802. p. 49.

This accident was far from proving " well-nigh fatal "
to the interests of vaccination ; it was, on the contrary,
the most fortunate occurrence for Jenner and his cause.
I regard it as having been productive of results which
completely turned the scale of opinion in favour of
the new inoculation. The variolous test, in Jenner's
cases, had been far from convincing. But here were
60 cases in which the variolous test appeared to settle
the question conclusively, for neither inoculation nor
exposure to infection produced any result. The Cow
Pox got the credit in these 60 and many similar cases,
and this constituted one of the stock arguments in
favour of the prophylactic power of Cow Pox. But
the fact that these patients had been variolated (and
perhaps Cow Poxed at the same time), and were therefore naturally protected from a subsequent attack of
Small Pox, was overlooked and forgotten. Many
wavering opinions were secured in favour of the new
inoculation by the immunity which was demonstrated
on applying the variolous test in these cases ; but, I
must repeat, *the immunity was produced by SMALL POX
which was introduced into the constitution as the result
of vaccinating in a variolous atmosphere or of employing
contaminated lancets.*[1]

It is not then surprising that Cow Pox inoculation
continued to gain ground, and that distinguished persons, in different parts of the kingdom, adopted the

[1] *Vide* vol. ii., pp. 137—147.

new practice, and exerted themselves to make it as widely known as possible. Ladies were particularly conspicuous in this work, becoming most energetic and successful vaccinators.

Jenner at this period resided at Berkeley and Cheltenham. His correspondence on the subject of vaccination so increased, that he had little leisure for other employment. It was at this time that various influential members of the profession opposed Cow Pox inoculation. But Jenner enlisted a powerful advocate in the person of Mr. Ring. Ring not only replied to the objections which were brought forward, but also collected together a number of medical men who, having satisfied themselves of the efficacy of Cow Pox inoculation, put their signatures to the following document :—

"Many unfounded reports having been circulated, which have a tendency to prejudice the public against the inoculation for Cow Pox : We the undersigned physicians and surgeons think it our duty to declare our opinion that those persons who have had the Cow Pox are perfectly secure from the future infection of the Small Pox."

Here followed the signatures of thirty-three physicians and surgeons.

In London, in the meantime, Dr. Pearson had determined to organise an Institution for inoculation of Cow Pox. He appointed a vaccine board, of which the chief place was occupied by himself, and the Duke of York consented to become a patron. In order that Jenner should be connected in some way with the

Institution, Pearson wrote offering to make him an extra corresponding physician. Jenner thought that sufficient consideration had not been shown him in the matter, and wrote a hasty letter to Pearson, declining the offer.

DR. JENNER TO DR. PEARSON.

"BERKELEY, *Dec.* 17, 1799.

"SIR,—I received your letter of the 10th instant, and confess I felt surprised at the information it conveys.

"It appears to me somewhat extraordinary that an institution formed upon so large a scale, and that has for its object the inoculation of the Cow Pox, should have been set on foot and almost completely organised without my receiving the most distant intimation of it. The institution itself cannot, of course, but be highly flattering to me, as I am thereby convinced that the importance of the fact I imparted is acknowledged by men of the first abilities. But at the same time, allow me to observe that if the vaccine inoculation, from unguarded conduct, should sink into disrepute (and you must admit, Sir, that in more than one instance has its reputation suffered), I alone must bear the odium. To you, or any other of the gentlemen whose names you mention as filling up the medical departments, it cannot possibly attach.

"At the present crisis I feel so sensibly the importance of the business that I shall certainly take an early opportunity of being in London. For the present I must beg leave to decline the *honour* intended me.

"I remain, Sir, your obedient Servant,

"E. JENNER."

Jenner left Berkeley for London on the 28th of January, 1800, in order to watch what was going on there, and shortly afterwards he published *A Continuation of Facts and Observations Relative to the Variolæ Vaccinæ.*[1] Soon after his arrival, Jenner wrote to Lord

---

[1] *Vide* vol. ii., p. 247.

Egremont, asking for an interview to enable him to submit a plan by which the country might derive the advantages of the new antidote, and to profit by his advice. Jenner had, also, an interview with the Duke of Clarence, and subsequently submitted the following proposals to Lord Egremont :—

PROPOSALS BY DR. JENNER FOR A PUBLIC INSTITU-TION FOR VACCINE INOCULATION.

(FOR LORD EGREMONT.)

" Having now pursued the inquiry into the nature of the Cow Pox to so great an extent as to be able positively to declare that those who have gone through this mild disease are rendered perfectly secure from the contagion of the Small Pox ; and being convinced from numberless instances that the occupations of the mechanic or the labourer will meet with no interruption during its progress, and the infected and uninfected may mingle together in the most perfect safety, I conceive that an institution for the gratuitous inoculation of the lower classes of society in the metropolis would be attended with the most beneficial conse-quences, and that it might be so constituted as to diffuse its benefits throughout every part of the British Empire.

" EDW. JENNER.

" LONDON, *March* 16*th*, 1800."

In order to diffuse the advantages of the institution for promoting the inoculation of the Cow Pox as widely as possible, it is proposed :

" 1st. That communications be made to the principal medical gentlemen in London and throughout the British Empire, acquaint-ing them with the nature of the Institution, and soliciting their associating as honorary members.

" 2ndly. That a Physician be appointed who shall superintend the medical department.

" 3rdly. That a house be appropriated in some convenient part of this metropolis, containing the necessary apartments for a medical attendant, a secretary, porter, etc. Apartments also for the reception of the patients sent for inoculation, and for the occasional reception of those who may choose to aid the charity.

"4thly. That virus for inoculating the Cow Pox be sent to all such honorary members as may make a proper application for it at the apartments of the Institution, and that none be sent forth without the signature of the superintending Physician, as a test of its being genuine.

"5thly. That the virus be accompanied with directions for its use, and (to guard against error) with some general observa-. tions on the nature of the disease.

"6thly. That the Institution be supported by voluntary contribution.

"7thly. That an annual subscriber of . . . . be a Governor.

"8thly. That the Governors meet at the apartments the first day of every month for the inspection of the reports relative to the general progress of the inoculation, etc., etc.

"9thly. That an abstract of the reports be published as often as it may be deemed proper."

Ultimately, Jenner succeeded in inducing the Duke of York and Lord Egremont to withdraw from the Vaccine Institution, formed by Pearson, and thus, according to Baron, Jenner defeated the ambitious designs of those who sought for high patronage.

A great piece of news for Jenner was the announcement that the King had permitted him to dedicate the second edition of the *Inquiry* to His Majesty; he was presented by Lord Berkeley, and later had an interview with his Royal Highness the Prince of Wales.

Concerning the progress of vaccination in London, at this time, Jenner wrote to Mr. Shrapnell :—

" Pray write without delay to Tierney, and tell him how rapidly the Cow Pox is marching over the metropolis, and, indeed, through the whole island. The death of the three children under inoculation with the Small Pox will probably give that practice the Brutus-stab here, and sink for ever the tyrant Small Pox. Would Tierney like to have a little virus, that the Cow Pox inoculation may be set going under his own eye at Edinburgh ? I should be happy to furnish him. Let him know that my new edition mentioning his name, with the appendix, is published. A very little attention would place the practice in its proper light in Edinburgh, a thing devoutly to be wished."

From this time until he left London, he was busily engaged in promoting the cause of the new inoculation, by meeting his professional brethren, and by discussions at the medical societies. And, finally, he left London with his nephew George, on the 23rd of June, for Oxford, where he had the gratification of obtaining the signatures of a number of learned scientists to the following testimonial drawn up by Sir C. Pegge :—

"We, whose names are undersigned, are fully satisfied upon the conviction of our own observation, that the Cow Pox is not only an infinitely milder disease than the Small Pox, but has the advantage of not being contagious, and is an effectual remedy against the Small Pox."

On the 13th of July, 1800, Jenner went to Cheltenham. His time was principally occupied in correspondence, in explaining the failures reported to him, and in collecting evidence in support of his theory. It was at this period that the Earl of Berkeley took the lead in advocating some practical expression of the public feeling in the county. He induced many to subscribe, and Jenner was presented with a service of plate.

Jenner took great interest in this testimonial. In a letter to his friend Hicks, he refers to it, as well as to the necessity of collecting cases of those who had resisted variolous inoculation after Cow Pox.

"Darke, when at Cheltenham, mentioned some strong cases to me of the preventive power of Cow Pox. He can also favour me with cases of those who have resisted variolous inoculation, because they had undergone the Cow Pox at some distant period of their lives. Evidence of this kind I cannot obtain too abundantly, as it is at this point the public mind makes a pause, from the early impression that was made of its proving a temporary preventive only. This must be the form : first state the evidence of the preventive powers of Cow Pox, and then add any comment you please upon the utility of the discovery. You may compare the anxiety you felt on the variolous inoculation in your family, with your feelings respecting the vaccine. Say nothing of Paul. It is time enough to determine how the subscription money shall be disposed of. A gold cup I should make choice of, in preference to anything else, if I may be allowed to name what it shall be. Have you thought of an appropriate device, etc. ? What think you of the *cow jumping over the moon ?* Is it not enough to make the animal jump for joy ? "

In 1801, Mr. Ring reported a case of Small Pox after Cow Pox, and Jenner replied—

"Your case would certainly have raised a clamour a year or two ago ; but now the phenomena of Cow Pox have been so fully examined, and are so well understood, none but the ignorant and illiberal will lay any stress on it for a moment."

But the way in which Jenner answered those who

reported *successful* cases of *inoculation* of Small Pox after Cow Pox, may be gathered from the following letters :—

DR. JENNER TO MR. BODDINGTON.

"LONDON, *April 21st*, 1801.

" DEAR SIR,—How a gentleman, following a profession the guardian angel of which is fame, should have so committed himself as to have called this a case of Small Pox after Cow Pox is not only astonishing to me, but must be so to all who know anything of the animal economy. He should have known that upon the skin of every human being that possesses a more than ordinary share of irritability, the insertion of the variolous virus (whether the person has previously had the Cow Pox or Small Pox) will produce either a pustule or a vesicle capable of communicating the Small Pox, and frequently attended with extensive inflammation."

DR. JENNER TO DR. EVANS, KETLEY-BANK.

" How little he (Mr. Cartwright) must have known of the agency of variolous matter, to have argued as he has done. Wonderful as it is, yet there are abundant facts to prove, that the insertion of variolous matter into the skin has produced a virus fit for the purpose of continuing the inoculation ; and yet the person who has borne it, and on whose skin it was generated, has subsequently been infected with the Small Pox, on exposure to its influence. Just so with the vaccine. . . .

" Vaccine inoculation has certainly unveiled many of the mysterious facts attendant upon the Small Pox and its inoculation. How often have we seen (apparently) the full effect on the arm from the insertion of variolous matter, indisposition, and even eruptions following it, and its termination in an extensive and deep cicatrix ; and yet, on exposure, the person who underwent this, has caught the Small Pox."

In the same year, Jenner published his account of

the origin of the vaccine inoculation. He maintained
that his inquiries commenced about 1776, and that
his attention had been drawn to the subject by the
failure to inoculate those who had had Cow Pox. He
said, a vague opinion prevailed that Cow Pox was
a preventive of the Small Pox, but this opinion was
comparatively new, and apparently originated at the
time of the introduction of the Suttonian method.
He added that in the course of the investigation
he had found some "*who seemed to have undergone
the Cow Pox*," and were inoculated with Small Pox
with success. "This," he says, "for a while damped,
but did not extinguish, my ardour." He was led to
assume the existence of a "true" and a "spurious"
Cow Pox, the latter possessing no specific power
over the constitution. Thus he "surmounted a great
obstacle." But soon there were instances of those
who had had true Cow Pox and yet received Small
Pox afterwards. "This," he adds, "like the former
obstacle, gave a painful check to my fond and aspiring
hopes." But he attributed it to the possibility of a
milker being infected one day and obtaining protection, while another milker infected the next day would
remain unprotected, the matter, having lost its *specific
properties*, producing sores and constitutional disturbance, instead of the particular change which was
necessary to render the human body insusceptible. This
observation ultimately led to the theory of spurious

vaccination. He was struck with the idea of propagating the disease by inoculation after the manner of the Small Pox, and he concluded by saying that Cow Pox was now proved to be a perfect security against the Small Pox ; and therefore that it was beyond the bounds of controversy, that the ultimate result of the practice would be the annihilation of the Small Pox.

At an early stage in the history of his observations, Jenner had hopes of his discovery proving a financial success. Baron, quoting from Jenner's diary, has given an account of his aspirations, after his successful communication of Cow Pox to Phipps.

" While the vaccine discovery was progressive, the joy I felt at the prospect before me of being the instrument destined to take away from the world one of its greatest calamities, blended with the fond hope of enjoying independence and domestic peace and happiness, was often so excessive, that in pursuing my favourite subject among the meadows I have sometimes found myself in a kind of reverie."

Jenner complained of impecuniosity when the *Inquiry* was published in 1798, but four years elapsed before a claim for remuneration was laid before Parliament. He went to London on December 9th, 1801, to prepare a petition, for which he obtained the promise of every assistance from Admiral Berkeley.

THE HON. ADMIRAL BERKELEY TO DR. JENNER.

" *Friday Evening.*

" Dear Sir,—I have arranged everything with respect to the Committee, and as I find Mr. White was employed by you to draw up the petition, I consulted him upon the best means of conducting it. He wishes to see you with the *heads* of the allegations you mean to prove, and I have therefore desired him to write to you upon the subject, because he will put us in the way of calling evidence with the least inconvenience ; as the respectable characters who are likely to appear will probably wish to be kept as little time as possible, and of course we ought to accommodate them as much as the nature of the case will admit. If you wish for any assistance which you may think me capable of affording before you see Mr. White, I hope you will believe you cannot afford me a greater satisfaction than employing me, being with great truth

" Sincerely yours,

" G. Berkeley."

Sir Henry Mildmay also promised his support, by either laying his claim for remuneration before the House or seconding it.

The petition was drawn up and duly presented, March 17th, 1802.

The following were the discoveries alleged :—

Firstly. That Cow Pox was inoculable from cow to man.

Secondly. That persons so inoculated were for life perfectly secure from Small Pox.

Jenner added that he had not made a secret of his discoveries, that the progress of Small Pox had already been checked, and that he had been put to much expense and anxiety ; therefore he prayed for remuneration.

" To the Honourable the Commons of the United Kingdom of Great Britain and Ireland, in Parliament assembled.

" The humble Petition of Edward Jenner, Doctor of Physic,

" Sheweth,

" That your petitioner having discovered that a disease

which occasionally exists in a particular form among cattle,
known by the name of the Cow Pox, admits of being inoculated on the human frame with the most perfect ease and safety,
and is attended with the singularly beneficial effect of rendering
through life the persons so inoculated perfectly secure from the
infection of the Small Pox.

"That your petitioner after a most attentive and laborious
investigation of the subject, setting aside considerations of private
and personal advantage, and anxious to promote the safety and
welfare of his countrymen and of mankind in general, did not wish
to conceal the discovery he so made on the mode of conducting
this new species of inoculation, but immediately disclosed the
whole to the public; and by communication with medical men in
all parts of this kingdom, and in foreign countries, sedulously
endeavoured to spread the knowledge of his discovery and the
benefit of his labours as widely as possible.

"That in this latter respect the views and wishes of your
petitioner have been completely fulfilled, for to his high gratification he has to say that this inoculation is in practice throughout
a great portion of the civilised world, and has in particular been
productive of great advantage to these kingdoms, in consequence
of its being introduced, under authority, into the army and navy.

"That the said inoculation hath already checked the progress
of the Small Pox, and from its nature must finally annihilate that
dreadful disorder.

"That the series of experiments by which this discovery was
developed and completed have not only occupied a considerable
portion of your petitioner's life, and have not merely been a cause
of great expense and anxiety to him, but have so interrupted him
in the ordinary exercise of his profession as materially to abridge
its pecuniary advantages, without their being counterbalanced by
those derived from the new practice.

"Your petitioner, therefore, with the full persuasion that he
shall meet with that attention and indulgence of which
this Honourable House may deem him worthy, humbly
prays this Honourable House to take the premises into
consideration, and to grant him such remuneration as to
their wisdom shall seem meet."

The king's pleasure was taken on the contents of the petition, and his Majesty recommended it to Parliament. It was referred to a Committee, presided over by Admiral Berkeley, and in June 1802, the Report was laid before the House. Admiral Berkeley moved for a grant of £10,000, which was duly seconded by Sir Henry Mildmay, and carried by a majority of three. After the conclusion of the Parliamentary inquiry, Jenner left London for Berkeley.

Once more, he had leisure to attend to his correspondence on the constant subject of failures of Cow Pox to protect from Small Pox.

To R. Dunning, Esq.

" 1802.

" My Dear Sir,—Our last letters crossed each other on the road, according to custom. Your letter of April the 22nd reached me at a time when my head was brimful of the bustles of the Committee, and was not, I think, sufficiently, at least properly, noticed in any subsequent letter of mine. What I allude to is your account of the inoculation of Mr. Courtney, Mr. Yonge, and the staggering cases of yourself and Mr. Lisle. Add to this, the case of the marine at Portsmouth. Now, my good friend, my mind having long since obtained what security it is capable of possessing, I request of you to tell me what time and enquiry have developed respecting these Plymouth cases. That of the marine at Portsmouth was clearly made out to have been imperfect. The people at this sea-port set up a kind of malignant shout (see the Letters of Hope in the Report of the Committee) at finding this case of supposed failure. They disliked vaccination because Plymouth adopted it; *tanta est discordia fratrum.*

" Mr. Bankes, who drew up the Report, was no friend either

to me or my cause, or he would have listened to my solicitations,
and inserted not only the certificates you mention, but your letter
also. Let any one read the Report of Dr. Smith, and compare
it with mine; then let them judge who had indulgences and who
had none. The indisposition of my chairman, Admiral Berkeley,
was a most unfortunate event. The whole merit Mr. Bankes
allowed me on the score of discovery in vaccination (considering
it abstractedly) was that of inoculating from one human being to
another. On this subject I remonstrated, but it was all in vain.
Cannot you contrive to get your papers into the Journal ? Surely
you might command my assistance whenever you please; they
would gain admittance with the most perfect propriety in reply
to Pearson's audacious assertion, and produce good effects in a
variety of ways."

After his return to Berkeley, several friends in London
resolved to endeavour to form a Jennerian Institution for
promoting universal vaccine inoculation. On January
19th, 1803, a public meeting was convened and presided
over by the Lord Mayor. It was proposed and
seconded, "that this meeting do form itself into a
society for the extermination of the Small Pox."
It happened that his Royal Highness the Duke of
Clarence was prepared to move, by deputy, a vote of
thanks to Dr. Jenner. So it was immediately resolved
that the Duke of Clarence should entreat his Majesty
to become patron of the proposed institution, and grant
permission for it to be called the Royal Jennerian
Society for the extermination of the Small Pox. His
Majesty graciously consented, the Queen became patron,
and other royal personages vice-patrons; many ladies
of rank also were induced to interest themselves in

supporting vaccination. A board of directors and a medical council were appointed.

Jenner remained at Berkeley until February 1803, when he went to London. On the 3rd of this month, he took his seat for the first time, as President of the Royal Jennerian Institution. At a subsequent meeting, Dr. John Walker was appointed resident inoculator. Thirteen stations were opened in the Metropolis, and in eighteen months they were able to announce that 12,288 inoculations had taken place, and 19,352 charges of Cow Pox virus supplied to different parts of the British Empire and to foreign countries. Events, however, did not continue to run smoothly. Jenner disapproved of Dr. Walker, and used all his influence to obtain his dismissal, which led to Dr. Walker's resigning his office. The Society lingered on for some time, but when the National Vaccine Institution was established in 1808, its finances were nearly exhausted, and it had practically collapsed.

Shortly after the formation of the Royal Jennerian Institution, Jenner was induced to take up practice in London. He settled for some years in Hertford Street, Mayfair, but the result was disastrous.

He therefore determined to leave London, and communicated his intention to one of his friends.

" I have now completely made up my mind respecting London. I have done with it, and have again commenced the village-doctor. I found my purse not equal to the sinking of a thousand pounds annually (which has actually been the case for several successive years), nor the gratitude of the public deserving such a sacrifice.

How hard, after what I have done, the toils I have gone through,
and the anxieties I have endured in obtaining for the world a
greater gift than man ever bestowed on them before (excuse
this burst of egotism), to be thrown by with a bare remuneration
of my expenses!"

Ten years afterwards, Jenner gave a detailed account
of his experiences.

"Elated and allured by the speech of the Chancellor of the
Exchequer, I took a house in London for ten years, at a high
rent, and furnished it; but my first year's practice convinced me
of my own temerity and imprudence, and the falsity of the minister's prediction. My fees fell off both in number and value; for,
extraordinary to tell, some of those families in which I had been
before employed, now sent to their own domestic surgeons or
apothecaries to inoculate their children, alleging that they could
not think of troubling Dr. Jenner about a thing executed so easily
as vaccine inoculation. Others, who gave me such fees as I
thought myself entitled to at the first inoculation, reduced them
at the second, and sank them still lower at the third."

In the year 1804, failures of the new inoculation had
multiplied to an alarming degree, and even some
of his friends began to lose confidence. His time was
again much taken up in correspondence, suggesting
fresh explanations to account for the numerous failures.

Nevertheless, some of Jenner's friends were of opinion
that this year formed a new era in the history of
Cow Pox, for, according to Baron, if the assertion that
Cow Pox afforded only a temporary security had
been correct, it would have deprived the discovery of
nearly all its value. Jenner had conceived that in cases
of Small Pox occurring after Cow Pox, the vaccination

could not have been properly performed; but Mr.
Dunning endeavoured to establish a belief in the
permanent protection of Cow Pox, by explaining
failures as the result of spurious vaccination. In the
course of the same year, Jenner published his tract
on the *Varieties and Modifications of the Vaccine
Pustule, occasioned by a State of the Skin,* which had
the same end in view.

Jenner, however, was fully aware that Small Pox had
occurred after perfect vaccination, and in his correspondence with Mr. Dunning, he was prepared
with various answers to meet these cases, though,
at the same time, he endeavoured to suppress their
publication.

"I have just received the Portsmouth paper of the 2nd of
April, sent to me, I suppose, by the printer. It contains, in
large letters, the following sensible paragraph : ' Reports of some
cases of Small Pox after vaccine inoculation were read at a very
full meeting of the Medical Society of Portsmouth on Thursday
last the 29th instant, which we are informed will be sent to the
press, and published in a few days.' Is Dr. Hope returned
to his old post? What a set of blockheads! How will our
continental neighbours laugh at us !"

His explanations, however, were ready to hand,
when he was applied to. Thus he wrote to Lord
Berkeley :—

"I expect that cases of this sort will flow in upon me in no
inconsiderable numbers; and for this plain reason—a great
number, perhaps the majority, of those who inoculate are not
sufficiently acquainted with the nature of the disease to enable

them to discriminate with due accuracy between the perfect and imperfect pustule. This is a lesson not very difficult to learn, but unless it is learnt, to inoculate the Cow Pox is folly and presumption."

Another correspondent pleaded with him to reply to the writings of those who opposed the Jennerian doctrine, the so-called anti-vaccinists. But Jenner declined to enter into the controversy.

"The post is just come in, and I have been entertaining Mrs. Jenner and my family with your dream. Some kind friend had perhaps thrown your stomach into disorder by tempting you to go too deep into an oyster-barrel; or had our friend P—— seduced you with the fumes of one of his favourite supper dishes? A devil, or a something, had certainly disordered your stomach; and your stomach shewed its resentment on your head; and your letter is the consequence. However, I will reason on it for a moment as if it were not a dream. You are imposed upon, and so is my friend Fox. Vaccination never stood on more lofty ground than at present. I know very well the opinion of the wise and great upon it, and the foolish and the little I don't care a straw for. Why should we fix our eyes on this spot only? Let them range the world over, and they must contemplate with delight and exultation what they behold on the great continents of Europe and America; in our settlements in India, where all ranks of people, from the poor Hindoo to the Governor-General, hail Vaccina as a new divinity. In the island of Ceylon, my account states that upwards of thirty thousand had been vaccinated a twelvemonth ago. I could march you round the globe, and wherever you rested you should see scenes like these. *There* I have honour, *here* I have none: and let me tell you, whatever my feelings may have been on this subject, they are now at rest. What I have *said on this vaccine subject is true. If properly conducted, it secures the constitution as much as variolous inoculation possibly can. It is the Small Pox in a purer form than that which has been current among us for twelve centuries past.*"

"You and my city friend suppose me idle—that I no longer employ my time and my thoughts on the vaccine subject. So very opposite is the real state of the case, that were you here (where I should be very glad to see you), you would see that my whole time is nearly engrossed by it. On an average I am at least six hours daily with my pen in my hand, bending over writing-paper, till I am grown as crooked as a cow's horn and tawny as whey-butter; and *you* want to make me as mad as a bull: but it won't do, Mr. D.; so good-night to you. I'll to my pillow, not of thorns, believe me, nor of hops; but of poppies, or at least something that produces calm repose."

Jenner had constantly to resort to the theory that if Small Pox occurred after Cow Pox, the vaccination could not have been properly performed.

DR. JENNER TO MR. DUNNING.

"*July 5th*, 1804.

"There is not a single case, nor a single argument, that puts the weight of a feather in the scale of the anti-vaccinist. That which seems to be the heaviest, becomes light as air, when we consider that the human constitution is at one time susceptible of variolous contagion, at another, not so; and this insusceptibility sometimes continues to a late period of life. Elizabeth Everet was a Small Pox nurse in this neighbourhood for forty years. She supposed she had had the Small Pox when a child. A few years since she was sent for to Bristol to nurse a patient, caught the disease, and died.

"Mr. Long, surgeon of St. Bartholomew's, had a similar instance in his own family.

"A thousand thanks to you and Dr. Remmet for your investigation of the Exmouth case. Never mind; you will hear enough of Small Pox after Cow Pox. It must be so. Every bungling vaccinist who excites a pustule on the arm, will swear like G. it was correct, without knowing that nicety of distinction which every man ought to know, before he presumes to take up the vaccine lancet."

But even after perfect vaccination, it was well known that after a little time, patients could be infected by inoculation. To meet this, Jenner urged that the inoculation test should be abandoned.[1]

"Had vaccination wanted firmer support than it has already, it would have obtained it from the very efforts made use of for its destruction. I will just remark that the fairest of all tests is exposure to variolous contagion; this is the natural test, inoculation is not. Who does not know (all medical men ought to know) that the insertion of the variolous poison into the skin of an irritable person will sometimes produce great inflammation, disturbance of the system, and even eruptions?

"Adieu, my dear sir. I write, as you must observe, in haste.

"Yours truly,

"E. JENNER.

"Just setting off with my family to Cheltenham.

"P.S. I am sorry to say I cannot send you advertisements to the cover of the Medical Journal. The review of G.'s book will tell you I have no interest there."

Mr. Dunning himself encountered failures, and his faith in vaccination was fast disappearing. He consequently was severely reprimanded—

"Vaccination calls imperiously for my attention, and to that I am determined all my other worldly concerns shall yield. But while I am fighting the enemy of mankind, it will be vexatious to see my aides-de-camp turn shy. Among the foremost in the field, I have always ranked *Richard Dunning*. No one has been more obedient to the commands of his general, or wielded the sword against the foe with greater force and dexterity. But shall I live to see my friend dismayed at the mere shadow of fortune on the side of the enemy;—will he who has led such hosts into the field and found them invulnerable,

---

[1] Extract from letter to R. Dunning. Baron, *loc. cit.*, vol. ii., p. 339.

start if, in the continuation of the combat, he should see a man
fall ? Enough of metaphor. The moral of all this is, that
I see you are growing timid ; the timidity so conspicuous towards
the close of your pamphlet, and that which is so manifest in
your letter of this evening, it would be wrong in me not to say
I was sorry to observe. More convincing or stronger facts
the public could never wish for than your pamphlet exhibits.
Had I been at your elbow, I should have certainly pulled back
your pen when you began reasoning upon them. The result
of your experiments authorised you to speak in tones the most
exulting and triumphant ; but most unfortunately, you almost
give up the field to the anti-vaccinists, by speaking of new and
better arrangements, IF *variolous inoculation should supersede the
vaccine !* Now, my good and valued friend, don't for a moment
think that I am out of temper with you,· or mean to speak
harshly. On the contrary, I attributed this oversight (such I must
call it) to the dreadful calamity that befell your family. Your
mind, I know, must have been oppressed, and you were bringing
your work to a conclusion under pressures scarcely bearable.
To those who made remarks upon what appeared so extraordinary, I communicated the circumstance which seemed to
me to account for it. The 115th page of your work, is that
which has occasioned the general surprise. The further I go
on with vaccination, the more I am convinced that the great
and grand impediment to the correct action of the virus on the
constitution, is the co-existence of herpes. I expected that my
paper on this subject, in the Medical Journal for August, would
have attracted more attention. Since my writing it, I have
detected a case of Small Pox after Small Pox inoculation, where
the cause of failure was evidently an herpetic affection of the
scalp. Are such cases as these—are such as Mr. Embling,
so circumstantially described in your pamphlet—are Mr. Tyre's
lately communicated in the Star—are Mr. Kite's of Gravesend,
and a thousand others, to go unnoticed by the public, while
failures in vaccination (a science far more difficult to understand
than variolation) are to make impressions so deep as even
to stagger the faith of those who are well informed upon the
subject ? Is common sense to be attached to one side of the

question only, and to have nothing to do with the other ? 'This case, connected with those in London at Fullwoods Rents, I grieve to say, appear extremely ugly.'—*Dunning.*

" Is it possible their ugliness can affright you ? What phantoms must they appear, if you will but look back and consider the period when those children were inoculated. Woodville at that time, and his coadjutor Wachsel knew nothing of the Cow Pox; this is clearly evinced by Woodville's first pamphlet, where he gives three hundred cases of Small Pox, and calls them Cow Pox. Surely his early inoculations are not to be regarded ; and does he not at this hour, in conjunction with a person whose dirty name shall not daub my paper, sanction the taking of virus from the pustule at any of its stages ? What are we to expect while such things as these are going forward ? Inclosed is the letter you requested me to return ; it is impossible for me to go into particulars on such cases. I can only go into general reasoning. My experience justifies me in saying that which I have said fifty times before, ' If the vaccine pustule goes through its stages correctly, the patient is secure from the Small Pox ; if not, security cannot be answered for.' There certainly is ·sometimes a nicety in discrimination, and it was this which in my early instructions occasioned me to say, ' When a deviation arises in the character of the vaccine pustule, of whatever kind it may be, common prudence points out the necessity of re-inoculation.' Cases may possibly. occur, where even you or I may (from the interposition of those events which medical men are always subject to) not have it in our power to catch opportunities of passing our judgment upon a pustule during those stages, whether it is or is not correctly defined. With respect to the doctrine of Mr. Moyle, I must candidly say, my experiments do not justify me in subscribing to them. Be of good cheer, my friend. Those who are so presumptuous as to expect perfection in man will be grievously disappointed. His works are and ever will be defective. Let people, if they choose it, spurn the great gift that heaven has bestowed, and turn again to variolation. What will they get by it ? Let them consult pages 67 and 68 of your decisive work on this subject, and they will know. Let them peruse the following extract from a letter which I have, within these few days, received from a medical gentleman of great respectability in this county.' 'A poor family belonging to Sudeley parish, consisting of a man, his wife, and five children, were vaccinated four or five years ago, except the eldest daughter, who had been before inoculated for the Small Pox by an eminent practitioner, and pronounced secure. This summer she caught the Small Pox when working among the rags at the paper mills, and had a very numerous and confluent eruption. The rest of the family have no fears, and have all escaped, though fully exposed to the infection.' Now had this case been reversed, what a precious morsel it would have been for an anti-vaccinist. Adieu my dear friend, and be assured of the unalterable regard of yours,

" EDW. JENNER.

For a time the letter had the desired effect upon Mr. Dunning, and it was soon followed by another, in which flattery was employed to smooth his ruffled feelings.

To RICHARD DUNNING, ESQ., PLYMOUTH.

"CHELTENHAM, 15*th Nov.* 1804.

" MY DEAR SIR,—The old occurrence of our letters crossing on the road has, I see, again taken place. If my writing frequently to you will afford you the least gratification, I shall not be slack in my correspondence.

"There is no one more entitled to my attention, and among all the vaccinists who have enlisted under my banner, there is no one who has a greater claim for my regard. There was no expression in my letter, I hope, which would bear the construction you seem to put upon it. You were rallied a little on your timidity respecting the *ugly* cases in town and country —on your glancing at a better regulation for the management of the Small Pox, *if* we are obliged to turn to it again—on your fear of reviews—and of a little shrinking, even, from the man whom you are opposing; but all was done in perfectly good humour, and now you will allow me triumphantly to exclaim, 'Richard's himself again!'"

Dunning was now ready to assert that the occurrence of Small Pox after Cow Pox, actually strengthened the theory. Even Jenner was puzzled and wrote :—

"Pray indulge me with a line or two very speedily, to put an end to a little perplexity. You tell me that you know Small Pox will sometimes follow Cow Pox, and nevertheless assert that a case of this sort, which has happened under your immediate observation, places vaccination on higher ground than it has yet stood on.

"Do pray explain, as soon as you can, your meaning. . . .

"I am pleased at seeing the friends of the vaccine cause showing themselves in the newspapers. These meet every eye, while the Journal meets that of medical men only, and has proved the tomb of many an impressive paper."

But Dunning was not yet completely subdued, for in a work which he wrote on vaccination, he was still willing to discuss doubtful cases. Jenner commended the pamphlet as a whole, while insisting upon the necessity for collecting all evidence in favour of vaccination and rejecting all criticism.

To R. Dunning, Esq.

"Berkeley, *Feb. 10th*, 1805.

"My Dear Friend,—Your *little* pamphlet contains many great and useful observations. I will now refer you to a few notes I made in perusing it. The book itself should have been printed in the more general shape and form of pamphlets. Page 16, concluding sentence of the first paragraph, pithy, and containing a complete reply to the anti-vaccinists, who may urge objections from a few solitary cases of Small Pox after

Cow Pox, or who might bring them forward if they were ten times as numerous.   100,000 cases of vaccination, by far too few to calculate upon.   Half that number I can reckon from extra-professional inoculations, 20,000 of which are. from my fair disciples ; and, to their credit be it spoken, I have not heard of one sinister event among this class of inoculations. And why ?   They implicitly obey vaccine laws.   Page 12, good reasoning on the subject of population.   I have often urged the following argument when too numerous a population has been thrown in my teeth, as one of the ill effects likely to attend vaccination. . . .

" Your manner of speaking of Goldson increases his arrogance. He obstinately holds the veil before his eyes, and will not behold the vaccine light.   I am about to make a stronger pull at this veil than has been done yet.   I have sent him an invitation to visit me at Berkeley, or to appoint a deputation from the Medical Society at Portsmouth ; I have gone further (perhaps too far), I have almost pledged my word that his conversion will be the consequence of the interview.   The fact is, he is totally ignorant of that wise discriminating power, without which no man can be a perfect vaccinist : and it is my wish to impart it to him.   One might as well contend with a blind man on the nature of the prism, as with a person in this situation, and entertain a hope of being successful ; but to proceed.   In another edition, pray take in Kite's cases of Small Pox after Small Pox inoculation.   They are the more forcible as they were published antecedent to the vaccine practice. Page 38.   Are you sure the pustule was variolated ?   Page 41. I do not see the necessity for your parenthesis.   Perhaps my feelings are too acute, but I do not like to see my darling child whipped even with a feather.   In your postscript, why not ask for cases of Small Pox after Small Pox inoculation, as well as cases of Small Pox after vaccination."

On March 1st, we find Jenner again writing on failures ; this shows how much his mind was occupied with them at this time.

" The security given to the constitution by vaccine inoculation,
is exactly equal to that given by the variolous.   To expect more
from it would be wrong.   As failures in the latter are constantly
presenting themselves, nearly from its commencement to the
present time, we must expect to find them in the former also.
In my opinion, in either case, they occur from the same causes ;
one might name for example, among others, some peculiarity
of constitution which prevents the virus from acting properly,
even when properly applied; from inattention, or want of due
knowledge in the inoculator; particularly in not being able to
discriminate between the correct and incorrect pustule."

Dunning wrote disapproving of the policy of setting
off cases of Small Pox after Small Pox, against those
of Small Pox after Cow Pox.   Jenner replied :—

" Think a moment of my situation before you censure me for
tardiness—the correspondence of the world to attend to.   The
pressure is often, I do assure you, so great, that it is more than
either my body or mind can well endure.   You say, 'let vaccination, for God's sake, rest on its own foundation.'   My dear sir,
that is exactly what I want, and the course I have been pursuing.
Neither the impudence of Pearson, the folly of Goldson, nor the
baseness of Moseley and Squirrel, to which I may add the stupid
absurdity of Birch, has put me out of my way in the least,—and
why ?   I placed it on a rock, where I knew it would be
immoveable, before I invited the public to look at it."

Some time afterwards, Dunning appears to have
spoken out freely.   Jenner replied:—

" A pretty sharp philippic, my good friend! but in such
veneration do I hold the man of feeling, that if it had been
ten times as sharp, I should have read it, though not without
emotion, yet certainly without a murmur.   Allow me just to
make one observation.   Should anything like the present occur-

rence ever happen again, let me entreat you not to indulge for a moment a fanciful speculation against your *friend*. As such I hope ever to be, and so to be considered by you."

Jenner continued to collect cases of Small Pox after Small Pox, and wrote for assistance to his friend, the Rev. John Clinch, Trinity, Newfoundland.

"Never aim, my friend, at being a public character, if you love domestic peace. But I will not repine. Nay, I do not repine, but cheerfully submit, as I look upon myself as the instrument in the hands of that power which never errs, of doing incalculable good to my fellow-creatures. You would do me an essential kindness in acquainting me with the state of vaccination in your island, as I shall appear again before the House of Commons next session, and I am collecting all the information I can from foreign parts. Write to me not as if your letter was to be shown to the House of Commons, and detail the real state of facts relative to the benefits derived from the new practice. Remember me kindly to Mrs. Clinch, and my old friend Edward, who I ardently hope is becoming useful to you ; and believe me, dear Clinch, ever truly, and sincerely yours,

"EDW. JENNER.

"Do you recollect any cases of persons catching the Small Pox after the Small Pox, either after casual contagion, or inoculation ? I have collected a great number of such cases, but want more."

We may now turn our attention for a moment to London. In the same year, 1805, a paper appeared in the *Gentleman's Magazine*, "the only publication that then would venture to insert anything adverse to the Vaccine System." This paper had been written by Birch,[1] in 1804, and circulated among his intimate

---

[1] John Birch, Surgeon Extraordinary to His Royal Highness the Prince of Wales, and Surgeon of St. Thomas's Hospital.

friends, in vindication of the opinion which he had given before the Committee of the House of Commons. Birch condemned vaccination as an unnatural experiment, unphilosophical, and unsafe.

" Magna est Veritas et prævalebit.

"Had the Inoculation for what has been called Cow Pox succeeded, agreeably to the sanguine promises and expectations of its advocates, I should have thought myself called upon to recant the opinion I gave to the Committee of the House of Commons, and to apologize for having persevered in it; but as the experiment has failed in several instances, and the truth can no longer be concealed from the public, I think it necessary to appeal to the judgment of discerning persons, whether I have not been treated with much injustice, for firmly maintaining an opinion for which I had such strong grounds.

"It was a maxim handed down to us while I was a Student at St. Thomas's Hospital, ' Never to sacrifice Experience to Experiment ;' and therefore in Diseases, for the treatment of which Time and Observation had laid down a rule of successful practice, I am cautious how I exchange this for new opinions.

"The judicious manner in which my excellent friend, Baron Dimsdale, managed the Inoculation for Small Pox, had long convinced me that if any man deserved well of his Country, he was entitled at least to the *thanks* of the Legislature ; and the opportunities I had of making myself acquainted with his opinions, taught me to listen with caution to any new practice, which was to overturn all I had made myself master of.

"When therefore it was proposed to me, to *introduce a new Disease into the human system*, I hesitated; but on the assurance given to me, that it was still milder than the Inoculated Small Pox, was productive of no ill consequences, and would equally arrest the progress of variolous Infection, I consented that Abraham Howard, the first Child mentioned at my Examination, should be vaccinated. The Cow Pox terminated successfully, but the Child afterwards sickened, and had an eruption, which I considered the Small Pox, though others called it an *Hybrid Eruption*, an appearance which I was told had been described as not un-common at the Small Pox Hospital, when the patient had been previously in a variolous Atmosphere.

" Two other Cases[1] however were followed by distinct and unequivocal Small Pox after Vaccination, and then it was admitted that the Cow Pox would not arrest the progress of *variolous* Infection ; although it is well known, Inoculation of the Small Pox within a limited period will *supersede* and *subdue* it.

" These Cases ascertained that there was no such thing as an Hybrid or. Mulish Eruption, but that what had been called so at the Small Pox Hospital was the real Small Pox.

" I appeal therefore to persons of Discernment, whether such mistakes, in the outset of a new practice, were not sufficient grounds for a cautious man to admit some doubts of the danger of introducing a new disease into the human system. The opinion which I gave to the Committee, was supported by such proofs, in the answers sent to their enquiries and published in their Report, from Messrs. Slater of Wycomb, Grosvenor of Oxford, Nooth of Bath, and Dr. Hope of Haslar Hospital, that what I have seen and heard since, has only served to determine me not to be misled by the fashionable rage.

" The steady and single opinion I have maintained in opposition to this practice, has brought me acquainted with some new Erup-tions, Abscesses and Disorders, which I had not before observed ; but these accidents are generally attributed to a *Spurious* sort of Cow Pox. This is a term I do not admit of ; I know of no such thing as *Spurious* Small Pox, *Spurious* Lues Venerea, *Spurious* Scrofula. We are yet left unsatisfied as to the nature and origin of what is called Cow Pox. It is a disorder known only to the Cow Doctor in *dirty* dairies, though we are taught to play with it as a blessing revealed from Heaven to this enlightened age.

" If I wished to corroborate the grounds for my doubts, I might mention an almost equally fashionable rage, which had seized too many of the faculty, previous to the appearance of Cow Pox, in favour of the Nitrous Acid, as a remedy for the Venereal Disease. Mercury was no longer to be called in aid, and the press teemed

---

[1] Will. Rinch, M. Solloway—*vide Report.*

with publications to prove the mistaken opinions of hospital Surgeons. This Novelty I resisted with equal firmness; here I was
unwilling to give up *Experience for Experiment,* wanting nothing
more safe or certain than Mercury, which for so many years, in
the practice of so many competent Judges, had proved an Antidote
to that malignant poison. The advocates for the Nitrous Acid
are now no longer heard of, the books on the subject no longer
regarded.

"Sacrificing, therefore, every consideration to my actual Opinion,
I have avoided the practice of Vaccination, but I have watched the
result of it. I do not mean to enter into the proof of its failures,
or mistakes: Mr. Goldson has published some, in a very candid
pamphlet—more are expected from another pen; and unless the
first Projectors have something better to say, than what has yet
been said, to reconcile the public mind to those Cases of Mr.
Hodges' children, in Fullward's Rents, Holborn, I shall continue
firm in the opinion I gave to the Committee of the House of
Commons, THAT WHAT HAS BEEN CALLED THE COW POX IS NOT
A PRESERVATIVE AGAINST THE NATURAL SMALL POX."

On the other hand, Dr. Lettsom came forward to
fight Jenner's battles. The Medical Society of
London conferred a gold medal upon Jenner in
honour of his discovery, and at the anniversary
festival, Dr. Lettsom delivered an oration on vaccination. Various honours and marks of distinction were
conferred upon Jenner about this time, both at home
and abroad. Clergymen warmly advocated the practice
of vaccination. The Rev. Dr. Booker, of Dudley,
printed sermons on the subject, and thus promoted
the practice. In a letter of his to Jenner, we read :—

"You will see, however, in the annexed address to parents on
the subject, that I have done more than recommend it from the

pulpit. One of these printed forms I give to every person who brings a child to be baptized either at church or at my own residence, or when sent for to baptize abroad. By this means I distribute about twenty a week, and have the satisfaction to learn that the expedient has produced the desired effect. It influences at a time when mankind are easily convinced of the precarious tenure of infantine existence."

The Rev. James Plumptre preached a sermon on vaccination at Cambridge, and, again, at the parish church, Hinxton, taking as his text, "And he stood between the dead and the living, and the plague was stayed."

The practice was still strongly opposed by an influential section of the medical profession; but while troubled with this hostility at home, Jenner derived very soothing consolation from the accounts which were received of the progress of vaccination abroad.

In 1805, Jenner was again in London, discussing with his friends "the establishment of vaccination and the advancement of his private fortune." Lord Henry Petty, who had taken up the cause of vaccination, had become Chancellor of the Exchequer; and the Duchess of Devonshire promised her influence. On the other hand, in 1806, Birch[1] published his reasons for objecting to the practice of vaccination. It was by far the most temperate of the arguments against the new practice, and deserves to be quoted *in extenso.*

---

[1] *Serious Reasons for uniformly objecting to the Practice of Vaccination, in Answer to the Report of the Jennerian Society.* 1806.

"That the enthusiasm with which Vaccination was at first adopted should subside, and that the Public should express regret that what ought to have been admitted as an experiment only, had been adopted as practice, are circumstances which, it was easy to foresee, would sooner or later occur. In all investigations, and in all inquiries, Truth must ultimately prevail. In the present, it would have long since prevailed, had not the patrons of Vaccination had recourse to such expedients to interest the passions, and mislead the judgment, of the Public as could hardly fail of obtaining for their system a temporary kind of success. But the triumph of prejudice and novelty will always be transient. The empire of Truth alone is permanent. I entertain no doubt, therefore, but that we shall soon see what yet remains of popular opinion favourable to the cause of Vaccination *vanish into thin air;* and that the speculatists in physic, like the speculatists in politics, will be brought back to the old standard of sober reason and experience.

"Impressed with this conviction, I should have patiently awaited the event; and, contenting myself with having declared my opinion publicly, should have forborne taking any part in the controversy, had it not been for considerations of humanity, which supersede every other.

"Wherever I go, I find the minds of parents distracted with doubt, and labouring under gloomy apprehensions. They tell me that the fluctuations of medical opinion concerning the origin and nature of the Vaccine disease fill them with alarm; and they say they are in the most fearful state of suspense, dreading lest what they were persuaded to do in the hopes of saving their children from one disease, may not prove the means of plunging them into another at once novel and malignant.

"Much as I lament their being in so distressing a state of suspense, I cannot wonder at it. For while, on the one hand, they hear of repeated instances of the failure of Vaccination, on the other, they find that reports from the Jennerian Committee, subscribed by names, some of the highest respectability, are widely circulated, full of seeming arguments and assertions in favour of the experiment; assertions which they have not the means of contradicting, and arguments just plausible enough to excite doubt, but not sufficiently strong to operate conviction. If, under these circumstances, I can adduce what may enable persons of this description to form a fixed opinion on the merits of Vaccination, and thus rescue them from the misery of uncertainty, I shall consider myself as having discharged one of the most important duties I owe Society.

"Such is the primary motive for my writing the following pages : a secondary motive is, that as the Jennerian Committee have sent me their Report of last January for my signature, I may candidly tell them why I have hitherto forborne to subscribe it, and why I shall never subscribe it. To this report therefore, and to a very ingenious pamphlet written by Mr. James Moore, certainly the ablest and most candid writer that has appeared in support of Vaccination, I shall confine as much as possible my remarks. The bitterness of invective, and the unhandsome sneers, with which the partisans of Vaccination have assailed their opponents, as they offer no argument, merit no reply.

"The Report opens by stating that the Medical Council appointed twenty-five members of the Jennerian Society as a Committee to inquire into the truth of various cases that had occurred, exciting prejudices against Vaccine Inoculation ; and it is the result of their inquiries that is submitted to the Public.

"Now, without calling in question the judgment of the Medical Council, I must observe that it became them, in a matter of such importance, to inform us who these twenty-five persons were. For as the Society is very numerous, comprehending many of both sexes, and of all professions, the Committee might have been formed of persons not altogether competent to the task : since evidently, besides what may be called a knowledge of Vaccination, it was necessary there should be likewise a thorough knowledge of medicine. In other words, the Public ought to have been assured that the Committee was composed of regular and experienced physicians and surgeons before they could be in reason expected to assent to its decisions : instead of which we have a Committee made up of persons whose very names we are unacquainted with. I confess that this circumstance, in my mind, throws as much suspicion over the Jennerian Reports, as it would over a verdict in a common court of law to be told, that it was the verdict of a jury, no one member of which the defendant was permitted to challenge; whose names, conditions and character were studiously concealed; and who had never so much as appeared in court during the trial.

" This, however, is not the only circumstance that makes me regard with an eye of suspicion the Reports of the Committee. The several articles of that Report are couched either in a style so dogmatizing, that the Committee seem more intent on imposing a law than on producing conviction ; or else in terms so vague, and ambiguous, that the reader must be at a loss to obtain any fixed and definitive idea of the subject. The former of these faults I will pass over, as it may be attributed to the force of the conviction entertained by the Committee of the justness of their positions : but the latter, as an honest man, I cannot, since it has a tendency to mislead, rather than direct the judgment of the Public. Surely the Committee are aware that nothing is more suspicious than the use of equivocal expressions ; and that there is nothing the candid disputant more scrupulously avoids. By means of these confessions of error, extorted by truth, may be made no confessions at all ; may be so worded as to produce no effect, and yet carry with them the appearance of candour, and concession. I will instance the truth of this remark in the Ninth and Tenth Article of the Jennerian Report.

" The Committee, being at last compelled to acknowledge that cases have been brought before them, in which it was incontestibly proved that persons having passed through the Cow Pox in a regular way, had afterwards received the Small Pox, contrive to destroy the effect of the concession, by the following ambiguous expressions.

" It is admitted that *a few* cases have been brought before them, of persons who had *apparently* passed through the Cow Pox in a regular way, etc.

" Now (not to remark on the use of the indefinite word *few*, which may mean five or six, or five or six dozen, for ought we know, when it was so obviously important, and easy to have specified the precise number), I must observe, that as the passage stands worded, it might seem as if the Committee, having seen all the cases of failure in Vaccination that could be produced, found only a *few* they could admit to be genuine. How many cases they did see, I will not take upon me to conjecture ; I suspect they did not wish to see many, for if they had, they might have seen, or have had unquestionable testimony of many hundred cases of failure, of which not a *few*, but far the greater part, if not the whole, would have been found conclusive against them.

"But it is said, '*apparently passed* through the Cow Pox.' What, only apparently ? If the Committee had not been satisfied the patients had *really* passed through the Cow Pox, they neither would, or ought to, have admitted the failure of what they call a *few* cases. Why then is the word 'apparently' introduced ? I can imagine no other cause, than that this equivocal word might serve to qualify the confession of the Committee, and thus make it *appear* less conclusive than it really is.

"But this is not all. The Committee proceed to say, that 'cases supported by evidence equally strong were brought before them of persons having had the Small Pox a second time by natural infection.'

"Will the Committee pardon me if I remark that they are here guilty of reasoning very unfairly, to say no worse of it. In the one instance they argue from cases *brought before them:* in the other, from the *evidence of cases* brought before them. That is, when a case makes against them, they admit no proof but the evidence of their own senses : when it is favourable to their cause, they admit it on the evidence of others. In fair reasoning, in both instances, a similar degree of proof ought to be required. If cases on the testimony of others are admitted to prove the failure of inoculation, cases on the testimony of others should be admitted to prove the failure of Vaccination ; and then the Committee will be compelled to state that not merely a few cases, but that many hundred cases of failure have occurred : for many hundred cases are already before the public of persons who have had the Small Pox after Vaccination, attested by the evidence, not of hasty observers and unscientific operators, but of able and experienced practitioners.

But this is not the only instance of unfair reasoning I am to complain of on the part of the Jennerian Committee.

"They say, '*In many of the cases* in which Small Pox has occurred after Inoculation!' *Many of the cases!* This expression I presume is to contrast with the *few cases of failure* admitted in Vaccination, and the reader is left to infer that cases of failure in Inoculation are of frequent recurrence ; than which inference nothing can be more unfounded, more contrary to truth.

For, in the first place, if we could grant all the cases that have been adduced on anything like proof, to attest the recurrence of Small Pox after Inoculation, these, during a period of more than half a century, would not amount to more than three.

"But, in the second place, the fact itself has been uniformly denied by the best and most able practitioners. They have always maintained that the Small Pox never has been known to recur after Inoculation ; and however the contrary may be assumed by those who have systems of their own to advance, it is considered as one of the invariable laws of nature, that (and if an exception could be proved, I should be justified in saying, *exceptio probat regulam*) a patient can suffer the Small Pox but once.

"I might quote in support of my opinion, that of the celebrated Baron Dimsdale, Dr. Archer, and many others ; but it will be of greater authority, in the present case, to quote the opinion of Mr. J. Moore, the candid supporter of Vaccination, who admits in his pamphlet, that Small Pox does not recur after Inoculation.

"I have dwelt longer on these two Articles, than I probably shall on any of the succeeding, that I might put the Reader on his guard against the false conclusions into which he might otherwise be led, by the ambiguous manner in which the Committee write. And I shall dismiss this part of the subject by saying, that the same inaccuracy of expression (whether accidental or studied, I presume not to decide) that reigns in this particular instance, reigns throughout the whole of the Report. So that the inference, drawn of old from the artful conduct of a single individual to the craftiness of a whole race, may be applied to the arguments of the Committee,

> "'Crimine ab uno,
> Disce omnes ————'

" Let us now follow the Committee to other particulars :—

"They proceed to assert, that most of the cases they examined were misstated, or unfounded.

"If they allude to the cases mentioned by Mr. Rogers in his Pamphlet entitled, ' Examination of the Evidence before the House of Commons,' I pledge my word as a man, and my character as a professional person, to prove them all. Nay, further, I pledge myself if more cases are necessary, to produce many, alas! too many more, of Variolous Infection caught after regular Vaccination. But of the abundant number of cases laid before the Public, the majority cannot be either misstated, or unfounded ; and if so, the cause of the Committee falls at once to the ground. For granting (what never can be granted) that only one-third of the cases adduced were substantiated, there would remain above one hundred and fifty instances of acknowledged failure : and surely these would be sufficient to convince any dispassionate person, that Vaccination is not, and cannot be, a preservative against the Small Pox. What shall we say then, when, in addition to this, it is proved, that several patients have died of the immediate consequences resulting from the puncture of Vaccination ; while on the other hand it never was, or could be with any truth, asserted that similar fatal consequences had in a single instance resulted from the puncture of Small Pox Inoculation ? The inoculated patient, if he dies (which is not one in three hundred in the general irregular mode of proceeding, and not one in a thousand among observant practitioners), dies of Small Pox, and of nothing but Small Pox ; the appearance of the punctured arm is uniformly the same ; and the treatment of it is one of those judicious points in surgery, peculiar to Baron Dimsdale's method of cure.

" The Committee, to exonerate the Society from the censures of repeated failures, state ; that many persons not acquainted with the Disease, have undertaken to vaccinate, and that much of the consequent ill success has resulted from this circumstance. But they forget that the principal evidence they themselves adduced to support their cause before the House of Commons was that of a Clergyman ; they forget too, that several of the Fanatical Preachers among the Sectaries, have been ever since the most zealous and approved champions of their system, both in their preachings, and practice; together with some Ladies, who have received their instructions from Dr. Jenner himself. So that the same set of people who are disowned, when it is convenient to disown them, are brought forward as good evidence, when it suits the cause. Is not this another instance of that *mala fides*, which throws a just suspicion over the cause altogether?

"But laying aside these equivocal practitioners, among the ignorant, the Committee, I presume, do not mean to class Mr. Wachsell, Apothecary to the Small Pox Hospital; or Mr. Ring, the Accoucheur; and yet from the patients vaccinated by these two persons, I would bring instances, if the House of Commons were again to demand it of me, of more failures, more deaths, and more diseases than have occurred in the practice of any other two persons who have come within my knowledge.

"It is further asserted by the Committee, that when the Small Pox occurs after Vaccination, it is more mild than usual, and loses some of its characteristic marks; but in many cases in which it recurs after Inoculation, or the natural disease, it is particularly severe, sometimes fatal.

"This article appears to me extremely objectionable and disingenuous. For, not to mention the improper use of the words, *many cases* of the recurrence of the Small Pox; the Committee here argue from an assumption of their own, which as fair and honest reasoners, as men having no other object than the investigation of truth, they never ought to have done. Their assertion is, that though Small Pox does sometimes recur after Vaccination, this circumstance is not to create any alarm; for when it does return, it is so mild that even its existence is doubtful; whereas in *many cases* in which it recurs after Inoculation, it is particularly severe and often fatal. Thus arbitrarily to assume the fact, that Small Pox does occur after Inoculation, a fact denied by the Advocates of Vaccination themselves, and then to build on it an argument in favour of their system, is in my mind a mode of proceeding bordering on criminality. For if the Committee were addressing their Reports to Medical Men only, no great mischief would ensue, since the fallacy would be immediately detected, and any argument built upon it would of course fall to the ground.

But as the Committee are addressing their Report to Parents, who, being ignorant of the history of Diseases, are compelled to rely implicitly on those who profess to tell them the truth, they ought to have remembered it was a solemn duty in their statement of the case, to have 'turned neither to the right hand, nor to the left.' They ought to have told their readers, that the recurrence of Small Pox after Inoculation was a fact, supported by such slender evidence, so contrary to the laws of nature, and so generally discredited, that when it does occur, as is supposed, a second time, this is considered as a proof that the disorder which the patient had in the first instance, was not the Small Pox. That the Committee therefore omitting all this should boldly beg the question, and argue from that as proved, which is one of the points in dispute, is such an instance of unfair reasoning as perhaps it would be difficult to parallel.

"The assertion of the Committee in the XXth article, that the [1] Diseases which are said to originate from Cow Pox are scrophulous, and cutaneous, and similar to those which arise from Inoculation, is according to my observation quite incorrect. Many of the eruptions are perfectly novel. As far as my experience and my information go, I will venture to affirm they are eruptions of a nature unknown before the introduction of Vaccination ; and peculiar to those who have been Vaccinated. Such was the case of the child in Jermyn Street : such was that of a child near Guildford, vaccinated by Dr. Elliot ; and of many more whose names, from respect to the parents, I forbear to mention.

"As for Latchfield's child, that case differed as much in every essential characteristic from Scrophula as possible. The first appearance, the increase, the colour of the suppurating part, and the indelible dark Eschar, all marked a new, and undescribed disease. Scrophula is a useful name on various occasions. But

---

[1] "The words of the Committee are—" Complaints represented as the effects of Vaccine Inoculation, when in fact they originated from other causes." This is another instance of the bold manner in which the Committee assert, to get rid of difficulties. What proof is advanced that the complaints did originate in other causes ? None but the *ipse dixit* of the writer.

its symptoms are well known and defined; they cannot long be
confounded with those of any other disease: and when a little
experience shall have made the distinction clear, then, if I mistake
not, many a babe whose parents transmitted to it the fibres of
health, and vigour, shall lament the dire effects of unsatisfactory
experiment; while those who may escape the ravages of any new
disorder, will still tremble lest that dreaded evil, the natural
Small Pox, which they sought to avoid, should in a luckless hour
overtake them.

"It is not my intention to pursue further the Report of the
Jennerian Committee. I have answered whatever applies materially to my argument: to expose all the errors and fallacies it
contains, would be a painful task: I should however be unjust
to the Public and myself, did I not state, that besides those I
have already noticed, there are in it assertions so unfounded,
and expressions so ambiguous, that these alone would have
deterred me from subscribing it.

"Thus in Article XVI. it is said, that by means of Vaccination, the Small Pox has in some populous Cities been wholly
exterminated.

"In Article XVIII. that the prejudice raised against Vaccination
has been, in great measure, the cause of the death of near 2,000
persons this present year, in London alone.

"In Article III. that the cases published to prove the failure
of Vaccination, have been for the most part fully refuted; and

"In Article IV. those Medical Men who dissent from the
Jennerian Committee, are stated *generally*, as acting perversely
and disingenuously; persisting in bringing forward unfounded,
and refuted reports; and even misrepresentations, after they have
been proved to be such.

"Of these Articles I am compelled to say, and am ready to
prove, that the three first are absolutely unfounded. Of the last
I must declare, that it seems to me conceived in a spirit of
illiberality and ungenerous censure, such as I should have
imagined a Committee formed of Gentlemen never would have
used; and which certainly no circumstances can justify.

"I presume not to judge the motives of action in others; I
know my own, and I am conscious of my sincerity. If I could

be actuated by party spirit, I should be unworthy the confidence of the Public. I seek for Truth, and Truth alone. With indignation, therefore, do I reject the charge of acting perversely, and disingenuously. When I am convinced of error, I shall take a pride in acknowledging my mistake; 'till then I shall consider it my duty to declare my opinion openly, and to state the reasons why I have from the first asserted, and why I still continue to assert, that I fear the experiment of Vaccination will be found injurious to the peace, the health, and the welfare of society.[1]

"But since motives of action are called in question, let me mention a few of the circumstances that have contributed to influence my conduct : they will be found to bear more upon the argument than may at first be imagined. I will afterwards proceed to offer a few strictures on Mr. J. Moore's pamphlet.

" The paper which I published in the *Gentleman's Magazine,* and which I shall here reprint, shews the ground I had to stand upon, in opposing the experiment at its very commencement. I have never changed my opinion ; I have uniformly maintained that it was a dangerous practice to introduce a new source of disease into the human frame.

" If I have been firm in my sentiments, it is because I have met with nothing in the sequel that has shaken my judgement.

---

[1] " Though I admit with the Committee, the impropriety of discussing subjects of serious investigation in any other than a serious style, I must object to the manner in which they have worded their Vth Article. Having said, some "printed accounts, adverse to Vaccination, have treated the subject with indecent and disgusting levity" (expressions I think much too strong, and coarse) they add, "as if the good or evil of society, were fit objects for sarcasm, and ridicule.' This seems to me an invidious, and an unfair manner of stating the question. The *good* and *evil* of society never were the objects of ridicule. But a system being advanced, which it was apprehended would ultimately prove an evil, not a good, it was thought proper to attack that system : and while * some chose the sober method of argument,† others preferred that of ridicule : still, however, it was the *system,* not the good or evil, that was ridiculed : and that system was ridiculed only so far as it was judged likely to injure, rather than benefit, society.

---

* Mr. Rogers, and Mr. Lipscombe.
† Dr. Moseley, *Lues Bovilla.*

" It is true the opinion of some of my colleagues was in direct opposition to mine. I, therefore, felt it incumbent on me, carefully and dispassionately to observe the result of the experiment. I did so : I read what was published ; and I found from time to time such contradiction in the Reports of the advocates for Vaccination ; such fluctuation in their opinion ; such inconsistency in their practice ; that the most favourable conclusion I could draw was, they knew not what they were doing. Surely this did not authorize me to alter my original position.

" To obviate the objections naturally raised from this extreme uncertainty, and which evidently affected the soundness of the principle on which the system rested, Vaccination was divided into Spurious and Genuine. I foresaw the consequences. I was satisfied that the Jennerian Society, having once embarked in the cause, would have recourse to any expedient, rather than abandon it : and finding I stood nearly single, and that the tide of Opinion set strong against me, I patiently submitted to have my judgement called in question for a season, resolving to wait a proper period to explain my reasons of dissent.

" The Cases of Mr. Hodge's Children occurred, confirming the truth of Mr. Goldson's Reports. I then thought it my duty to print my opinions in support of what that Gentleman had advanced. What I then wrote, and all I have written since, has been couched in the language of Seriousness, and. Candour, not of levity or prejudice. Never shall I be ashamed that I was the first to express a doubt whether Inoculation, so perfectly understood, and so successfully managed as it was, ought to be abandoned for a mere Experiment ; holding the change too serious a matter, to be trifled with : neither shall I ever be ashamed to say, that I viewed with indignant scorn the ungenerous artifice adopted by the Jennerian Society, of sticking up in every Station-house, in the Vestries of fanatical Chapels, and in Sunday Schools, that false, *Comparative View of the Effects on Individuals, and Society, by the Small Pox, and the Cow Pox,* ornamented with tablets like a School-boy's writing-piece, representing to the gaping multitude a frightful picture of Inoculation, with the supposed misery attendant on it ; and exhibiting representations equally false, and exaggerated, of the blessings of Vaccination. When I saw this, and afterwards understood that these disgraceful Pictures were intended for the use of our distant Colonies, where the Truth would long be concealed, and Argument be totally lost, I was compelled to suspect, still more and more, not only the goodness of the cause itself, but the Candour of those who stooped to such means in its support.

"Soon after this, I heard with great surprise that an application had been made to the late Archbishop of Canterbury, persuading his Grace to direct the Clergy of the Church of England to recommend Vaccination from their pulpits.

" I received a letter from the Palace at Lambeth, desiring to know if I had changed the opinion I had originally advanced; and a respectable Clergyman waited on me from his Grace, to talk with me on the subject. Without entering into any argument, I contented myself with relating to him all I knew : shewed him my correspondence with other medical men on the subject, and left him to judge for himself. He retired from me, saying, ' *His Grace must not commit the Church.*'—This transaction is perfectly well known, I believe, to all the Partisans of Vaccination. Why it has never been hinted at by any of the writers in favour of the Cause, and why it has been concealed, is a secret best known to themselves, and the Jennerian Committee.

"These circumstances occasioned an increased degree of distrust in my mind ; and called more loudly for care and circumspection ; especially when I recollected the Anniversary dinner of Mr. Guy's hospital in 1802, where I expected to meet the Professors, the Medical Gentlemen, and the Students, on the same terms as usual. What was my surprise then to find, that the sole business of the meeting was to begin a canvass for names to a petition to Parliament, in support of Dr. Jenner's bill ? it was presented to me, and I refused to sign it.

" My surprise was increased after the dinner, to find that toasts, songs, and compliments from one Professor to another in honour of Vaccina, were the *order of the day.*

" As I had seen, among the various business of life, some political manœuvres, and the management of some party schemes, I was not at a loss to conjecture in what manner the cause of Vaccination would be carried on.

" The Royal Patronage, the authority of Parliament, would be made use of, beyond what the sanction given warranted : the command of the Army and Navy would be adduced, not merely as the mean of facilitating the experiment, but as proof of the triumph of the cause : and above all, the monopoly of the press, and the freedom of the Post Office would be employed to circulate the assertions of the friends of Vaccination, and to suppress the arguments of their opponents.

" What I foresaw happened : and such was the influence of the Jennerian Society, that many publishers and booksellers refused to print, or sell such works as might be deemed adverse to Vaccine Inoculation : in consequence of which it was hardly possible, at the first moment, to contradict any thing the Society chose to assert. It was in vain to argue against the system ; for even the Ladies themselves were prejudiced, were influenced, and employed in its defence. Men midwives found their interests were essentially connected in its success ; and they foresaw that if they could vaccinate at the breast, without danger of conveying infection, they should secure to themselves the nursery, as long as Vaccination lasted : no one could enter to interfere with them ; they would prescribe for the Apothecary, and hold him at a distance ; the Physician and Surgeon would be set aside ; and if any accident occurred that rendered a dissection after death necessary, some anatomist, friendly to the cause, might be called in to quiet the alarms of a family.

" The College of Physicians seem at last to have opened their eyes to the innovations of these practitioners, who, like the Jesuits of old, through the medium of the female branches, aim at managing the whole family.

" They have therefore forbidden them to prescribe in future for children above two years old ; that safe age, before which, unless in peculiar cases, according to Baron Dimsdale, Inoculation ought not to be performed ; and that for self-evident reasons. For if the loss of beauty, or the probability of danger are proportionate to the crop of pustules on the face, who, but one ignorant of Surgery, would advise that bed of roses, the blooming cheeks of an infant, during the eruptive fever of Small Pox, to be applied to the warm breast of a well-fed nurse ? What maturating poultice is more likely to invite the pustules to that part ? Against this practice, every notion of sound sense revolts ; and I will venture to affirm that the majority of children who suffer from Inoculation, are those inoculated at the breast.

"When, therefore, such pains are taken to magnify the numbers that fall victims to Small Pox, why is not this pernicious custom, which every sound practitioner reprobates, taken into the account? and why is it not remembered that in the populous parts of the Metropolis, where the abundance of children exceed the means of providing food and raiment for them, this pestilential disease is considered as a merciful provision on the part of Providence, to lessen the burthen of a poor man's family ?

"Let the College of Physicians, who examine the Apothecaries' shops in the narrow streets, and suburbs of London, report the state of the medicines, the scales and measures, and the annual reproofs they are constrained to make to many, where,

> " '———— among the shelves
> A beggarly account of empty boxes,
> Green earthen pots, bladders, and musty seeds,
> Remnants of packthread, and old cakes of roses
> Are thinly scattered to make up a show,'

and then, we shall in some measure be able to determine, how little can with justice be urged against any particular mode of practice, from the frequency of deaths among the poorer classes of mankind.[1]

"Enough has been said to explain why, from the first, I was led to regard with a certain degree of suspicion, the conduct of the friends of Vaccination ; and why I have uniformly disapproved their proceedings. It remains to make some observations on an

---

[1] "One of the most prevalent causes of death among infants is the loss of their mothers' milk. Women who abandon their own children, to sell their milk to a stranger, will be found too frequently to have destroyed their deserted babes. An Hospital under the Queen's patronage, was settled at Bay's-Water, to receive the children thus deserted, but it subsisted a very short period, for all the children died. The Foundling Hospital, the Enfant trouvé at Paris, and the registers of large parishes, will elucidate this fact ; but it is never mentioned in the Bills of Mortality.

ingenious pamphlet written by Mr. J. Moore, hitherto the best defender of the Jennerian cause. What Dr. Thornton will produce, who has announced himself employed by the Committee, to answer the wit of Dr. Moseley, and the sober arguments of Mr. Lipscombe, the event will prove. I doubt not but that Dr. Moseley will be able to answer all that Dr. Thornton shall advance.

" With respect to Mr. J. Moore, he certainly deserves some praise for the pleasant manner in which he has treated the subject, but much more for the candour he has shown. I must do him the justice to point this out, least the Reader, seduced by his pleasantry, should suffer himself to misconstrue the Author's intentions.

" I cannot, however, discover in Mr. J. Moore's pamphlet, any answer to the arguments of Mr. Rogers, or any thing like a reply to the five questions in my printed Letter. A particular reply, indeed, I was not to expect, for he chuses to unite all the writers against Vaccination in one class, as if he wished that a censure applicable to any one of them individually might attach to them all generally. As I do not approve this method, which is unfair and sophistical, I shall not follow it, neither will I pay his ingenuity so bad a compliment as to couple him with Mr. Ring, to whom, perhaps, Mr. Squirrel is a more than equal antagonist.

" Mr. Moore, in the beginning of his book, for what reason I cannot discern, pays a studied compliment to the humanity of the Faculty of Medicine at the expence of Surgeons. But he must allow me to say, it is the peculiar boast of Surgery to have softened the malignity, and to have discovered the cure of two of the greatest evils that afflict mortality, in the judicious practice of Inoculation and by the improved treatment of Lues Venerea.

" Surgery has positive grounds to rest upon, which will for ever secure to it the gratitude and the support of mankind ; if it ever should lose any part of its due estimation, this will be owing to the unwarrantable presumption of some who practise it without being properly educated in its principles.

" Every Apothecary's journeyman, lectured for six months to pass an examination for the lower ranks of the Army and Navy, now pretends to be a proficient in this art.

"The fatal consequences that result from uneducated practitioners in every branch of medicine, assuming the province of the Surgeon, and experimenting on Inoculation, is justly depicted in the Report of the Jennerian Society. Mr. Moore makes the same observation, and tells us that the results from this general practice were so different to the accounts of Mr. Jenner and his friends that many experiments were set on foot in order to establish a permanent theory. By these it was ascertained that Dr. Jenner's account of the origin of the disease was unfounded, and untrue. This was a distressing circumstance to befal the great Father of the Experiment, as he was called, who ought certainly to have been, morally speaking, sure of his principle of action, before he ventured to propose it to the Public, or petition Parliament for a reward for his discoveries. It was now asked, what had he discovered? What had he recommended? What were his principles as well in Theory, as Practice? These were awkward questions; to answer them was difficult: therefore, to avoid the perplexing appeals that were daily made to him, and the messages that were perpetually sent requesting him to visit untoward cases, the Doctor retired from London. Had matters gone on smoothly, the Doctor would have found it his interest to have remained in the Metropolis.

" The horrible description which Mr. Moore paints of the Confluent Small Pox, and of the Lues Venerea, may be just: but as they happily are not often seen, if ever, where proper treatment can be procured, and will be followed, they stand as extreme cases, on which the rhetorician may declaim, indeed, but from which the sound reasoner can draw no conclusive argument. I see not, therefore, what Mr. Moore gains to his cause by the description. I must however, thank him for it, as he thus affords me an opportunity of saying, that it is the pride of Surgery, to have reduced the mortality consequent on the first of these disorders, to one in a thousand ; and that attendant on the last, to nearly the same proportion.

" The Natural Small Pox might almost always be avoided, if Inoculation were duly performed : and instances of persons dying of Lues Venerea, except in ill-conducted Workhouses, are almost unknown to regular Surgeons.

"Mr. Moore asserts, that Vaccination was opposed before any facts could be alleged against it. But in so early a stage of the business as when before the Committee of the House of Commons, I brought *three* cases, and named *four* others, of Small Pox following Vaccination. Was this opposing without facts? Nay, it was these very cases that taught Dr. Woodville, what he had mistaken for an Hybrid Eruption, was real Small Pox; and which made Mr. Cline acknowledge, that Vaccination would not prevent Small Pox, where the patient had breathed variolous atmosphere.

"Our Author goes on to relate the rapidity with which Vaccination was spread through every part of the world. That the progress of Vaccination was rapid, beyond almost belief, I readily admit: that this circumstance is a proof of the merits of the System I deny. We live in a capricious age; an age that is fond of believing paradoxes, and of grasping at novelty. And this alone might account for the wonderful avidity with which the experiment was adopted. But there were other causes that co-operated, and I have already specified them. So long as the liberty of the Post Office was allowed, and the Press was in possession of the Society, had their scheme been more objectionable than it is, it would with facility have been at home propagated; and as for the Continent, English faith stood so firm there about that period, that any thing from England was received as sterling. Yet I had accounts even from the Continent, very different to Mr. Moore's representation; accounts which lamented the too easy faith of some Hanoverian parents, whose children were the victims of this new experiment.

"Mr. Moore's candour begins to shew itself about the ninth page, where he admits this Cow Pox to be erroneously attributed to that gentle Animal. 'No Cow that is allowed to suckle her own Calf, untouched by the Milker, ever had this complaint.' He concludes therefore, that the Vaccine Disease is some pollution, imposed upon the harmless Animal by contact of the Milker. This I can readily believe to be the case. We do not understand indeed by what law of Nature the corrupt humour of an human disease acting on the teats of an harmless animal, can generate a new disorder; but it seems to be the only rational way of accounting for the phænomenon; and nothing remains for us but to inquire what that disease is, which being communicated from the Milker, produces the Vaccine Matter.—Is it the Itch? the Lues Venerea? or the Small Pox itself?—It evidently must be something common among the lower orders, for with them it originates: I could almost be tempted to think it was often the Itch.

"A man applied to me at St. Thomas's Hospital to examine his hand and arm, which were full of ulcerations. He said he belonged to a milk house near the end of Kent-street; that several of the milkers were in the same condition with himself; and that most of the cows' teats, belonging to the house, were affected in a similar manner; he added, he had been told it was Cow Pox.

"As I had not been accustomed to see the natural Cow Pox, I asked one of my Pupils from the country what he thought of the case. He replied, that the patient exhibited every symptom of having the itch, in that stage, which is commonly called the Rank Itch. On farther examination, the appearance about the fingers confirmed his observation; I directed the man to use Jackson's Itch Ointment, and he appeared again at the end of a week, quite cured.

"From this accidental circumstance, and from the tormenting itching which some children, when vaccinated, are afflicted with, it will be worth while for the Committee to inquire whether the itch may not be one of the diseases that form the base of the Vaccine Matter.—At all events, since the Cow is proved innocent, and the Milker alone guilty, it will be proper to ascertain what the complaints are, to which the Milkers in Glostershire, and in Holstein are liable.

"Dr. Jenner's theory of the grease of the horse is now given up, even by his best friends: but surely, it is time either for himself or them to find us some just criterion, that may enable us to distinguish the genuine source from which it originates. Why however are we forbidden to inoculate from the Cow herself? Does her simple food increase the virulence of that disease with which the foul milker contaminates her teats? or again, must the disease be meliorated by passing through some human victim, who is perhaps to be sacrificed in consequence, before it can be fit for general use?

What the Small Pox is, we know; and we know also, that

when given properly by Inoculation it will communicate a mild
disease to the human frame.   I say we are fully acquainted with
the benefits and the management of that meliorated contagion ; a
management so simple, that we have little to apprehend even from
the unskilfulness of ignorant Practitioners ; and a benefit so
unalloyed, that the experience of now near a century, has proved,
that the use of it does not contribute to swell the catalogue of
human woes by new disorders.   I see not therefore what wisdom
there is in wishing to drop Small Pox Inoculation altogether (for
that is the clamorous demand of the Jennerian Society), and
inoculate from a disease, the nature of which we know not : a
disease so varying, and so ambiguous in its appearance and effects,
that even the most skilful Vaccinator, even Dr. Jenner himself,
who has proudly suffered himself to be called, ' The man destined
to expel contagion,'[1] cannot be certain when it is communicated,
and when not ; when it is genuine, when spurious ; a disease that
has already given suffering mortality a new malady, which,
whether it shall be called the Cow Evil, from the animal, or the
Jennerian Evil from the inventor, posterity will determine.

"But why do I say the inventor ?   I beg pardon of this ' expeller
of contagion,' if I state, that the Cow Pox has been known for
generations.   If it has not been brought forward before, the
reason is, that the Physicians of former days, less confident, and
less empirick than some of the present, thought it unbecoming
their character, and what they owed Society, to obtrude any
experiment, which they were not fully satisfied was a salutary

---

[1] " When Dr. Jenner's Bust was exposed at the Exhibition last year, it
was subscribed, if I mistake not, with the following lines of the Œdipus
Tyrannus of Sophocles.

The Man—

    By great Apollo's high command ordain'd
    T'expel the foul contagion from this land :
    Nursed there too long, but to be nursed no more.

Dr. J. was, I understand, wonderfully pleased with the application ; which
certainly was very ingenious, and only wanted truth to be really admirable.   If a second Bust were to appear, I apprehend a more appropriate,
though less splendid motto would be

    Davus sum, non Œdipus.

one. They therefore tried it in silence; they found, notwithstanding an apparent success at first, that it failed ultimately, and they dropped it. I shall instance no other name than that of Sir George Baker, who had Dr. Jenner's *invention* mentioned to him forty years ago; it was tried, it failed, and no more was said of it. Mr. John Hunter did not give the Experiment much credit. The event justifies their conduct: for surely it does not do much honour to the cause, much less does it accord with the positive assurances given Parliament, for Dr. Jenner to lay down a Theory, to be obliged to recant it, and to leave the Public nothing satisfactory in its place: it does us nationally no great honour to have the Cow Pox make so much noise all over the world, and then to be declared no Cow Pox: neither does it argue much in favour of the wisdom of the Faculty, to adopt so blindly a practice, which the first Leaders seem to know nothing about after seven years experience, except, that it fully contradicts the evidence they produced in the House of Commons in its favour.

" It is allowed by all the writers among the Vaccinists, that from the Cow is to be got a genuine and a spurious matter. I cannot understand this doctrine; it seems contrary to the general Laws of Nature; she has given us a genuine but no spurious Small Pox; a genuine but no spurious Measles. More merciful in her operations, than Vaccinators; she gives us a specific evil, that we may know how to administer specific remedies; and when we may be securely freed from the dread of its recurrence.

" But since a genuine and a spurious Cow Pox is admitted by Vaccinists, how do they account for it? 'Till wiser heads than mine have determined this point, I will suggest the following conjecture :—

" It is allowed on all hands, that Cow Pox is generated by some disorder imparted by the milker. Now if that disorder should happen to be the Small Pox, then the Pustule so occasioned, and the matter coming from it, may inoculate Small Pox, and the patient thus inoculated, may be for ever secure from that disease, for in fact he will have received Small Pox Inoculation. But if the disorder generated on the Cow's teats, have for its base, Itch, as I apprehend has sometimes happened, then the patient will be inoculated with a disorder, which, though it may suspend the capacity for Small Pox for a season in the constitution, will ultimately prove no security.

"Notwithstanding Mr. Moore's pleasant way of treating the subject, he cannot laugh away this simple argument.

"If there is no such disease belonging to the Animal as Cow Pox, if she must be subject to infections from the hand of him to whom she spares her milk, and sacrifices her calf, let us be acquainted with the nature of these infections, and do not let us so inhumanly submit our babes, while smiling in the mother's face, to, *we know not what!*

"In the Smal Pox, and other infectious disorders, I repeat, we know of nothing spurious ; the matter inoculated from a patient who may die afterwards of the Confluent Small Pox, will produce nothing but a mild disease ; nothing but Small Pox.

"When the Societies quarrelled, and parted, they were almost upon the point of declaring, that one was the genuine, the other the spurious, Society for exterminating the Small Pox. This would have been a death blow to the whole system. The friends of both parties saw this ; an accommodation was effected : like the contending heroes on the stage, they said, *"Brother, Brother, we are both in the wrong;"* they shook hands, and agreed at all events to support the Experiment.

"I shall not take notice of that part of our Author's pamphlet which attacks the Physicians; not only because I conceive it beside my immediate subject, but because I consider 'The Commentaries on the Cow Pox,' lately published by Dr. Moseley, to contain a full answer to all that Mr. Moore has asserted on this head.

"Those pages which are employed in describing the nature of Small Pox, and other infectious diseases, are well worth attending to; though they are written with such affectation of wit, that if hastily perused, they may be mistaken.

"However, I admire Mr. Moore's candour, as I collect from these pages, that he is of opinion the *Small Pox cannot be twice received;* and observe, that he admits some cases to have occurred, where the Small Pox has appeared on persons who had apparently passed through the Cow Pox, in a regular way. He then concludes, 'A true Philosopher knows there is no real exception to the Laws of

Nature; apparent deviations are common, but the Laws of Nature are immutable.' And again he observes, 'If Medical men were as ready to own their errors as Chemists, they would not so often accuse Nature of being so capricious as they do.

"'To admit that a few individuals organised like others, are susceptible of having certain diseases twice, while the flood of mankind can only have them once, is almost a contradiction in the uniformity of the Laws of Cause and Effect.'

"These are sentiments so just in themselves, and conceived in such a spirit of candour and liberality, that although Mr. Moore discovers sometimes a little flippancy of wit he had better have spared, and although he sometimes deals too much in authoritative assertion which does not sit well on him, I nevertheless sincerely wish he had been employed earlier in the controversy: the question then probably would have been more easily decided.

"I lament, however, that he will not suffer his own principles to produce with himself that conviction I apprehend they ought.

"If a true philosopher knows there are no real exceptions to the Laws of Nature, then a patient *cannot have the Small Pox twice.* But Mr. Moore admits that patients have had the real Small Pox after Vaccination; the disease therefore which the Vaccine matter excited, could not have been Small Pox; and consequently, those patients (except in the cases suggested in page 45) remain liable to it, as soon as the suspending power of the Vaccine disease shall have ceased.

"This argument is so simple a one, and the conclusion in my mind so just, that I feel confident its force must be felt by every impartial person.

"What Mr. Moore says of the primary and secondary Small Pox, in which all sound Practitioners will readily concur with him, proves everything I could wish in favour of my argument.

"Whoever has read the Report of the Committee of the House of Commons, would conclude from the multitude of evidence there adduced, that the practice of Vaccination was at that time perfectly settled and understood. But Mr. Moore informs us, 'All the peculiarities of this curious complaint were not *detected* at once. In the first two or three years it was not to be expected that the Art of Vaccination should be brought to perfection. It is therefore not to be wondered at, if among the multitude of Surgeons, Apothecaries, *Clergymen*, and *Ladies*, who practised, a few mistakes have happened.'

"That no experiment is perfected at once, even where the principles are just, I readily allow : it is no more than what must be expected from the imperfection of human wisdom. What I complain of, is, that while Vaccination was nothing more than an experiment it should have been, not merely recommended to the public notice, but authoritatively imposed on the public practice. If it should be argued that Inoculation was urged with nearly as much earnestness ; I shall reply that the cases are altogether different. Inoculation when brought into England was no longer a mere experiment : it was a practice confirmed by the experience of generations in foreign countries ; and as the laws of Nature could not be supposed to be different here, and in Turkey, the opposition made to Inoculation might be fairly said to have been the result of ignorance, and prejudice.

"I must be permitted however to observe, in answer to Mr. Moore's statement, that among the *multitude of Surgeons*, hardly any of the Court of Assistants of the College are to be found. That Parliament should have omitted to consult the College of Surgeons, seems to me an oversight hardly to be accounted for. As Parliament could not be supposed to act from any knowledge of their own ; the merits of the case not depending on the science of politics, or legislation, but on that of surgery and medicine, common prudence should have dictated the propriety of consulting the Colleges of these two professions, who might be supposed competent to give them the information they wanted. When the College of Physicians were applied to, they gave a negative answer. Had the College of Surgeons been consulted, they would have discovered a truth, which has not yet been revealed. The only surgeons of that court, whose names appear in the Report of the Jennerian Society, are Mr. Ford and Mr. Home.

"But the apothecaries are men of experience ; how came their *multitudes* to join so readily in the experiment ? ' Why, they came into the new practice, because they early discovered it was the plan of the men-midwives to seclude them, by this manœuvre from the nurseries ; and finding they could not fight them fairly on their own ground, they resolved, by forming an alliance, to share, if possible, the conquest.

" 'The co-operation of the Clergy (I speak of those · of the Established Church, and I speak of them with that reverence due to so learned, and so respectable a body), may be accounted for, from that solicitude to benefit the bodies, as well as the souls of men, which forms part of the ministerial character. I think however that they would have done wiser, to have waited till the experiment was so firmly established that they could not have stood committed by any subsequent failure ; for in proportion to the sacredness of any character, ought to be the scrupulous desire of avoiding what might expose it to censure.

" As for Sectarian preachers, whether in or out of the church, they saw it was an easy way of securing acceptance to their peculiar tenets, by stealing, under the specious appearance of Charity, and Philanthropy, into the bosom of maternal tenderness ; while the tender sex, who from innate benevolence are ever ready to assist in doing good, were flattered, were soothed, and were instructed, ' to insinuate the plot into the boxes.' Dr. Jenner took so much pains to teach some ladies to vaccinate with a light hand, that one of them declared she only brought blood from two in the village ; and that only one family among her patients had shewn any symptom of the Cow Pox disorders.

" Mr. Moore tells us that all the misfortunes have happened about Chelsea, and in London ; and that there has hardly been a suspicion of any failures in opulent families.

" There is something very insidious and unjust in these assertions ; they afford almost the only instance of disingenuous reasoning to be found in Mr. Moore's book. By stating the failures to have occurred round Chelsea, I presume he aims at one of the opposers of Vaccination, whose practice lying much in that part of the country, if it could be shewn that no cases came from other quarters, he would infer that those adduced were the result either of the want of candour, or want of skill in a prejudiced individual : and by asserting that there is hardly any suspicion of failure among the opulent, he would insinuate that those cases instanced from among the poor are not to be credited ;

the poor not having the means of contradicting, what may be asserted of them.

"To the first of these insinuations I reply, by saying, that there are few parts of the kingdom from which I will not pledge myself to bring instances of failure in Vaccination, as notorious as any mentioned in the vicinity of Chelsea, and London.

"To the second I reply, by asserting that it is unfounded. There is a degree of respect due to the superior orders of society which exacts from us, when speaking of them, an increased degree of delicacy. To proclaim that an afflictive malady has befallen an individual in the lower orders of society, can be productive of no great inconvenience; to proclaim the same of persons who perhaps may be connected with some of the first families in the kingdom, would be a serious evil. I think Mr. Moore therefore highly to blame, in using an argument which he must be aware from a sentiment of delicacy could never perhaps be answered as it ought. I trust, however, I am not infringing the rule I wish to observe when I say, that if Dr. Jenner were again to apply to Parliament for support, he would find from many members of both Houses that marked opposition to his pretensions, which would prove a full answer to this assertion of our Author.

"Mr. Moore acknowledges one benefit to have arisen from the opposition made to Vaccination, namely, the improvement of the Practice; and he says, a little more time will dispel the prejudices of the inferior Practitioners, and the vulgar.

"If the lower orders of society have conceived prejudices against Vaccination, it will not be easy to root them out; for not only do they know from sad experience that it does not answer; but they have been so ungenerously deceived and imposed on by the Inoculators at the Small Pox Hospital, and other places, where Cow Pox was inserted when they were told they were to be inoculated with Small Pox, that they do not know where to put their trust. This is such an instance of *bad faith*, as, I hope, will never occur again; every principle of humanity revolts against it. Was it not sufficient to have had recourse to every possible means of perverting the judgment of the poor by every artifice ingenuity could suggest, but, when still unconvinced of the efficacy of Vaccination, they demanded to be inoculated with Small Pox, must they be systematically deceived? and implicitly relying on the honour of the Operator, must they be clandestinely contaminated with the very disease they were anxious to avoid?

> " '—— Speak it in whispers lest a Greek should hear !
> Lives there a man so dead to fame, who dares
> To think such meanness, or the thought declares :
> And comes it ev'n from him, whose Sov'reign sway
> The banded Legions of all Greece obey ? '

" Mr. Wachsel I have understood is not to be blamed for this imposition on their good faith ; he is but a servant of the charity, and must follow orders. Where do these orders originate? Who is to blame? Let us know where to fix the stigma.[1]

" It has been asserted, that more children have died within the last twelve months of Small Pox, than in any former year : and from this circumstance, an argument has been raised to discredit Inoculation : but in my mind a conclusion exactly opposite ought to be drawn from it.

" If the fatality of Small Pox has been greater during the last year, than for several years preceding, this is owing to the suspension of Inoculation, having left more subjects open to its infection. For many with whom the suspending power of Vaccination had subsided, fell unsuspecting victims to the Natural Disease : and many others perished by it, who had been left open to its attack, because their parents justly objected to the unfair proceedings of those Practitioners who substituted Cow Pox for Small Pox ; and having thus lost all confidence in the integrity of the Faculty, and not knowing whom to trust, they suffered the natural disease to take its fatal course.

" Let us put things upon the old footing ; let us drop Vaccination altogether for seven years, and practise only Small

---

[1] " Small Pox Hospitals, *if properly conducted*, appear to me such useful charities in a great Metropolis, that I could wish to see them maintained even at the public expence ; since from such Institutions, every Parish might be supplied, at stated periods, with proper Medical men, who should inoculate the poor gratis. By this means, and by compelling the parents to abstain from public exposure, the evils of Natural Small Pox would in a short time be easily subdued.

Pox Inoculation, and if the mortality in Small Pox do not return to its old standard, I will be content to give up my opinion, and become as devout a worshipper of the Cow, as any idolater within the realms of Hindostan, or the precincts of Salisbury Court.

"That there always has been a mortality attendant on Small Pox, even when Inoculation alone was adopted, no one can deny. I deny however, that this mortality ever has been as great as Mr. Moore asserts, or as the friends of Vaccination, eager to establish their own system by discrediting the other, have wished to make the Public to believe. But what makes more to the argument is, that it will be easy to point out the flagrant error to which the mortality may be referred: namely, the public exposure of patients during the eruptive state of the disorder. A common error, which has been made use of to raise a prejudice against Inoculation, but which, so far from forming a necessary part of the treatment, has been expressly forbidden by that able and successful Practitioner, Baron Dimsdale. I cannot help therefore humbly suggesting, that the Legislature would do well thus far to interfere, and by prohibiting under penalty such improper exposure, remedy an evil, which otherwise society must continue to suffer from the ignorance, or perversity of unskilful Practitioners.

"The last objection I shall notice is one on which it seems to have been the aim of Vaccinators to lay great stress, viz. that what is called the King's Evil, generally takes its rise from Inoculation: this is particularly depicted in some of the engravings of that disgraceful production I have mentioned in a former page, 'The View of the Comparative Effects of Inoculation, and Vaccination.'

"I shall answer this assertion, not by entering into any discussion on the nature of Scrophula in general; to do this satisfactorily I should be obliged to swell my pamphlet beyond the size calculated for general circulation; but by simply adducing matters of fact: a mode of arguing to plain and unsophisticated minds always the most agreeable, and certainly the most conclusive.

"I must therefore remind Mr. Moore, and the partisans of

Vaccination, that Scrophula was far more prevalent before, than after the introduction of Inoculation.

"Who now ever hears of crowds of people flocking from the most distant counties to be cured by the supposed virtue of the Royal Touch? Who now sees those pieces of gold, which in the reign of King James the First, and long after, were suspended so generally as amulets, endued with sovereign power to cure the Evil?

"But this I shall be told is only a presumptive argument. I grant it : a more positive one is, that I could adduce several large families of children, where this glandular complaint has for generations been acknowledged to be hereditary, who, having been all regularly Inoculated by able practitioners, have grown up to full maturity without suffering from Scrophula, or so much as ever exhibiting symptoms of this disorder.

"I have now noticed all that Mr. Moore has brought forward in any shape relevant to the question ; and the result is, that I am still more than ever convinced of the propriety of adhering to those opinions, I from the first entertained, of the inefficacy of Vaccination.

"I am willing to pay this Author the compliment, that if the cause could have been defended satisfactorily, it would have been so defended by him,

> "'Si Pergama dextra
> Defendi possent, etiam hâc defensa fuissent,'

but, my conviction is, that the system does not rest on any solid foundation ; that it never can stand. For let us candidly and impartially sum up all that has been established, after the experience of now above seven years ; let us compare the result, with the promised advantages, and let us come fairly to our conclusion.

"When the Committee of the House of Commons recommended Dr. Jenner to the munificence of Parliament, it was for a discovery in practice which was never to prove fatal ; which was to excite no new humours, or disorders in the constitution ; and which was to be, not only a perfect security against the Small Pox, but would, if universally adopted, prevent its recurrence for ever.

"Here then are three distinct points on which Dr. Jenner stands pledged to give the public the fullest satisfaction; otherwise, not only will he fail in his part of the contract, but the experiment itself will fail of having any claim to public notice or support.

"Let us see what Dr. Jenner has done to establish the justness of his several positions in favour of Cow Pox.

"And first he was called upon, as might naturally be expected, to give an account of the origin of the disease itself.

"This could not be considered as a difficult task; for surely Dr. Jenner would not propose to inoculate from a disorder without knowing what that disorder was. He therefore assured the world, that it originated from the grease of the horse's heel, communicated by the hands of the milker to the teats of the cow.

"This theory, which in itself was suspicious, by subsequent experiments was proved to be erroneous: however from that hour to the present, Dr. Jenner has been able to advance nothing satisfactory, and he has left us at this very moment in the dark as to the real nature and origin of the Vaccine Disease.

"But though Dr. Jenner could not tell us what the Cow Pox was, he soon came forward to inform us that it was of two sorts, the one genuine, and harmless, the other spurious, and hurtful.

"This was a discovery so much the more alarming as at the same time no criterion but the effect was given, by which the two sorts could be distinguished. Here then was a direct failure, on the part of Dr. Jenner in his agreement, if I may so call it, with the Houses of Parliament.

"But yet further. In cases where Vaccination did not produce fatal consequences, it gave rise to new, and painful disorders. It was followed sometimes by itchy eruptions; sometimes by singular ulcerations, and sometimes by glandular swellings of a nature wholly distinct from Scrophula, or any other known glandular disease. Here, again, was a failure in the second point stipulated: and finally,

"It was ascertained that even when Vaccination was performed, from what was called the genuine matter, it would not always prove a preservative against the Small Pox: as several patients, who had been pronounced by the most experienced Vaccinators to have passed regularly through the Cow Pox, were nevertheless attacked with the genuine Small Pox.

"These points being established, and they are established by the most uncontested facts, facts which the public are not called upon to believe on the assertions of those who oppose Vaccination, but on the confession of those who support it, how can Dr. Jenner be said to have fulfilled what he stood pledged to Parliament to execute? and not fulfilling his agreement, how can his system claim reasonably any longer its support.

"Were an architect to undertake to build an edifice which he engaged should be firm, and unshaken in its foundations; all its rooms wind and water tight; and such as might be inhabited with perfect security: if before the edifice were well finished the foundations were discovered to be rotten; and if in less than seven years, several apartments had fallen in and killed those who occupied them, while in a great number of rooms, the wind or rain was perpetually beating in, could I be blamed for declaring that the architect had broken his contract, and that the edifice ought to be no longer tenanted? should I deserve the opprobrium of acting perversely, and disingenuously, if I advised my friends not to quit their own houses, where they had lived securely for generations, to occupy apartments where they could never be free from danger? Certainly not. Every body would say, that in giving this advice I was acting the part of a real friend! Why then am I to be told I am acting *disingenuously*, or *perversely*, when I remonstrate against the general practice of the Cow Pox? for, such an edifice as I have described above, so rotten in its foundation, so ill-built, so ruinous, is Vaccination.

"Has the conduct of the friends of Vaccination in supporting and recommending their system been such as to impress me with a favourable opinion of the system? No! Their conduct has been marked with so much art, and trick, and contrivance, nay, so much deceit has been resorted to, that this circumstance alone would make me suspect the goodness of the cause altogether, and the motives that influence its partisans.

"Or again, have the writers in favour of Vaccination been able

to produce any thing that has operated conviction ?   Certainly
not.   They have disproved no well attested fact: they have confined themselves for the most part to raillery and contemptuous
sneers at their opponents ; and the Jennerian Society itself, when
it publishes a report, advances such unfounded assertions, and
uses such equivocal language as I think never could have been
employed had the system been a good one.

"Why then, or on what grounds, am I to come into the
opinions of the Jennerian Society ?   Is there any thing in their
conduct that can prepossess me in their favour ? any thing in
their practice to recommend them ?

" But arguments may be fallacious—let us come to facts. Can
any one disprove the three following :

"That Vaccination has been too often fatal :

" That Vaccination has introduced new disorders into the
human system :

"That Vaccination is not a perfect security against the Small Pox.

"These facts I maintain can never be disproved.

" That Vaccination is sometimes fatal may be shewn, not
vaguely by assigning to it the subsequent death of the patient,
as the only probable cause, but from destructive inflammation
which, in some instances, has arisen immediately from the puncture of Cow Pox Inoculation ; a case that never did occur in
Small Pox Inoculation.

" That Vaccination introduces new disorders, is proved from a
new genus of disease, unknown to any former practitioner ; unknown till after the introduction of the Cow Pox : and never to be
found but in those subjects who have had that disorder.

"That Vaccination is not a perfect security against the Small
Pox—*we have the confession of the Jennerian- Committee itself.*

" Let these facts be considered, and then let the concluding
sentence of the report of the Jennerian Committee be read.

" How after all that has been established, and admitted, can it
be said 'that mankind have already derived great and incalculable
benefits from the discovery of Vaccination ?' how can it be maintained there is full cause for believing, that Cow Pox Inoculation
will ultimately succeed in extinguishing the Small Pox ?

" And yet this conclusion is subscribed by a list of many

respectable names. I really could almost be tempted to believe that some of those signatures have been applied further than was intended : and that there are those among the subscribers, who, only wishing to encourage the experiment, have been made to appear to support the system.

" However this may be, one thing is certain : those names convey in reality only the opinion of so many practitioners. Now, the opinion of the wisest men that ever lived, if in opposition to facts, must be erroneous, and consequently of no authority. Besides which on the very score of opinion, something ought to be taken into consideration.

" There are persons in the list whose abilities, whose character, and knowledge I revere ; I might instance Dr. Baillie, and some others ; but there are those among them, whose abilities, whose character, and knowledge I do not revere : whose opinions consequently, have no weight with me, and ought not, I think, to have any with the public.

" These then are the grounds on which I feel myself justified in adhering to the opinion I first declared before the Committee of the House of Commons ; and these are the reasons for which I do not hesitate to pronounce, that I think the high sanction that has been given to the Cow Pox Experiment, as well from the Royal Name, as from the protection of Parliament, ought to be withdrawn : for that sanction is deservedly of such weight, that remote . practitioners do not even give the subject a consideration, but conclude that a system so recommended must be unexceptionable.

" I trust it will not be supposed, from what I have said, that I am presuming to censure either that August Personage, or the Houses of Parliament, for the support they have afforded the cause of Vaccination. What they did arose from that parental solicitude which they feel, and never can cease to feel, for the welfare of individuals, and the happiness of the community : and though I may think the experiment was not sufficiently tried before it was recommended, still they did but exercise that principle, which has been so often exerted for the public good ; and which has procured us blessings, eminently greater than any enjoyed by the other nations of the world.

" That Dr. Jenner should have been remunerated by the munificence of Parliament I conceive to be no more than just ; on this general principle, that he who neglects his own private interests, in order to promote the public benefit, has some claim for public compensation.   That the experiment itself should have been made, I likewise think wise ; because it is only from experiment that we can ascertain what is, or what is not, beneficial to society. But I can neither think it just, nor wise, that when Vaccination has failed in so many points of accomplishing those ends it promised to accomplish : it should still continue to receive that degree of sanction and support, which a completely successful, and unobjectionable, practice, alone, is entitled to enjoy."

In July 1806, Lord Henry Petty again brought the subject of vaccination before the House.

He moved the following address to his Majesty :—

" That the Royal College of Physicians should be requested to inquire into the progress of vaccine inoculation, and to assign the causes of its success having been retarded throughout the United Kingdom, in order that their report might be made to the House of Parliament, and that we may take the most proper means of publishing it to the inhabitants at large."

Lord Henry Petty was of opinion that if the result of such proposed inquiry resulted (as he was strongly disposed to think it would) in a corroboration of the beneficial effects, which other nations were inclined to regard as the result of vaccine inoculation, it would afterwards be for the House to consider whether a sufficient reward had been bestowed on the original discoverer of vaccine inoculation.

The Royal College of Physicians having received their commands, applied themselves to the inquiry, and corresponded with the Colleges of Physicians in Dublin and Edinburgh, the Colleges of Surgeons in London, Edinburgh, and Dublin, and having reported in favour of Dr. Jenner, the question of a further grant was put to the House, and £20,000 was agreed to by a majority of thirteen.

The subject which then occupied Jenner's attention was the prohibition of Small Pox inoculation, for Baron says,

" He knew that vaccination would be comparatively powerless while its virulent and contagious antagonist was permitted to walk abroad uncontrolled."

Jenner had an interview on this subject with the Minister, Mr. Perceval, but his mission was unsuccessful. He communicated the result in a letter to Dr. Lettsom, July 1807.

" You will be sorry to hear the result of my interview with the Minister, Mr. Perceval. I solicited this honour with the sole view of inquiring whether it was the intention of government to give a check to the licentious manner in which Small Pox inoculation is, at this time, conducted in the metropolis. I instanced the mortality it occasioned in language as forcible as I could utter, and showed him clearly that it was the great source from which this pest was disseminated through the country, as well as through the town. But, alas! all I said availed nothing; and the speckled monster is still to have the liberty that the Small Pox Hospital, the delusions of Moseley, and the caprices and prejudices of the misguided poor, can possibly give him. I cannot express to you the chagrin and disappointment I felt at this interview."

The State having been committed to the policy of

supporting vaccination, the Government was now called
upon to found an establishment, in place of the Royal
Jennerian Institution, which had almost collapsed, from
want of funds and from bad management. Vaccination
would then be conducted under the countenance and
support of Government, and employed throughout the
empire.

Jenner drew up a plan, and prepared an estimate of
the expenses. The illness of his son necessitated his
return to Berkeley, but the warrant for instituting a
National Vaccine Establishment was obtained in his
absence, and he was appointed Director. Jenner
nominated his friend, Mr. Moore, as Assistant Director,
and his faithful advocate, Mr. Ring, as Principal Vaccinator and Inspector of Stations. The Board assembled
to appoint the principal officers, and Mr. Ring was set
aside and another candidate selected. At the next
meeting of the Board to appoint subordinate officers,
Jenner sent in the names of seven whom he wished to
be elected, but the appointments were first reduced to
six, and out of six persons nominated by Jenner, four
were rejected.

The board appointed him Director, but they soon
contrived to let him feel that he was a "*Director
directed.*" The danger of a Director with the patronage
of all the appointments was obvious, for the public
would soon have lost confidence in Reports emanating
from a ring of officials bound, by the circumstances of

their appointment, to support the credit of the Institution and of Vaccination.

Jenner, however, considered that he had been very badly treated, and wrote to Mr. Moore:—

"It was stipulated between Mr. Rose, Sir Lucas, and myself, that no person should take any part in the vaccinating department, who was not either nominated by me, or submitted to my approbation, before he was appointed to a station. On my reminding Sir Lucas of this, he replied, 'You, Sir, are to be the whole and sole director. We (meaning the board) are to be considered as nothing: what do *we* know of vaccination?'"

Under these circumstances, Jenner felt himself obliged to withdraw from the establishment, although his friends thought the step was uncalled for. But Jenner was not influenced by their advice, and Mr. Moore was therefore appointed in his place.

Jenner communicated his reasons to Mr. Moore in the following letter:—

FROM DR. JENNER TO JAMES MOORE, ESQ.

"MY DEAR FRIEND,—At the time I informed you of my intention to come to town, believe me I was quite in earnest. But while I was getting things in order, came a piece of information from a Right Hon. Gentleman which determined me to remain in my retirement. It was as follows. *That the Institution was formed for the purpose of a full and satisfactory investigation of the benefits or dangers of the vaccine practice, and that this was the reason why Dr. J. could not be admitted as one of the conductors of it, as the public would not have had the same confidence in their proceedings as if the board were left to their own judgment in doubtful cases.* This is the sum and substance of the communication; —'What do we know of Vaccination? We know nothing of Vaccination.'

"And yet, my friend, these very *we* are to be the sole arbitrators in doubtful cases! Alas, poor Vaccina, how art thou degraded!

"You intimated something of this sort to me some time since, and now I get it from the fountain head. An institution founded on the principle of inquiry seven or eight years ago, would have been worthy of the British nation; but now, after the whole world bears testimony to the safety and efficacy of the vaccine practice, I do think it a most extraordinary proceeding. It is one that must necessarily degrade me, and cannot exalt the framers of it in the eyes of common sense. I shall now stick closely to *my own Institution*, which I have the pride and vanity to think is paramount to all others, as its extent and benefits are boundless. Of this, I am the real and not the nominal director. I have conducted the whole concern for no inconsiderable number of years, single handed, and have spread Vaccination round the globe. This convinces me that simplicity in this, as in all effective machinery, is best.

"I agree with you that my not being a member of the British Vaccine Establishment will astonish the world; and no one in it can be astonished more than myself. An establishment liberally supported by the British Government,—its arrangements harmonious and complete,—every member intimately acquainted not only with the ordinary laws and agencies of the vaccine fluid on the human constitution, but with its extraordinary or anomalous agencies,—all fully satisfied from the general report of the civilized part of the world and their own experience of the safety and efficacy of the vaccine practice,—all cordially uniting in directing that practice to one grand point, the extermination of the Small Pox in the British Empire:—a society so formed, was a consummation devoutly to be wished. But instead of this, taking away yourself and a few others, an assembly, which from well-known facts must appear discordant in the eyes of the public, is packed together. However, incongruous as it is, it would have been still more so, had I mingled with it; and what is above all other considerations, and which would have proved a source of perpetual irritation, I must have gone in with a sting upon my conscience.

"Though resolved on not incorporating myself with the Society, be assured I shall be ever ready to afford it any assistance in my power.

> " Believe me, my dear Friend,
>> " Most truly yours,
>>> " EDWARD JENNER.

" BERKELEY,
  "*April 4th,* 1809."

Jenner had also turned his attention to the prevention of distemper in dogs. Having successfully inoculated dogs with Cow Pox, he concluded that they would be thereby protected from distemper, and several fox-hunters availed themselves of the suggestion, and had their hounds vaccinated. Together with his nephew, George Jenner, he vaccinated about twenty of his Majesty's staghounds. But in this year, 1809, Jenner seems to have abandoned the idea, for he published a paper on distemper in the *Medico-Chirurgical Transactions*, and omitted any reference to the effects of vaccination. Baron, however, believed that the protective influence was established, and relates that a friend of Dr. Jenner's, Mr. Skelton, a sporting gentleman in Yorkshire, made some " very decisive " trials.

" Having selected three couples of healthy pups of six weeks old, I inoculated three of them with the Cow Pox under the left arm, a little above the elbow, which regularly matured. The other three with those inoculated were sent out to quarters. At a proper age they were all brought to the kennel. The former with other hounds were soon attacked with and died of the distemper, whilst the latter remained perfectly healthy, though surrounded by their infected companions, becoming the strongest hounds in the pack, and having certainly the best noses."

Jenner was also much interested in the treatment of hydrophobia. He corresponded with the Rev. Dr. Worthington on this subject :—

" BERKELEY, 4th May, 1810.

" MY DEAR SIR, —I have been favoured, since my last dispatch to Southend, with your neat little essay on Vaccination and your observations on *dipping*. Have you seen an account of some bold Vaccine transactions now going forward among the medical men of the county ? Their resolutions appear in the Gloucester and Cheltenham papers. Your county I hope will soon follow this laudable example. The Small Pox will never be subdued, so long as men can be hired to spread the contagion by inoculation.

"With regard to the other subject you mention, be assured my thoughts have not been idle upon it, having lived man and boy much beyond half a century in a dipping country. Pyrton Passage, four miles only from this place, has been noted for this practice from time immemorial ; and true it is, I never saw or heard of a single case of hydrophobia after dipping in the Severn, or as our friend Westfaling has it, drowning ; for so it is, as you shall hear. I once asked a long-experienced professor what length of time he kept his patients under water ? His reply was, 'As to that I can't tell, but I keep them under till they have' done kicking, when I bring them up to recover their senses, and get a little breath, and then down with them again, and so on to a third time, observing the same rule, not to take them up till their struggle is over.'

" You see then what a shock the vital principle receives from this process. The modus operandi let us not trouble our heads about, if the fact can be established that it deadens the action of the inserted virus. I have wished to see how far it can be supported by analogy, by getting some vaccinated patient dipped within a few days after the insertion of the vaccine lymph. At all events an inquiry so highly important should be taken up, and it cannot be in better hands than yours."

A month later, Dr. Worthington appears to have

encountered a failure, and communicated the information to Jenner. He received a ready-made explanation in reply.

"I told Westfaling, in a conversation on dipping, that there might be bad dippers as well as bad vaccinators, for which there seems at present to be no allowance. Pray do not be deterred from prosecuting your inquiry. He also proposed a trial with snake poison as an antidote, and that failing, he advised Vaccination.

"Yesterday I dined with Professor Davy. I wish you had been with us. His mind is all in a blaze. He seems to be one of those rare productions which nature allows us to see once in a score of centuries. We touched on hydrophobia. He started an ingenious idea, that of counteracting the effects of one morbid poison with another. What think you of a viper? Not its broth, but its fang, as soon as the first symptom of disease appears from *canination.* If this should succeed, we must domiciliate vipers as we have leeches. But from this hint I should be disposed to try, under such an event, Vaccination; as it can almost always be made to act quickly on the system, whether a person has previously felt its influence or not, or that of the Small Pox.

"An answer to one of your questions. I am sure the cuckoo has nothing to do with hatching, as all the adults *are off,* while a great number of their eggs remain unhatched. I should put dogs quite out of the question in the new research, and confine myself totally to the human animal; I mean, with respect to dipping."

During 1809, and for some years afterwards, Jenner corresponded with Mr. Moore, supplying him with details in support of vaccination, for the Reports of the National Vaccine Establishment and for a work on the subject.

To James Moore, Esq.

" Dear Moore,—Depend upon it there are many such cases
as those which have occurred in Mr. Wingfield's family in reserve
for us. Vaccination at its commencement fell into the hands of
many who knew little more about it than its mere outline. One
grand error, which was almost universal at that time, was making
one puncture only, and consequently one vesicle ; and from this
(the only source of security to the constitution) as much fluid
was taken day after day as it would afford : nevertheless, it was
unreasonably expected that no mischief could ensue. I have
taken a world of pains to correct this abuse ; but still, to my
knowledge, it is going on, and particularly among the faculty
in town. Mr. Knight's cases were first made known to me by
Lady Charlotte Wrottesley. This lady was one of my early
pupils, and is an adept at vaccination, as thousands of her poor
neighbours in Staffordshire can testify. She saw at once the
true state of the children in question. I do not presume to say,
that these children are examples of any improper practice ; they
might have been affected with herpetic eruptions at the time of
vaccination, which are so apt, without due attention, to occasion
a deviation from the perfect character of the vaccine vesicle. I
think it must be the paper on this subject you allude to as wishing
to see. I have, therefore, sent it to you ; and a copy of that
paper you saw in manuscript, on secondary variolous contagion.
If you should want any more of the latter, you may draw upon
Gosnell the printer for them. By the way, it might be right to
send one to the National Vaccine Establishment ; determine this
point yourself. Willan, in his Treatise on Vaccination, has spoken
much to the purpose respecting Small Pox after Cow Pox ; you
cannot quote a better author. His word will go further than
mine, as he must be supposed to be less interested. I do not
think enough has yet been said of the Small Pox after supposed
security from Small Pox inoculation. Blair told me, when I left
town, he was collecting these cases with a view to publication.
Thousands might be collected ; for every parish in the kingdom
can give its case. I fear your materials for the year are more
scanty than could be wished for your Report ; but they are in

gccd hands to make the most of. Addington will not be an improper addition to your establishment. He has talents; and will be always ready to assist you with his pen and ink when you are hurried."

" BERKELEY, *February 26th*, 1810.

"I have made a great blunder, it seems, in my reply to your inquiry respecting my opinion of what you call papulary[1] eruptions after Cow Pox. I really thought you alluded to that appearance which I mentioned; but finding myself set right, I have no hesitation in saying, that what Willan has said on this subject is correct.[2] My friend Dr. Parry, of Bath, has made some interesting observations on these modifications or varieties of variola; and I am sure he would readily furnish you with them on an application for that purpose. Creaser, of Bath, could also give you some good facts, with observations on the same subject. By the way, have you his pamphlet respecting P———'s bad conduct? You should have it. I have myself seen but one solitary case of this secondary Small Pox, and that was in a child of Mr. Gosling's vaccinated by a Mr. Armstrong. This went through its course in the usual rapid way.

"You spoke of a print for your intended work. There are several about the town. The best, I think, is from a painting of Northcote's, done some years since for the Medical Society at Plymouth. I believe this is rather scarce; but you are acquainted with Northcote, and I daresay he has one in his possession. When I was last in town, my friends urged me to sit to Lawrence, and I complied. If you approved of it, and he had no objection, that might suit you. He talked of getting a print from the painting for himself. It will never do for me to go to the pencil now; for if my countenance represents my mind, it must be beyond anything dismal.

"I cannot refer to your pamphlet, as it is among my books at Cheltenham. If you have one to spare, pray send it to Harwood's,

---

[1] " Or was it secondary that you called them? I cannot at this moment refer to your letter."

[2] " The College, in their Report, have expressed themselves very well on this subject."

the bookseller, in Russel Street, who will soon send me some books from town.

"Do you not intend mentioning cases of Small Pox after supposed security from Small Pox inoculation? Such cases are innumerable. I think there are thirteen on record among the families of the nobility. Blair, I believe, has collected the greatest number of them. You know my old opinion on the matter; that they occur, for the most part, through the interference of herpetic affections at the time of inoculation. One decisive proof you will find in Willan's vaccine book, given by me. From facts I go to hypothesis; and conceive that the appearance of the Small Pox twice on the same individual arises from the same cause. On this subject I could write a long chapter; but as it would necessarily be theoretical, you would not thank me for it. I must just touch upon it. We see that variolous matter may be generated by inoculation on the arms of one person in that degree of perfection, as to communicate the Small Pox by transferring it to those of another; yet the person, whose constitution shall in the first instance have been exposed to it, shall remain unprotected from future infection, although the system has been deranged during its presence on the skin. Where, then, is the difference, whether the morbid poison was confined, or limited to a point or two, or spread universally in the form of pustules? If the change required to give security could not take place in this one instance, why should it in another, under the same existing circumstances? The *peculiarity of the action* [I do not like to call it *morbid*, because it is generally salutary], is often too strong to be overcome, yet I am ready to conclude that this is not a frequent occurrence. . . .

"What is your Establishment about? I fear little or nothing; but you will soon hear that a spirit of activity has shown itself in this county, which will do more to serve the cause of vaccination than anything which has yet started up. Its advantages will be so self-evident, that it will soon run the kingdom over. You shall know the full particulars as soon as they come out. The great feature of the scheme is this, to place every man in a questionable point of view who presumes to inoculate for the Small Pox, with such a mass of evidence as will be held up to him in favour of vaccination. A general association will be formed of all the medical men, in the county, favourable to the plan; and I really think, to avoid the ignominy of resistance, nearly the whole will come in. Some of the variolo-vaccinists have already abjured their old bad habits and joined the standard before it was half hoisted. . . .

"You don't like my style when I write for the public eye, nor do I; but I cannot mend it, for I write then under the impression of fear; and it must be remembered, that when I write in London my brain seems full of the smoke. My great aim is to be perspicuous, and I got credit for succeeding in the papers first sent out; but some of the others might be more obscure through my taking greater pains with them: an error I shall be happy to avoid in future; for you know I am not fond of much work."

In 1810, Jenner was afflicted with domestic trials. He lost one of his sons from phthisis, and the occurrence affected him so deeply that he became melancholic. His symptoms, says Baron, became so distressing, that active means were necessary to obviate them. He was sent to Bath, and returned with health and spirits restored. On his return he was called upon to attend the Earl of Berkeley up to the time of his death, and shortly afterwards Jenner lost his sister.

In the year 1811, Jenner was destined to experience "the most unpleasant event that had befallen him in his vaccine practice." There had been numerous reports of Small Pox occurring after Cow Pox, but they were, for the most part, silenced by the usual apologetics, and had therefore failed to produce a lasting impression.[1]

---

[1] Brown, *An inquiry into the antivariolous power of Vaccination.* Pp. 14, 151, *et seq.* 1809.

But it was very different with the case now to be
described.   Jenner had been summoned to London
in the first week in June; for on the 26th of May,
the Hon. Robert Grosvenor was seized with a; violent
attack of Small Pox.   In four days, he became
delirious, and an eruption appeared on the face; but
the Small Pox was not expected, because he had
been vaccinated by Jenner only ten years previously.
The following day, the eruption " increased prodigiously,
and some of the worst symptoms of a malignant and
confluent Small Pox showed themselves."   Master
Grosvenor was attended by Sir Henry Halford and
Sir Walter Farquhar, and was also visited by Jenner
in company with the latter.   The boy recovered,
although, from the severity of the attack, a fatal
termination had been regarded as inevitable.

A report of the case appeared, in which it was
stated that the latter stages of the disease were passed
through more rapidly in this case than usual, and that
it was a question whether this extraordinary circumstance, as well as the ultimate recovery of Master
Grosvenor, were not influenced by previous vaccination,
—an explanation which later gave rise to the theory
of Small Pox being modified, if not prevented, by
previous vaccination.

But this was not all.   There were several other cases
of the same description, and these events created so
much excitement that the National Vaccine Establish-

ment was obliged to publish a special report to explain them away. The state of feeling in London may be gathered from the following letter from Jenner to Moore.

"COCKSPUR STREET, CHARING CROSS,
"*June 11th*, 1811.

"MY DEAR FRIEND,—I should be obliged to you to send me, by the first coach, some of the Reports of our association. It will probably be my unhappy lot to be detained in this horrible place some days longer. It has unfortunately happened that a failure of vaccination has appeared in the family of a nobleman here; and, more unfortunately still, in a child vaccinated by me. The noise and confusion this case has created is not to be described. The vaccine lancet is sheathed; and the long concealed variolous blade ordered to come forth. Charming! This will soon cure the mania. The town is a fool,—an idiot; and will continue in this red-hot,—hissing-hot state about this affair, till something else starts up to draw aside its attention, I am determined to lock up my brains, and think no more *pro bono publico;* and I advise you, my friend, to do the same; for we are sure to get nothing but abuse for it. It is my intention to collect all the cases I can of Small Pox, after supposed security from that disease. In this undertaking I hope to derive much assistance from you. The best plan will be to push out some of them as soon as possible. This would not be necessary on account of the present case, but it would prove the best shield to protect us from the past, and those which are to come.

"Ever yours,
"EDWARD JENNER."

There was a panic among those who had had their children vaccinated, and many resorted at once to variolous inoculation. Jenner's friends applied to him for advice in the matter. The following is an example of the reply which was received:—

To Miss Calcraft.

"Take a comprehensive view of vaccination, and then ask yourself what is the case? You will find it a speck, a mere microscopic speck on the page which contains the history of the vaccine discovery. In the very first thing I wrote upon the subject, and many times since, I have said the occurrence of such an event should excite no surprise; because the Cow Pox must possess preternatural powers, if it would give uniform security to the constitution, when it is well known the Small Pox cannot; for we have more than one thousand cases to prove the contrary, and fortunately seventeen of them in the families of the nobility. We cannot alter the laws of nature; they are immutable. But, indeed, I have often said it was wonderful that I should have gone on for such a series of years vaccinating so many thousands, many under very unfavourable circumstances, without meeting with any interruption to my success before. And now this single solitary instance has occurred, all my past labours are forgotten, and I am held up by many, perhaps the majority of the higher classes, as an object of derision and contempt. There is that short-sightedness among them (I will not use a harsher term) which makes them identify a single failure with the general failure of the vaccine system. Before their dim eyes, stand two cases in the family of Lord Grosvenor, which they cannot see, or will not. There are two children vaccinated ten years ago, who have been constantly exposed to the infection of the other child, and inoculated for the Small Pox also; but all without effect. The infected child would have died,—that is universally allowed, —but for the previous vaccination. There was but little secondary fever; the pustules were much sooner in going off than in ordinary cases; and, indeed, the whole progress of the disease was different. It was modified, mitigated, and the boy was saved. What if ten, fifty, or a hundred such events should occur? they will be balanced an hundred times over by those of a similar kind after Small Pox. That is what I want to impress on the public mind; but there will be great difficulty in bringing this about because the multitude decide without thinking. No less than three cases of this description have happened in the family of one nobleman (Lord Rous). But I must check myself, lest I should tire you by going too far into the subject. I should not have said so much, had it not appeared to me that even your judgment was carried down the tide of popular clamour. I beg my compliments to Mrs. St. Quintin. I daresay her children are very secure ; but, if she has the weight of a feather on her mind, the safest and best test is vaccination with matter taken in its limpid state. I have stated my reasons for this over and over, in print and out of print.

"*June 19th.*"

The Grosvenor case, and a summons to give evidence before the House of Lords on the Berkeley peerage, thoroughly unnerved Jenner.

"I can compare my feelings to those of no one but Cowper the poet, when his intellect at last gave way to his fears about the execution of his office in the House of Lords. It was reading Cowper's Life, I believe, that saved my own senses, by putting me fully in view of my danger. For many weeks before the meeting, I began to be agitated, and, as it approached, I was actually deprived both of appetite and sleep, and when the day came I was obliged to deaden my sensibility, and gain courage by brandy and opium. The meeting was at length interrupted by a dissolution of Parliament, which sent the leading people to the country ; and what was at first merely postponed was ultimately abandoned, to my no small delight and satisfaction."

The Special Report of the National Vaccine Esta blishment, and the succeeding Reports of that Institution, which contained many striking accounts (supplied by Jenner) of the alleged extirpation of Small Pox by vaccination in the Caraccas and in Spanish America, and of the results in foreign countries generally, were greatly instrumental in gradually restoring the shattered credit of the new inoculation.

Jenner not only continued to supply information for the press, but while declining to enter into controversy with the anti-vaccinists, he encouraged the use of the newspapers as a channel for " cheering and persuasive reports."

" I have always thought that the subject of vaccination should be kept before the eyes of the public by means of the newspapers. This was never well done, and now it is scarcely done at all. Can you stimulate the Board to think of this ? It would be very easy to give extracts from reports.

" I have very lately received from Italy, a Poem 'Il Trionfo della Vaccinia,' by Gioachino Ponta, who, I hope, is a bard of celebrity, for he has spun it out to between 4,000 and 5,000 lines. It is beautifully printed, at the famous press of Bodoni at Parma.

" Knowing nothing of the language in which it is written, it lies before me in a tantalising shape. I shall bring it to town. If it is a good thing, cannot we transform it into English ?

" I shall say something on the *Report* in my next. That part of it which points out the happy results of vaccination among our troops must make the country feel, if they have any feeling in them. I am hurt to think the Small Pox again rages. That must be the case, till inoculation is conducted in a different way, if conducted at all. It does not appear in vaccinating districts ; for example, in this. As no particular notice has been taken of the foreign communications, I am thinking of sending them to one of the periodical journals. The Edinburgh Quarterly Journal is the most respectable.

" You do not seem to have understood me clearly respecting *newspapers*. It would certainly be *infra dig.* to go into controversy ; but not so to lay cheering and persuasive reports before the public through this widely flowing channel. This is what I meant, and I hope you will agree with me in the propriety of the measure.

"Make my affectionate regards to Mrs. Moore, and believe me

"Truly yours,

"EDWARD JENNER."

"Mrs. Moore saw my copy of the poem, and I do not think liked it much. Perhaps she might think the thread spun a little too fine. The poet's fancy has certainly flown in all manner of directions, and if you would like to judge for yourself, my daughter bids me tell you she will with pleasure copy for you a faithful analysis presented to me by a lady here, a complete mistress of the Italian language. I do not mean the whole poem, but its outline. The fact, as you have an excellent knack at managing these things, would perhaps find admittance with some advantage in the work you are now engaged in, as a *rub* to the British Bards, not one of whom, whose voice has obtained celebrity, has sung one single note in honour of Vaccina. Anstey, perhaps, may be considered as an exception, who piped up a Latin Ode about a dozen years ago, which the indefatigable John Ring translated neatly into English verse."

Jenner continued to assist Moore not only with his National Vaccine Establishment Reports, but also with his History of Vaccination, and he was particularly anxious to influence Moore to utterly discredit Dr. Pearson's labours. Thus he wrote to Moore :—

"I should much like to see your paper containing the History of Vaccination, and the exploits of the man who brought it up. In looking over my papers, I have found a great many which will throw a strong light on the conduct of Dr. P. Is there any chasm in this part of your history? It is a very important part, and justice demands the exercise of severity. It must begin with the Petworth business. This is given by Lord Egremont. Next his uniting with Woodville, and forming (without mentioning the matter to me) his institution. His cajoling the Duke of York to be patron. The Duke's disgracing him. His spreading the Small Pox through the land and calling it the Cow Pox, explaining *mechanically* the reason why it had changed its character. His treatment of me before the Committee of the House of Commons, attempting to prove that there were papers found in an old chest at Windsor, which anticipated my discovery. The portrait of the farmer from the Isle of Purbeck, with the farmer's claim to reward, as the discoverer at the foot of it, with a thousand minor tricks; and finally, finding all tricking useless, his insinuations that vaccination is good for nothing. The *Anti-Vacks* are assailing me, I see, with all the force they can muster in the newspapers. The Morning Chronicle now admits long letters. Birch has certainly much the worst of it there. Can you tell me who my friend and defender is in the Sun, who signs himself Conscience ?"

It is evident from a paragraph in the same letter that the ardour of his friend Ring had somewhat diminished.

"Do you ever see anything of your neighbour John Ring ? He writes but seldom to me now, and when he does write, it is not in his old pleasant strain. Nothing is going wrong with him I hope. I wish you would find out; for, with all his peculiarities, he is an honest fellow, and I have a great regard for him. He has been paying money for me to some of the institutions, and the enclosed draught, if you would have the goodness to take it to him, would be an excuse for your calling on him."

In some later correspondence with Moore, we again find Jenner cutting the ground from his critics and dwelling on explanations of Cow Pox failures.

"MY DEAR MOORE,—Before you make a comparative calculation of failures between the vaccine and variolous inoculations, you must consider the immense disparity between the numbers inoculated with the one and the other. If you calculate on a period of forty years, I should conceive that in the course of the last twenty years there have been at least five times as many vaccinated as have been variolated. . . .

"Then you must take into account the *failures* attributable to ignorance, neglect, etc., etc., etc. Why is not the list of failures from Small Pox brought forth? My friend, John Ring, had this in progress some years ago; but nothing appears in a compact form from any quarter. No less than seventeen of such cases have been found in the families of the nobility. The late Mr. Bromfield, whom you must recollect was surgeon to the Queen, abandoned the practice of inoculation in consequence of his failures, one of which was at the palace, from an inoculation with a portion of the same thread as was used on the arms of the Duke of Clarence and Prince Ernest, the Queen's brother. Is not this a precious anecdote for your new work?"

In 1814, Jenner was received by the Grand Duchess of Oldenburg, who presented him to the Emperor of Russia, on the occasion of their visit to London.

He explained to these royal personages his theory of the origin of phthisis from hydatids, and also pointed out to the Emperor that in whatever country vaccination was conducted in a way similar to that which his Majesty had commanded, in the Russian Empire,[1] Small Pox must necessarily become extinct.

---

[1] Jenner had a theory that both scirrhus and tubercle originated in a hydatid. "I long since discovered that the ordinary source of scirrhus is the hydatid, when passed on to its secondary stage." In another letter he repeats the same of tubercle. "What dreadful strides pulmonary consumption seems to be making over every part of our island. I trust

Jenner also had an interview with Count Platov, who remarked, " Sir, you have extinguished the most pestilential disorder that ever appeared on the banks of the Don." After this interview, Jenner returned to Cheltenham, where he had the misfortune to lose his wife, and a short time after this event he removed to Berkeley, where he continued to reside " in elegant retirement."

---

some advantage may, one day or another, be derived from my having demonstrably made out that what *is* tubercle in the lungs *has been* hydatid." At an interview with the Duchess of Oldenburg, sister of the Emperor of Russia, he again propounded this theory, but " as we had not yet dis. covered the means of absorption of these bodies in which phthisis pulmonalis originates, it therefore remains at present an incurable disease." The story of this interview is thus related by Fosbrooke. " The Duchess, who had lost a much valued friend by this malady, then took her handkerchief from her pocket and dropped a tear. She resumed her conversation, and remarked, ' Though you say it knows no remedy at present, yet think what a great point is gained.' "

Dr. Jenner presented the Emperor with a volume of his works, and " he (the Emperor) observed how pleasant must be his feelings when he contemplated what services he had rendered to mankind—' to the world, sir !' with emphasis. Dr. Jenner replied that when he reflected upon the benefit of which Providence had made him the instrument nothing could exceed his satisfaction. After a short pause the Emperor said, ' You have received, sir, the thanks, the applause, the gratitude of the world.' Dr. Jenner answered, ' Your Majesty, I have received the thanks and the applauses of the world.' But he did not echo the third position from a regard to truth. The Emperor then fell back a little, drew himself up with an altered countenance, and his face became suffused. A pause ensued ; and Dr. Jenner resumed the conversation by observing that local gratitude he had experienced abundantly ; but (pointing to a diamond ring upon his finger) never in a more gratifying form than in the token then before his Majesty's view, as being presented by his august mother, the Empress Maria. The Grand Duchess had just joined, and her tender feelings always permanent, said, ' Ah ! my mother !' and then dropped a tear. .She added, ' I wish, Dr. Jenner, that you would give the Emperor an account of your discovery respecting pulmonary consumption' Dr. Jenner made the effort, but feeling a little embarrassment, did

In 1818-19, there was a severe outbreak of Small
Pox in Edinburgh, and in 1819, a very fatal epidemic
at Norwich. There was increased opposition to
vaccination, which was supported by many eminent
members of the profession. But Jenner only regarded
these cases as the result of badly performed vaccination, or explained that some circumstances had
interrupted the proper influence of vaccination, such
as the existence of cutaneous disease.

"With regard to the mitigated disease which sometimes follows
vaccination, I can positively say, and shall be borne out in my
assertion by those who are in future days to follow me, that it is
the offspring entirely of incaution in those who conduct the
vaccine process. On what does the inexplicable change which
guards the constitution from the fang of the Small Pox depend?
On nothing but a correct state of the pustules on the arm excited
by the insertion of the virus ; and why are these pustules sometimes incorrect, losing their characteristic shape, and performing
their office partially ? But having gone pretty far on this subject
in my former letter, I shall not trouble you with a twice-told tale."

Others, unable to believe in the occurrence of Small
Pox after Cow Pox, were inclined to regard the

not do it in so perfect a manner as he could have wished. Upon this her
Imperial Highness observed in her usual good-natured tone, ' Dr. Jenner,
you do not make this so clear to my brother as you did to me at our late
interview.' He replied, ' Madam, it is my misfortune to be of a nervous
constitution ; and your Imperial Highness must not be surprised if a feeling of this sort should assail me at the present moment.' The Emperor
then exhibited the most amiable condescension and knowledge of the
human mind. Taking Dr. Jenner by the hand with a good-natured smile,
he held it till the doctor's embarrassment had disappeared. Dr. Jenner
then resumed his narrative concerning hydatids, and made it particularly
clear to his Majesty."

outbreak as one of malignant Chicken Pox. But this explanation had to be abandoned, and it was acknowledged even by Baron as only a way "of getting rid of the difficulty by giving the disorder a new appellation." At last, Small Pox was imported into Berkeley, and Henry Jenner was himself infected. Jenner wrote to Dr. Worthington :—

"We have at last imported the disease into this place. Henry Jenner, who, though he has seen nearly half a century fly over his head, has not yet begun to *think*, perched himself in the midst of a poor family pent up in a small cottage. It was the abode of wretchedness, had the addition of pestilence been wanting. He was infected, of course ; and his recovery is very doubtful. I am told to-day that he is very full of an eruption, the appearance of which stands midway between Small Pox and Chicken Pox. This has been spoken of by some of the Dublin and Edinburgh authors."

The outbreaks of Small Pox in various parts of the country, and the failures of vaccination, led Jenner to send a circular letter, early in 1821, to the profession, endeavouring to arouse attention to those points in vaccination which he considered essential to afford protection. Even the most ardent supporters of vaccination would now only claim that vaccination modified an attack of Small Pox in future, but Jenner's original opinion remained unchanged. Nothing would shake his belief that persons vaccinated were for ever after secure from the infection of Small Pox. On the back of an envelope dated January 14th, 1823, he wrote :—

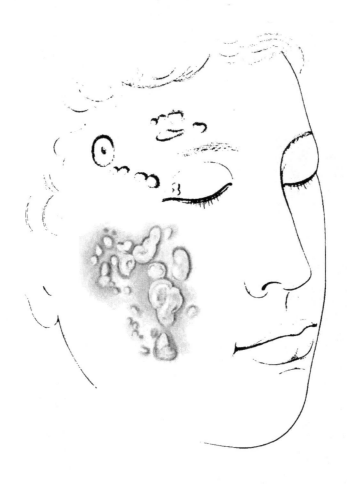

SMALL POX AFTER PERFECT VACCINATION (MONRO).

"My opinion of vaccination is precisely as it was when I first promulgated the discovery. It is not in the least strengthened by any event that has happened, for it could gain no strength ; it is not in the least weakened, for if the failures you speak of had not happened, the truth of my assertions respecting those coincidences which occasioned them would not have been made out."

On January 23rd, he wrote to his friend Gardner :—

"I have an attack from a quarter I did not expect, the Edinburgh Review. These people understand literature better than physic ; but it will do incalculable mischief. I put it down at 100,000 deaths, at least. Never was I involved in so many perplexities."

Two days afterwards, he had an attack of apoplexy, which proved fatal the following morning, January 26th, 1823.

Before I make any further remarks upon the history of Cow Pox inoculation, especially the continuance of the practice after Jenner's death, I will devote a few chapters to the discussion of Jenner's original paper and of his published *Inquiry*, together with an account of the various diseases which have been resorted to for a supply of lymph for the purposes of "vaccination."

CHAPTER VII.

JENNER'S REJECTED "INQUIRY."

In the autograph manuscript of Jenner's original paper, we have a record of the evidence upon which he was prepared to recommend inoculation of Cow Pox, and we are enabled to judge for ourselves whether the Royal Society was justified in refusing the communication.[1]

This paper[2] bears the modest title, *An Inquiry into the Natural History of a Disease known in Gloucestershire by the Name of the Cow-Pox.*

It opens with the following statement :—

" The deviations of Man from the state in which he was originally placed by Nature seem to have proved a prolific source of Diseases. From the love of Splendor, from the indulgences of Luxury and from his fondness for amusement, he has familiariz'd himself with a great number of animals, which may not originally have been intended for his associates."

Jenner mentions the horse as an example, and proceeds to describe a disease called by farriers "the Grease."

---

[1] Presented in 1796, or early in 1797, *vide* p. 138, and vol. ii., p. 20.

[2] *Vide* vol. ii., p. 1 *et seq.*

An

History

3

The devia

in which he u

seem to hav

source of Di

Splendor, fo

from his fon

familiariz

of animals.

been intend

dis arm'd of

the Lady's

✳ The late M

that the Dog

"*It is an inflammation and swelling in the heel, from which issues matter possessing properties of a very peculiar kind. It is capable of generating a disease in the Human Body (after it has undergone the modification which I shall presently speak of) which bears so strong a resemblance to the Small Pox, that I think it highly probable it may be the source of that disease.*"

Then follows a suggestion of a possible relation between this disease and Cow Pox.

"*In this Dairy Country, a great number of Cows are kept. The office of milking is here performed indiscriminately by both Men and Maid-servants. One of the former having perhaps been appointed to apply dressings to the heels of a Horse affected with the Grease, and not paying due attention to cleanliness, incautiously bears his part in milking the cows, with some particles of the infectious matter adhering to his fingers. Should this be the case it commonly happens that a disease is communicated to the Cows, and from the Cows to the Dairymaids, which pretty rapidly spreads until most of the cattle and domestics of the farm feel its unpleasant consequences.*"

Thus Jenner accounts for the origin of Cow Pox, the characters of which he proceeds to describe :—

"*It first appears on the nipples of Cows in the form of distinct pustules. They are seldom white, but more commonly of a palish blue, or rather of a colour somewhat approaching to livid, and are generally surrounded by more or less of an erysipelatous inflammation. These pustules, unless a timely remedy be applied, are much disposed to degenerate into phagedenic ulcers, which prove extremely troublesome.*"

The eruption on the hands of the milkers is more fully given :—

"*Several inflamed spots appear on different parts of the hands of the domestics employed in milking, and sometimes on the wrists, which quickly run on to suppuration, first assuming the appearance of the small vesications produced by a burn Most commonly they appear on the joints of the fingers, and at their extremities ; but whatever parts are affected, if the situation will admit, these superficial suppurations put on a circular form, with their edges more elevated than their centre, and of a colour distantly approaching to blue. Absorption takes place, and tumours appear in each axilla. The system becomes affected—the pulse is much quickened, and shiverings with general lassitude and pains about the loins and limbs with vomiting, come on. The head is painful, and the patient is now and then even affected with delirium. These symptoms, varying in their degrees of violence (for they rarely attack so severely), generally continue from one day to three or four, leaving ulcerated sores about the hands which from the sensibility of the parts, are very troublesome, and frequently becoming phagedenic, like those from whence they sprung, commonly heal slowly. The lips, nostrils, eyelids, and other parts of the body, are sometimes affected with sores ; but these arise from their being heedlessly rubbed or scratched with the patient's infectious fingers. No eruptions on the skin have followed the decline of the feverish symptoms in any instance that has come under my inspection, one only excepted, and in this a very few appeared on the arms. They were of a vivid red colour, very minute, and soon died away without advancing to maturation ; so that I cannot determine whether they had any connection with the preceding symptoms, but am inclined to think they had not.*"

We should naturally expect to hear some details of the history of these observations, and still more to be told that the country folk believed that the disease would prevent the Small Pox, but Jenner introduces the alleged prophylaxis thus :—

" *Morbid matter of various kinds, when absorbed into the system, may produce effects in some degree similar ; but what renders the Cow Pox virus so extremely singular, is, that the person who has been thus affected is for ever after secure from the infection of the Small Pox ; neither exposure to the variolous effluvia nor the insertion of the matter into the skin producing this distemper.*

" In support of this assertion, I shall produce many instances. I could produce a great number more, but the following, I presume, will be fully sufficient to establish the fact to the satisfaction of this very learned body."

We may get a better idea of the history of these instances, if we arrange them according to the years in which the patients presented themselves to be inoculated with Small Pox. It is impossible to give the exact sequence of all, as in some cases the dates are not given.

TEN COW POX CASES.

Date of Inoculation with Small Pox.			Name.			Ascertained to have had Cow Pox.
1. 1778	.	.	. Mrs. H——	.	.	. When very young.
2. 1791	.	.	. Mary Barge	.	.	. 31 years previously.
3. 1792	.	.	. Sarah Portlock .		.	27 ,, ,,
4. } 1795	.	.	. { Joseph Merret .	.	.	25 ,, ,,
5. }	.	.	. { William Smith .	.	.	1, 5, 15 ,, ,,
6. }	.	.	. { Elizabeth Wynne	.	.	10 months ,,
7. } 1797	.	.	. { Sarah Wynne	.	.	9 ,, ,,
8. }	.	.	. { William Rodway	.	.	38 years ,,
9. After 1782	.	.	. Simon Nichols		.	Some years previously.
10. Not stated	.	.	. John Phillips .	.	.	53 years ,,

We learn from other sources that Jenner was busily employed in 1778, in inoculating Small Pox by the method of Sutton ; but when he wrote his paper, he mentions only one case, that of Mrs. H., in whom, in that year, the failure of inoculation was attributed to a previous attack of Cow Pox. It appears, further, from the dates given, that it was not

until 1791, that Jenner seriously turned his attention
to collecting the histories of similar cases.

During twenty years of country practice, Jenner had
been called upon to inoculate with Small Pox, a number
of persons who had had Cow Pox. For the purposes
of his paper, ten instances were selected in which the
Small Pox inoculation produced its minimum effect. In
these cases, Cow Pox had been contracted at times
varying from nine months to fifty-three years previously.
No cases of really successful inoculation after Cow Pox
were included, and no allowance was made for individual
insusceptibility to Small Pox.

In addition, Jenner adds three cases of persons who
had been infected with "grease." In one case only, the
inoculation produced its minimum effect; in a second,
eruptions followed; and the third caught Small Pox
in the natural way.

THREE HORSE GREASE CASES.

Date of Inoculation with Small Pox.	Name.	Ascertained to have had "Grease."
1. Not stated .	. Thomas Pearce	. 6 years previously.
2. ,,	. James Cole .	. Some years ,,
Date of Infection with Small Pox.	Name.	Ascertained to have had "Grease."
3. Not stated .	. Abraham Riddiford .	. 20 years previously.

This presented a difficulty. Jenner believed that
Cow Pox arose from "grease," and that it protected
against Small Pox, yet persons directly infected with
"grease" enjoyed no such immunity. Jenner is
ready with an explanation. These cases, in his
opinion, decisively proved that the grease could not

be relied upon *until it had been passed through*
the cow.

Another difficulty for which no explanation was
forthcoming, was encountered in the case of William
Smith, who had Cow Pox in 1780, in 1791, and again
in 1794; the disease being as severe the second, and
third time, as it was in the first. Jenner simply states
the case without attempting to explain it.

"*Although the Cow Pox shields the constitution from the
Small Pox, and the Small Pox proves a protection against its
own future poison, yet it appears that the human body is
again and again susceptible of the infectious matter of the
Cow Pox.*"

Jenner, we must remember, was inquiring into the
natural history of the disease, and he was anxious to
observe more accurately the progress of the infection.

He selected a healthy boy about eight years old,
with a view to inoculate him with Cow Pox. On
the 14th of May, 1796, matter was taken from a
"suppurated sore on the hand of a dairymaid" and
inserted by means of two superficial incisions in the
arm, each about three-quarters of an inch long.

"*On the seventh day, he complained of uneasiness in the
axilla, and on the ninth, he became a little chilly, lost his
appetite, and had a slight headache. During the whole of this
day, he was perceptibly indisposed, and had rather a restless
night, but on the day following, he was perfectly well. The
appearance and progress of the incisions to a state of
maturation were pretty much the same as when produced in
a similar manner by variolous matter. The only difference*

which I perceived was that the edges assumed rather a darker . hue, and that the efflorescence spreading round the incisons took on rather more of an erysipelatous look than we commonly perceive when variolous matter has been made use of in the same manner."

The next stage of this experiment was, to apply the variolous test. On the 1st of July (less than seven weeks after the insertion of the Cow Pox), this boy was inoculated with matter taken immediately from a Small Pox pustule.

" Several punctures and slight incisions were made on both his arms, and the matter was well rubbed into them, but no disease followed. The same appearances only were observable on the arm as when a patient has had variolous matter applied after having either the Cow Pox or the Small Pox."

Jenner appears to have anticipated as an objection, that the test had been applied less than seven weeks after the original operation. The statement that the boy felt " so slight an affection of the system" after Cow Pox, that he was "perfectly well" on the tenth day, leads the reader to conclude that the test was not applied until five or six weeks had elapsed *after recovery*.[1] In the accompanying table [pp. 258, 259] I have made an analysis of the cases which Jenner described, and we can see what was the material which he had collected for a paper for the Royal

---

[1] *Vide* p. 136.

Society. He had put together a few cases which seemed to support the tradition of the dairymaids; he showed by ONE EXPERIMENT that the disease could be communicated from the cow to the human subject, after the manner of variolous inoculation, and that in this case the attempt a few weeks afterwards to inoculate with Small Pox, had proved abortive. This he considers to be quite sufficient.

"*I presume it would be swelling this paper to an unnecessary bulk, were I to produce further testimony in support of my assertion that the Cow Pox protects the human constitution from the infection of the Small Pox. I shall proceed then to offer a few general remarks upon the subject, to some others which are connected with it. Though I am myself perfectly convinced, from a great number of instances which have presented themselves, that the source of the Cow Pox is the morbid matter issuing from the newly diseased heels of horses, yet I could have wished, had circumstances allowed me, to have impressed this fact more strongly on the minds of this Society by experiments.*"

Jenner assumes that the virus from the horse's heels is intensified by being passed through the cow, on the ground that the horse so rarely affects his dresser with sores, while a milkman rarely escapes infection from the cow. He could not positively determine, if the disease from the horse or cow could affect the sound skin, but thought that it probably did not.

"*The hands of the farm servants in this neighbourhood, from the nature of their employments, are constantly exposed to those injuries which occasion abrasions of the cuticle, to punctures from thorns and such like accidents.*"

I.—Ten Cases

	Occupation.	Date of Cow Pox.	Date of Inoculation with Small Pox
I. *Joseph Merret*	Farm-servant and milker	1770 (Several sores on his hands).	April 1795
II. *Sarah Portlock*	Farm servant	1765	1792. In both arms
III. *John Phillips*	Tradesman	At 9 years of age	At the age of 62, with matter just before the commencement of the eruptive Fever, and instantly inserted.
IV. *Mary Barge*	Farm servant	1760	1791
V. *Mrs. H——*	Respectable gentle-woman.	"When very young contracted by contact with some of the servants of the Family who were infected by Cows. Her hands were extremely sore and her Nose was inflamed and very much swoln."	1778. "With active variolous matter."
VI. *Sarah Wynne*	Dairymaid	May 1796.	March 28th, 1797. "By carefully rubbing variolous matter into two slight incisions made upon the left arm."
VII. *William Rodway*	Servant at a Dairy	Summer of 1796	Feb. 13th, 1797. "Variolous matter was inserted into both his arms; in the right by means of a slight incision and into the left by punctures."
VIII. *Elizabeth Wynne*	Dairymaid	1759 ("In a very slight degree, one very small sore only, breaking out upon the little finger of her hand, and scarcely any indisposition following")	March 28th, 1797. "By making two superficial incisions on the left arm in which the matter was cautiously rubbed."
IX. *William Smith*	Farm servant	1780 ("One of his hands had several ulcerated sores upon it, and he became very ill" with such symptoms as have been before described. In the year 1791 . . . he became affected with it the second time, and in the year 1794 he was so unfortunate as to catch it again ").	In the spring of the year 1795. Twice.
X. *Simon Nichols*	Farm servant	1782. Later at another farm his hands were "affected in the common way, and he was much indisposed."	Some years afterwards.

II.—Three Cases

	Occupation.	Date of Cow Pox.	Date of Inoculation with Small Pox
I. *Thomas Pearce*	Farrier	No date. (Sores on his fingers which suppurated and which occasioned a pretty severe indisposition).	Six years afterwards variolous matter inserted into his arm repeatedly.
II. *Mr. James Cole*	Farmer	No date	Some years afterwards was inoculated with variolous matter.
III. *Mr. Abraham Riddiford*	Farmer	No date. (Very painful sores in both of his hands, tumours in each axilla, and severe and general indisposition).	[Not stated.]

III.—One Case

	Occupation.	Date of Cow Pox.	Date of Inoculation with Small Pox
I. *A Boy* (about 8 years old)		Inoculated by Jenner on the 14th May, 1796, with matter taken from a suppurated sore on the hand of a dairymaid . . . by means of two superficial incisions each about ⅞-in. long.	

Casual Cow Pox.

Result.	Exposure to Infection of Small Pox.	Result.
"An efflorescence only taking on an erysipelatous look about the centre, appearing on the skin near the punctured parts."	"During the whole time that his family had the Small Pox, one of whom had it very full."	"Received no injury from exposure to the contagion."
> in preceding case	"Nursed one of her own children who had accidentally caught the disease."	"No indisposition ensued."
"A sting-like feel in the part; an efflorescence appeared which on the 4th day was rather extensive, and some degree of pain and stiffness were felt about the shoulder, but on the 5th day these symptoms began to disappear, and in a day or two after went entirely off without producing any effect on the system."	[Not stated.]	— —
"An efflorescence of a palish-red colour soon appeared about the parts where the matter was inserted, and spread itself rather extensively, but died away in a few days without producing any variolous symptoms."	"Repeatedly employed as a nurse to Small Pox patients."	"Without experiencing any ill consequence."
The same appearance followed as in the preceding cases; an efflorescence on the arm without any effect on the constitution.	Soon after infection with Cow Pox. "Mrs. H—— was exposed to the contagion of the Small Pox, where it was scarcely possible for her to have escaped it, as she regularly attended a relative who had the disease in so violent a degree that it proved fatal to him."	"No indisposition followed."
"A little inflammation appeared in the usual manner around the parts where the matter was inserted, but so early as the 5th day it vanished entirely without producing any effect on the system."	[Not stated.] . . .	— —
"Both were perceptibly inflamed on the 3rd day. After this the inflammation about the punctures soon died away, but a small appearance of erysipelas was manifest about the edges of the incision till the 8th day, when a little uneasiness was felt for the space of half an hour in the axilla. The inflammation then hastily disappeared without producing the most distant mark of affection of the system."	[Not stated.] . . .	— —
"A little efflorescence soon appeared, and a tingling sensation was felt about the parts until the 3rd day, when both began to subside, and so early as the 5th day it was evident that no indisposition would follow."	[Not stated.] . . .	— —
"No affection of the system could be produced."	"Since associated with those who had the Small Pox in its most contagious state."	"Without feeling any effect from it."
"With not the least effect on the constitution." .	With several other patients inoculated at the same time "he continued during the whole time of their confinement."	"With not the least effect on the constitution."

Casual Horse Grease.

Result.	Exposure to Infection of Small Pox.	Result.
"Without being able to produce anything more than slight inflammation, which appeared very soon after the matter was applied."	"And afterwards exposed him to the contagion of the Small Pox."	"With as little effect."
"A little pain in the axilla and feet; a slight indisposition for three or four hours. A few eruptions showed themselves on the forehead, but they very soon disappeared without advancing towards maturation."	[Not stated.] . . .	— —
. . . .	"Was assured that he never need to fear the infection of the Small Pox. But this assertion proved fallacious; for on being exposed to the infection upwards of twenty years afterwards,	"He caught the disease, which took its regular course, in a very mild way. . . . There was no room left for suspicion as to the reality of the disease as I inoculated some of his family from the pustules who had the Small Pox in consequence."

Inoculated Cow Pox.

"On the 1st of July this boy was inoculated with matter immediately taken from a small-pox pustule, several punctures and incisions were made on both his arms, and the matter was well rubb'd into them, but no disease followed. The same appearances only were observable on the arms as when a Patient has had variolous matter applied after having either the Cow Pox or the Small Pox."

Having assumed that his theory of the origin of
Cow Pox was correct, he continues the argument until
it ultimately culminates in the theory of the origin,
ex animalibus, of all infectious fevers and many other
communicable diseases of man.

*" It is curious to observe that this matter acquires new
properties by passing from the horse through another medium,
that of the cow ; not only is its activity hereby increased, but
those specific properties become invariable which induce in the
human constitution symptoms similar to those of the variolous
fever, and effect in it that peculiar change which for ever renders
it unsusceptible of the variolous contagion.*

*" May we not then reasonably infer that the source of the
Small Pox is the matter generated in the diseased foot of a horse,
and that accidental circumstances may have again and again
arisen, still working new changes upon it, until it has acquired
the contagious and malignant form under which we now
commonly see it making its devastations among us ? And from
a consideration of the change which the infectious matter from
the horse has undergone after it has produced a disease on the
cow, may we not conceive that many contagious diseases now
prevalent among us, may owe their present appearance not to a
simple, but a compound origin ? For example, is it hard to
imagine that the measles, the scarlet fever, and the ulcerous sore-
throat with a spotted skin have sprung from the same source,
assuming some variety in their forms according to the nature of
their new combinations ? The same question will apply respecting the Yaws and the Syphilis, and indeed many other diseases."*

Jenner adds that he believes in varieties of Small Pox,
and mentions that seven years previously an outbreak,
which the nurses and the common people called the
Swine or Pig Pox, appeared in many towns and
villages in Gloucestershire ; a fatal case was scarcely

heard of, and the people had only as mild and light a disease, as if they had been inoculated with variolous matter in the usual way.

Jenner then proceeds to give a "cautionary hint" with regard to "*management* of the variolous matter previously to its being used for the purpose of inoculation." He gives the instance of a fellow-practitioner who employed matter not unfrequently, after it had been taken several days from the pustules. When inoculated it produced inflammation of the incised parts, swelling of the axillary glands, and, as he had been informed by the patients, eruptions. "But," says Jenner, "what was this disease? Certainly not the Small Pox."

"*The same unfortunate circumstance of giving a disease, supposed to be the Small Pox, with inefficacious matter, having come under the direction of some other practitioner, and probably from the same incautious method of securing the variolous matter, I avail myself of this opportunity of mentioning what I conceive as of great importance; and as a further cautionary hint I shall take the liberty of adding another observation on this subject of inoculation.*

"*Whether it be yet ascertained by experiment that the quantity of variolous matter inserted into the skin makes any difference with respect to the subsequent mildness or violence of the disease, I know not; but I have the strongest reason for supposing that if either the punctures or incisions be made so deep as to go through it, and wound the adipose covering beneath, that the risk of bringing on a violent disease is greatly increased. I have known an inoculator whose practice was to go deep enough, to use his own expression, to see a bit of fat and then to lodge the matter. The great number of bad cases, and the fatality which attended this practice, was almost inconceivable, for let it be recollected that it is only from a different mode of receiving the infectious particles that the difference between inoculation and the natural Small Pox arises.   Though it is very improbable that any one would inoculate in this way by design, yet this observation may tend to place a double guard over the Lancet, when infants fall under the care of the inoculator, as the skin is comparatively so very thin.*

In other words, any one disposed to apply the variolous test after Cow Pox, was cautioned to employ the Suttonian method, and if an eruption followed, it was not to be hastily concluded that genuine Small Pox had resulted.

As to how long Cow Pox had been known among the farmers, Jenner says that the oldest among them were acquainted with it, and had heard their forefathers speak of it, but a connection with Small Pox was unknown to them, and his belief that the disease arose from the heels of horses, was new to most of them.[1]

" But it has at length produced conviction, and probably from the precautions, which they now seem disposed to adopt (for a farmer is not the most flexible of human beings), the appearance of the Cow Pox here may either be extinguished or become extremely rare."

In conclusion, Jenner proposes to substitute Cow Pox inoculation for Small Pox inoculation, and this is the answer which he is prepared to give, should any one ask whether this " discovery," or rather investigation,

---

[1] Compare Jenner's MS. notes, p. 376.

were a matter of mere curiosity or tended to any beneficial purpose.

"*I should answer, that notwithstanding the happy effects of Inoculation, with all the improvements which the practice has received since its introduction into this country, we sometimes observe it to prove fatal, and from this circumstance we feel at all times somewhat alarmed for its consequences. But as fatal effects have never been known to arise from the Cow Pox, even when expressed in the most unfavourable manner, that is, when it has accidentally produced extensive inflammations and suppurations on the hands; and as it clearly appears that this disease leaves the constitution in a state of perfect security from the infection of Small Pox, may we not infer that a mode of Inoculation might be introduced preferable to that at present adopted, especially among those families which, from previous circumstances, we may judge to be predisposed to have the disease unfavourably? It is an excess in the number of pustules which we chiefly dread in the Small Pox; but in the Cow Pox no pustules appear, nor does it seem possible for the contagious matter to produce the disease by effluvia or by any other means, as I have before observed, than contact; so that a single individual in a family might at any time receive it without the risk of infecting the rest, or of spreading a disease that fills a country with terror. Without further research, I should therefore not in the least hesitate to inoculate Adults, and Children not very young, with the matter of Cow Pox in preference to common variolous matter. How far it may be admissible on tender skins of infants further experiments must determine. I have no other scruples than such as arise from the darkish appearance of the edges of the incisions on the arm of the Boy whom I inoculated with this matter, the only experiment I had an opportunity of making in that way. But in this case the incisions, though perfectly superficial, were made to a much greater extent than was necessary for communicating the infection to the system. However it proved of no consequence, as the arm never became painful nor required any application. I shall endeavour still farther to prosecute this Inquiry, an Inquiry*

I trust not merely speculative, but of sufficient moment to inspire the pleasing hope of its becoming essentially beneficial to Mankind."

Such was the evidence on which Jenner had first proposed to introduce vaccination ; a proposal which was rejected, in not very flattering terms, by the Council of the Royal Society.

I was struck by the substitution, in a different handwriting, of the word *investigation* for *discovery.* Some friendly critic had evidently read the manuscript and made this correction among others. Had Jenner made a discovery, and, if so, what was it? He had not discovered that Cow Pox produced an immunity from Small Pox ; for, assuming such to be the case, it was the discovery of the dairymaids. He had not discovered that Cow Pox could be intentionally communicated from cow to man, for this had been practised by Jesty and others. He was not the first to employ the test of variolous inoculation after Cow Pox, for this had been performed upon Mrs. Jesty ; and as for the test of exposure to infection, this had been carried out repeatedly. The correction of his critic was therefore fully justified. Jenner had made no discovery, but he had carried out an investigation from which he was led to observe a similarity between inoculated Cow Pox and inoculated Small Pox, and to express a belief in the origin of Cow Pox and Small Pox, and many other diseases, from horse grease. Apart from these speculations, a Dorsetshire surgeon [1] had done almost as much as Jenner. Both had proposed to introduce Cow Pox inoculation as a substitute for Small Pox inoculation, for which the surgeon was threatened with the loss of his practice, and Jenner with the loss of such scientific credit as he had hitherto possessed.

[1] *Vide* p. 116.

CHAPTER VIII.

JENNER was by no means discouraged by the verdict of
the Royal Society, and he had no intention of abandoning his project. He proceeded to amplify his original
paper [1] by inserting the cases of William Stinchcomb and
of the paupers of Totworth, between Cases X. and XI.,
and he also added the case of Sarah Nelmes, from
whom he had taken matter to inoculate the boy Phipps.
Her case was inserted between Cases XIII. and XIV.
Jenner also re-inoculated Phipps with Small Pox, but
" no sensible effect was produced upon the constitution."

Jenner was most anxious to see his pamphlet in
print, but he appears to have resolved, in June 1797,
not to risk a second rejection by the Royal Society.
Thus he wrote to a friend :—

"I have shown a copy of my intended paper on the Cow
Pox to our friend Worthington, who has been pleased to express
his approbation of it, and to recommend my publishing it as
a pamphlet instead of sending it to the Royal Society."

But Jenner wished to add some more original
material to the paper, and he therefore kept it in hand

---

[1] *Vide* vol. ii., pp. 1-33.

in the hope that he might meet with some more cases
of the Casual Cow Pox in the dairies, and that he
might have time to fulfil his intention of proving, by
experiment, its origin from "grease." On the 2nd
of August, he wrote :—

"The simple experiment of applying the matter from the
heel of the horse, in its proper state, to the nipples of the cows,
when they are in a proper state to be infected by it, is not so
easily made as at first sight may be imagined ; after waiting with
impatience for months in my own neighbourhood, without effect, I
sent a messenger to Bristol, in vain, to procure the true virus.
I even procured a young horse, kept him constantly in the stable,
and fed him with beans in order to make his heels swell, but to
no purpose. By the time the Pamphlet goes to a second edition,
I hope to be able to give some decisive experiments."

But no Cow Pox appeared in the dairies, and his
researches were thus interrupted until the spring of 1798,
when an outbreak occurred which afforded him the
much-wished-for opportunities for further observations.

A mare, the property of a dairyman in a neighbouring parish, began to have "sore-heels" in the
latter part of February 1798. The horse's heels were
dressed by the farm servants, Thomas Virgoe, William
Wherret, and William Haynes who, in consequence,
contracted sores on their hands, followed by inflamed
lymphatic glands in the arms and axillæ ; and constitutional symptoms, shiverings succeeded by heat,
lassitude, and pains in the limbs. Haynes and Virgoe
had both previously been successfully inoculated with
Small Pox, but Wherret had not had Small Pox.

"Haynes was daily employed as one of the milkers at the farm, and the disease began to shew itself among the cows about ten days after he first assisted in washing the mare's heels. Their nipples became sore in the usual way, with bluish pustules; but as remedies were early applied they did not ulcerate to any extent."

The Cow Pox was raging in several dairies, but Jenner confined his attention to this one outbreak. Whether it was the only one in which there happened to be a horse with "greasy" heels, we are not told.

Jenner's mind was occupied with the opportunity of making a double experiment; inoculation of one child with humanised horse-grease, and of another child with matter from the cow's teats.

With regard to the horse-grease inoculation, Jenner says :—

"This experiment was made to ascertain the progress and subsequent effects of the disease when thus propagated."

The object of this experiment is thus clearly stated. Jenner had already condemned horse-grease, for he had committed himself to the statement that it had been *decisively proved that grease could not be relied upon as a protective against Small Pox.*[1] The object of studying the progress and effects may have been a double one. First, to ascertain whether an attack of Small Pox would follow. For Jenner was firmly of opinion that the grease was the source of Small Pox; it was after it was transmitted through the cow, that it appeared in the modified form known as

---

[1] Vol. ii., pp. 18 and 160.

Cow Pox. This outbreak, therefore, afforded him an opportunity for testing his theories. He could inoculate one child with the matter of the grease, and another with the matter of Cow Pox, and study the results side by side. And if he could experimentally generate Small Pox in the one case, and carry on Cow Pox in the other, what an interesting addition to his paper it would prove. Secondly, he may have wished to ascertain, whether by successive cultivation in the human subject, protective properties would be gradually assumed by the horse-grease virus.

For his experimental purposes, Jenner selected a child five years old, John Baker by name, and on March 16th, 1798, he took matter from a pustule on the hand of Thomas Virgoe, one of the servants who had been infected from the mare's heels.

"He became ill on the sixth day, with symptoms similar to those excited by the Cow Pox matter. On the eighth day, he was free from indisposition.

"There was some variation in the appearance of the pustule on the arm. Although it somewhat resembled a Small Pox pustule, yet its similitude was not so conspicuous as when excited by matter from the nipple of the cow, or when the matter has passed from thence through the medium of the human subject."

The result had little in common with inoculated Small Pox; but it so far corresponded with inoculated Cow Pox, that Jenner was encouraged to apply the variolous test to ascertain whether, in spite of his previous conclusions, the system had been rendered insusceptible of Small Pox.

"We have seen that the virus from the horse, when it proves infectious to the human subject, is not to be relied upon as rendering the system secure from variolous infection, but that the matter produced by it on the nipple of the cow is perfectly so. Whether its passing from the horse through the human constitution, as in the present instance, will produce a similar effect, remains to be decided."

Jenner, of course, intended to apply the test of variolous *inoculation*, and to watch the results.

Now, in the historical case of James Phipps, the Cow Pox was inoculated on the 14th of May; on the tenth day, he was said to be perfectly well. On the 1st of July following, that is to say, in less than seven weeks after inoculation, he was inoculated with Small Pox. We may therefore conclude that, as John Baker had been inoculated on the 16th of March, and was said to be free from indisposition eight days afterwards, that it was Jenner's intention to inoculate him on or about the 1st of May.

"This would now have been effected, but the boy was rendered unfit for inoculation from having felt the effects of a contagious fever in a workhouse soon after this experiment was made."

The question naturally arises, whether the fever might not have been the result of the inoculation with horse grease. What was the meaning of "contagious fever," and why this vagueness of expression? Jenner was well acquainted with measles, scarlet fever, ulcerous sore-throat with spotted skin, erysipelas, swine pox, chicken pox, and other fevers. We are

therefore left to suppose that it was some unrecognised form of " fever," from which the boy
ultimately recovered ; but as the variolous inoculation
had been prevented at the time, the history of the
fever was not worth tracing, although further details
might have been given, for the *Inquiry* was not
published until June 21st.

It is not until we read Jenner's *Further Observations*
that our attention is again drawn to this matter. In a
reference[1] to this case, Jenner insists upon the "similarity
to the Cow Pox of the general constitutional symptoms
which followed," and in a footnote we read :—

" The boy unfortunately **died** of a fever at a parish workhouse,
before I had an opportunity of observing what effects would have
been produced by the matter of Small Pox."

The fact, then, of the boy's death was omitted
in the first account, and this is the full meaning of
the boy being " rendered unfit for inoculation."

But why should the fact of the boy's death have
been omitted ? Did the boy die from the effects of
inoculation ? Let us revert to the history of the case.
What was the state of the progress of the vesicle on
the boy's arm ? No description is given in the *Inquiry*;
all that we learn is that the *symptoms* were similar to
those excited by Cow Pox matter, and on the eighth
day, he was free from indisposition, and the pustule
" somewhat resembled a Small Pox pustule." On

[1] Vol. ii., p. 169.

referring to the coloured illustration, it is hardly
credible that the lad was free from indisposition on
the eighth day [Plate IV.]. A vesicle is depicted with
the appearances which indicate that the "vaccination"
had taken severely. Another casual reference[1] in
Further Observations, throws additional light on this
case. Jenner says he was led to assume the origin of
Cow Pox from the grease, partly "from the *progress
and general appearance of the pustule* on the arm of
the boy inoculated with matter taken from the hand
of a man infected by a horse." Now, if it progressed
in the same way as the Cow Pox inoculation on
Phipps, it must have been a vesicle surrounded by
an efflorescence, with "rather more of an erysipelatous
look than we commonly perceive when variolous
matter has been made use of in the same manner . . .
leaving on the inoculated parts scabs and subsequent
eschars." The progress of the vesicle having been
compared to that of inoculated Cow Pox, we may
conclude that it ran on to ulceration, the bane of
Jenner's early inoculations. This supposition is verified
by an abstract, published by Baron, from Jenner's
manuscript notes, in which he alludes to "the peculiar
appearance of the pustule, and *its disposition to run
into an ulcer,* in the arm of the boy who was inoculated with matter taken from the hand of a man, who
received the infection from dressing a slight spontaneous

---

[1] *Vide* vol. ii., p. 169.

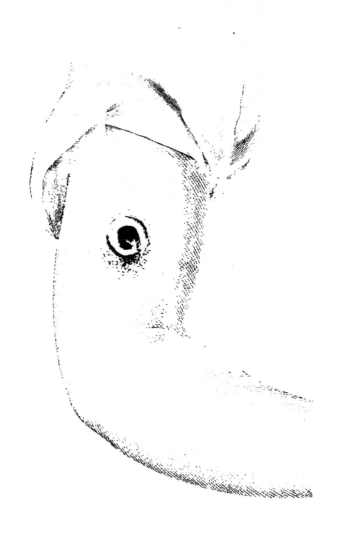

INOCULATED HORSE POX (JENNER).
CASE OF JOHN BAKER.

sore on a horse's heel." It is evident that in the published account of this boy's case, Jenner had suppressed all details of the progress of the vesicle, the ulceration, and the erysipelas, as well as the fatal termination of the case, and he inserted instead that " on the eighth day he was free from indisposition," but " was rendered unfit for inoculation from having felt the effects of a contagious fever."

It would seem most probable that in this boy, five years old (selected by Jenner as a suitable subject for testing his speculations as to the progress and effects of horse grease), a large vesicle was produced which ran on to ulceration, that the angry blush developed into erysipelas, and the boy died.[1] But his death was attributed to a contagious fever *caught* in the workhouse.

Jenner considered that his former cases had so satisfactorily withstood the subsequent inoculation of Small Pox that it was unnecessary to test all the subjects of these later experiments. He, however, inoculated William Summers, but the date of the operation and the local results are not mentioned. All that we are told is, that the system did not feel the effects of it. Two other children, Barge and Pead, were inoculated by his nephew, Henry Jenner, who reported as follows :—

"On the second day, the incisions were inflamed, and there was a pale inflammatory stain around them. On the third day, these

---

[1] Compare Creighton. *Cow Pox and Vaccinal Syphilis*, p. 32.

appearances were still increasing, and their arms itched considerably. On the fourth day, the inflammation was evidently subsiding, and on the sixth, it was scarcely perceptible."

William Summers had been inoculated from the cow, the same day as Baker.

" He became indisposed on the sixth day, vomited once, *felt the usual slight symptoms* till the eighth day, when he appeared perfectly well."

From William Summers the disease was transferred to William Pead, after the manner of arm to arm variolation. From William Pead, several children and adults were inoculated ; three suffered from extensive erysipelatous inflammation. From one of these patients, Hannah Excell, matter was taken and inserted into the arms of John Marklove, Robert F. Jenner, Mary Pead, and Mary James. From Mary Pead lymph was taken to inoculate J. Barge.

PEDIGREE OF JENNER'S FIRST STOCK OF LYMPH
(EQUINE INDIRECT).

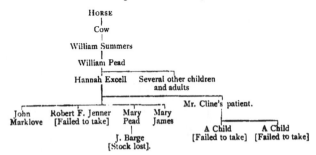

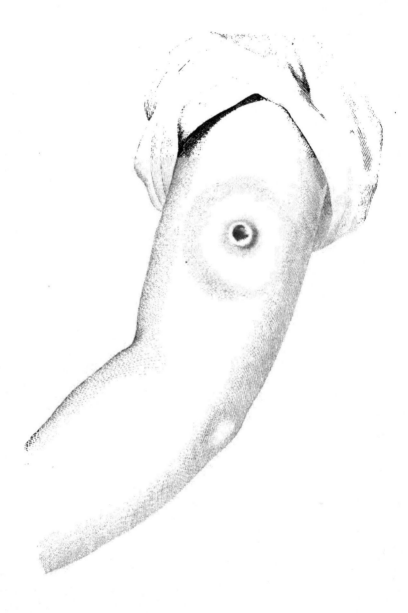

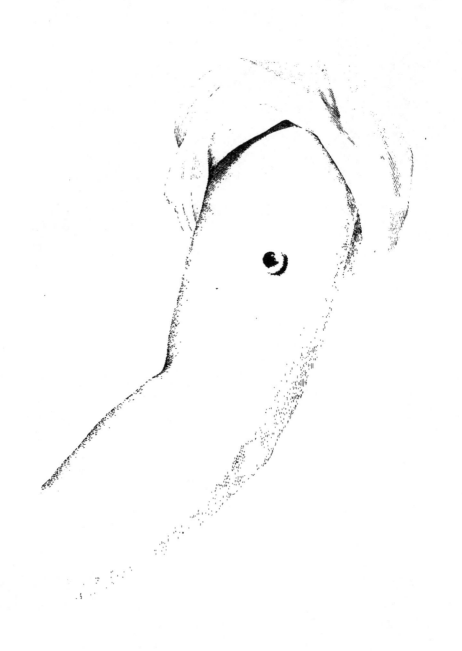

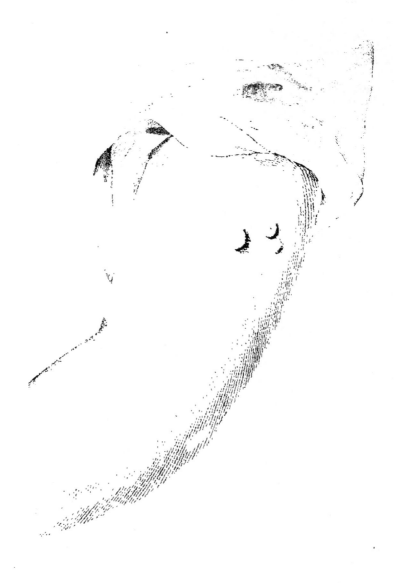

INOCULATED HORSE POX (JENNER).
Case of Hannah Excell.

Besides adding fresh cases, the whole manuscript was carefully revised. With regard to the horse grease theory, Jenner now felt himself in a position to speak more positively, for in referring to the possible transference of infectious matter from the horse's heel to the cow's teat, he substituted the words *when this is the case* for *should this be the case.*

Several expressions are modified in his description of Cow Pox. In his paper, he had written that the pustules were "seldom white, but more commonly blue, and generally surrounded by more or less of an erysipelatous inflammation," but the published *Inquiry* reads :—

"At their first appearance, they are commonly of a palish blue, or rather of a colour somewhat approaching to livid, and are surrounded by an erysipelatous inflammation."

And in the third edition of the *Inquiry* the word *erysipelatous* is omitted.

Another instance of modifying original statements occurs in the description of the case of Sarah Wynne. The account in the original paper may be compared side by side with the revised version in the published *Inquiry.*

ORIGINAL PAPER.	PUBLISHED " INQUIRY."
"She caught the complaint from the cows, and was affected with it [Cow Pox] in so violent a degree that she was incapable of doing any work for the space of ten days."	"She caught the complaint from the cows, and was affected with the symptoms described on the 8th page, in so violent a degree, that she was confined to her bed, and rendered incapable for several days of pursuing her ordinary vocations on the farm."

Now if we turn to *the symptoms described on the 8th page* we are referred to a foot-note, in which it is stated that these symptoms arise from the irritation of the sores, and not from the primary action of the vaccine virus upon the constitution. The meaning of this correction is now apparent. Jenner's idea, at this period, was to provide a *mild* substitute for Small Pox inoculation, and these severe symptoms described in the original paper as an essential part of the Cow Pox are now attributed to accidental causes.

This system of modifying his original observations is adhered to throughout the paper. The sentence " pustules which *are most disposed to* degenerate into phagedenic ulcers," now reads "pustules which *frequently* degenerate into phagedenic ulcers."

But one of the most important alterations is the suggestion of a *spurious Cow Pox.*

ORIGINAL PAPER.

" But first it is of importance to remark that there are other causes besides contagious matter which produce pustules and sometimes ulcerations on the nipples of the cows, and instances have occurred of the hands of the servants, employed in milking, being affected with sores in consequence, and even of their feeling an indisposition from absorption. But instances are very rare. This complaint

PUBLISHED " INQUIRY."

" It is necessary to observe that pustulous sores frequently appear spontaneously on the nipples of cows, and instances have occurred, though very rarely, of the hands of the servants employed in milking being affected with sores in consequence, and even of their feeling an indisposition from absorption. These pustules are of a much milder nature than those which arise from that appears at various seasons of the year, but most commonly in the spring, when the cows are first taken from their winter food and fed with grass. It is very apt to appear also when they are suckling their young. But this disease is not to be considered as having any kind of connection with that of which I am treating, as it is incapable of producing any specific effects on the human constitution. This distinction between the two diseases becomes the more important as the want of it might occasion an idea of security from the infection of the Small Pox which would prove delusive."

contagion which constitutes the **true** Cow Pox. They are always free from the bluish or livid tint so conspicuous in the pustules in that disease. No erysipelas attends them, nor do they show any phagedenic disposition as in the other case, but quickly terminate in a scab, without creating any apparent disorder in the cow. This complaint appears at various seasons of the year, but most commonly in the spring, when the cows are first taken from their winter food and fed with grass. It is apt to appear also when they are suckling their young. But this disease is not to be considered as similar in any respect to that of which I am treating, as it is incapable of producing any specific effects on the human constitution. However, it is of the greatest consequence to point it out here, lest the want of discrimination should occasion an idea of security from the infection of the Small Pox which might prove delusive."

Jenner was obviously referring in the original paper to the Blister Pock, though he does not name the disease. But in the paragraph inserted in the published *Inquiry*, he used the term *true* Cow Pox for the first time, which leads the reader to suppose that

the disease "of a milder nature" was a *false* Cow
Pox. And at the conclusion of the paper, Jenner has,
no longer, any hesitation on this point, but uses the
terms *true* Cow Pox and *spurious* Cow Pox, with
a reference to the foot-note which has been quoted
above.

I wish to insist upon the gradual assumption of
the existence of a *spurious Cow Pox*. The farmers
and cow doctors knew nothing of this *spurious Cow
Pox*. They distinguished, from other eruptions such as
blistered teats, a disease which produced troublesome
ulcerations on the cow's teats, and ulcerations on the
hands, enlarged glands, and constitutional symptoms in
milkers, and this disease they called the Cow Pox.
Jenner was alone responsible for assuming the existence
of two kinds of Cow Pox, a true and a spurious. And
this assumption was extended in *Further Observations* to
include not' *one* but *several kinds* of so-called spurious
Cow Pox.

In a subsequent publication, entitled *The Origin of
the Vaccine Inoculation*, Jenner has given the history
and full meaning of this innovation :—

"In the course of the investigation of this subject, which, like
all others of a complex and intricate nature, presented many
difficulties, I found that some of those **who seemed to have
undergone the Cow Pox**, nevertheless, on inoculation with the
Small Pox, felt its influence just the same as if no disease
had been communicated to them by the cow. This occurrence
led me to inquire among the medical practitioners in the
country around me, who all agreed in this sentiment, that the

Cow Pox was not to be relied upon as a certain preventive of the Small Pox.

" This for a while damped, but did not extinguish, my ardour; for, as I proceeded, I had the satisfaction to learn that the cow was subject to some varieties of spontaneous eruptions upon her teats; that they were all (*sic*) capable of communicating sores to the hands of the milkers, and that, whatever sore was derived from the animal, was called in the dairy the Cow Pox.

" **Thus I surmounted a great obstacle,** and, in consequence, was led to form a distinction between these diseases; one of which only I have denominated the **true,** the others the **spurious,** Cow Pox, as they possess no specific power over the constitution."

In some concluding remarks,[1] in the published *Inquiry*, Jenner relates the cases of Hannah Pick and Elizabeth Sarsenet, who contracted Cow Pox, with all the other servants, at a farm in the parish of Berkeley.

It puzzled Jenner still more to find an explanation for these cases, for Hannah resisted variolous inoculation, so the Cow Pox was pronounced to be " true; " and yet when Elizabeth Sarsenet was exposed to variolous infection, she caught the disease.

" This impediment to my progress was not long removed, before another, of far greater magnitude in its appearances, started up. There were not wanting instances to prove, that when the true Cow Pox broke out among the cattle at a dairy, a person who had milked an infected animal, and had thereby apparently gone through the disease in common with others, was liable to receive the Small Pox afterwards. **This, like the former obstacle, gave a painful check to my fond and aspiring hopes;** but reflecting that the operations of nature are generally uniform, and that it was not probable the human

---

[1] *Vide* vol. ii., p. 32.

constitution (having undergone the Cow Pox) should in some instances be perfectly shielded from the Small Pox, and in many others remain unprotected, I resumed my labours with redoubled ardour.

The result was fortunate ; for I now discovered that the virus of Cow Pox was liable to undergo progressive changes, from the same causes precisely as that of Small Pox, and that when it was applied to the human skin in its degenerated state, it would produce the ulcerative effects in as great a degree as when it was not decomposed, and sometimes far greater ; but having lost its specific properties, it was incapable of producing that change upon the human frame which is requisite to render it unsusceptible of the variolous contagion ; so that it became evident a person might milk a cow one day, and having caught the disease be for ever secure ; while another person milking the same cow the next day, might feel the influence of the virus in such a way as to produce a sore or sores, and in consequence of this might experience an indisposition to a considerable extent ; yet, as has been observed, the specific quality being lost, the constitution would receive no peculiar impression."

Jenner adds a few additional notes. He reiterates his conviction that Cow Pox alone arises from the grease, and states that true Cow Pox was occasionally absent, because the farmer's horses had not, from the dryness of the season, been affected with grease.

In another paragraph, he repeats his belief that Cow Pox is not self-protective, and gives the case of Elizabeth Wynne, who had Cow Pox in 1759, was inoculated with Small Pox without effect in 1797, and caught Cow Pox again in 1798.

Jenner adds to his remarks on the precautions to be observed in applying the variolous test, and advocates the more moderate method of Sutton.

The horse grease theory was supported by another case.

"An extensive inflammation of the erysipelatous kind appeared on the upper part of the thigh of a sucking colt, and terminated in the formation of abscesses. Those who dressed the inflamed parts milked the cows. They all had Cow Pox, and the milkers were infected also."

Jenner adds:—

"That the disease produced upon the cows by the colt, and from thence conveyed to those who milked them, was the *true* and not the *spurious* Cow Pox there can be scarcely any room for suspicion; yet it would have been more completely satisfactory had the effects of variolous matter been ascertained on the farmer's wife, but there was a peculiarity in her situation which prevented my making the experiment."

The *Inquiry* concludes with the following paragraph:—

"Thus far have I proceeded in an inquiry founded, as it must appear, on the basis of experiment; in which, however, conjectures have been occasionally admitted, in order to present to persons, well situated for such discussions, objects for a more minute investigation. In the meantime, I shall myself continue to prosecute this inquiry, encouraged by the hope of its becoming essentially beneficial to mankind."

We may now sum up the cases which were added to the original paper.

CASUAL COW POX.

Name.	Inoculated with Small Pox.	Date of Cow Pox.
William Stinchcomb . . .	1792 . .	. 10 years previously.
Hester Walkley	1795 . .	. 13 ,, ,,
Seven paupers of Totworth .	1795 . .	. "different period: .
Sarah Nelmes	—— . .	. May 1796.

CASUAL HORSE GREASE.

Name.								*Date of Horse Grease.*
Thomas Virgoe	.	.	.	.	.	.	.	February 1798.
William Wherret	.	.	.	.	.	.	.	
William Haynes	.	.	.	.	.	.	.	

INOCULATED HORSE GREASE (EQUINE DIRECT).

John Baker	.	.	.	.	.	.	.	March 16th, 1798 (Died).

INOCULATED HORSE GREASE (EQUINE INDIRECT).

William Summers . . . . March 16th, 1798.

William Pead . . . . March 28th, ,,

Hannah Excell (and several other children and adults) } . . . . . . April 5th.

John Marklove   Robert F. Jenner   Mary Pead   Mary James   . . April 12th.

J. Barge

In the previous chapter, I have analysed the contents of Jenner's original paper, and concluded that the Council of the Royal Society was perfectly justified in rejecting it. It is true that in the original paper, Jenner could lay claim to priority of *publication* of an account of the symptoms of the casual Cow Pox in the cow and in man, but he could not lay claim to the theory of the origin of Cow Pox from grease. He could lay claim to being the first *to publish* the experimental transmission of Cow Pox to the human subject. We have now to consider whether the additions to the paper, when published, contained anything which could be claimed as a discovery. This was undoubtedly the case. He could lay claim to the discovery that Horse Pox, like Small Pox, could be

carried on from arm to arm, through a number of
individuals, a fact which, so far as we know, was new to
the traditions and experience of the country people.

That this is a just estimate of what was original
in his work, is verified by the fact that when Jenner
published his account of the origin of the vaccine
inoculation, he laid no claim to the discovery of Cow
Pox or of its alleged protection against Small Pox,
but only that it could be experimentally inoculated in
the human subject.

"During the investigation of the casual Cow Pox, I was struck
with the idea that it might be practicable to propagate the disease
by inoculation after the manner of the Small Pox, first from the
cow, and finally from one human being to another."

In the propagation, by inoculation, from the cow to
the human subject, he had been anticipated by Jesty
and others ; so that the two main points of the inquiry
were, that he was the first to carry on a series of
arm to arm equinations, and he was the first to
advocate *in print* the adoption of this new inoculation.

We are now in a position to estimate what Jenner's
researches amounted to, up to the time of the inquiry.
Jenner himself gives 1776 as the date of the commencement of his inquiry, and says nothing of the
Sodbury incident. In this year, inoculation by the
Suttonian method became very general in Gloucestershire. Jenner's attention was drawn to a case of
insusceptibility which, in accordance with the provincial

rumour, was attributed to a previous attack of Cow Pox.
But he does not appear to have paid much attention to
the subject until 1780, when he repeated the provincial
tradition in London, and showed a drawing of the
eruption on the hand of a milker. But about
1791 (about seven years before the publication of the
Inquiry), he had again turned his attention to Cow
Pox, and between 1791 and 1795, he had collected
four more cases of insusceptibility to the inoculated
Small Pox.

In 1790, Cow Pox broke out in a dairy near Berkeley,
and Jenner took the opportunity to inoculate Phipps.
Then his inquiries were stopped until 1798, when horse
grease broke out at a neighbouring farm, and John
Baker was inoculated and died. William Summers,
inoculated with horse grease passed through the cow,
survived, and the virus was carried on from arm to
arm through several patients.

The cases are carelessly jumbled together ; important
details are often missing ; dates are omitted ; facts unfavourable to the project are suppressed ; and excuses
for failures are ingeniously incorporated. All that the
Inquiry contained was known to dairymaids and farriers,
with the exception of the doctrine of spurious Cow
Pox, and certain speculative comments. All that was
added experimentally, to what had been previously
practised, was the inoculation of Horse Pox from arm
to arm, in imitation of arm to arm variolation. Up to

the year 1796, Jenner had simply collected notes of
a few cases of milkers and others, who had had
either Horse Pox or Cow Pox, and had resisted inoculation with Small Pox, and Fosbrooke tells us that
up to this date he was not burdened with work. In
the same year, he made ONE EXPERIMENT of inoculation
on the human subject, and hurriedly wrote a paper
which was rejected by the Royal Society. Two years
later, he carried on a series of arm to arm inoculations,
and then published the *Inquiry* on his own account.

These are the dry facts of the case, which Baron
sums up as follows :—

" If we look at the origin of this discovery from its first dawning
in his youthful mind at Sodbury, and trace it through its subsequent stages—his meditations at Berkeley—his suggestions to his
great master, John Hunter—his conferences with his professional
brethren in the country—his hopes and fears, as his inquiries and
experiments encouraged or depressed his anticipations—and, at
length, **the triumphant conclusion of more than thirty years' reflection
and study, by the successful vaccination of his first patient, Phipps ;
we shall find a train of preparation never exceeded in any scientific
enterprise ;** and in some degree commensurate with the great
results by which it has been followed.

And in more recent times this extraordinary out-
burst of rhetoric has been officially endorsed.[1]

" Among the dairy-folks of Gloucestershire there was a curious
tradition . . . that persons who had suffered from this Cow Pox,
as it was called, were by it rendered insusceptible of Small Pox.

Simon. *History and Practice of Vaccination.* 1857.

Words to this effect were once spoken in the hearing of EDWARD JENNER, then a village doctor's apprentice in the neighbourhood of Bristol. They were never afterwards absent from his mind. **Thirty years elapsed before their fruit was borne to the public; but incessantly he thought and watched and experimented on the subject**; and the work on which at length he recorded the incomparable results of his labour may well have commanded the confidence of reflecting persons.

"Little would ever be heard of objections to vaccination if all who undertake the responsibility of its performance, and all who feel disposed to resist its adoption would but thoroughly study that **masterpiece of medical induction**, and imitate the **patience and caution and modesty** with which Jenner laid the foundation of every statement he advanced.

CHAPTER IX.

HUMAN SMALL POX AS A SOURCE OF " VACCINE LYMPH."

SYDENHAM was the first to distinguish different varieties of Small Pox. Adams[1] experienced outbreaks of what the nurses called the *white sort*, which he believed to be the same as a variety mentioned by Sydenham, which left no marks. A similar outbreak which prevailed in Gloucestershire was referred to by Jenner. The attack was as mild as in the inoculated Small Pox, and the lower classes of people were so little afraid of it that social intercourse was maintained as usual. The nurses and common people called it the Swine or Pig Pox.

According to Adams, the pustules of this variety are never very large, but round and uniform in proportion as the disease is well marked. As they increase, the upper surface extends over the base, and as they dry, the scab becomes nearly globular. The scab is of a pale amber colour, and dries much harder than in the common distinct disease. From the figure,

---

[1] Adams. *A Popular View of Vaccine Inoculation.* 1807.

colour, and other properties preserved throughout the whole progress, Adams called this variety the *pearl sort*.

In the chapters on Small Pox inoculation, I have drawn attention not only to the various methods of inoculation, but also to the different results which followed the employment of virus of different strengths.

Inoculators had learnt by experience that it was not advisable to take matter from the confluent Small Pox, as a severe attack would probably follow ; and, therefore, in the directions given, it is constantly recommended that *a mild sort of Small Pox* should alone be used. In the hands of the Suttons, inoculation became still milder, because they were always careful to inoculate with variolous *lymph ;* and as Sutton was said to have been more successful in his early practice, it is probable that the success largely depended upon the accidental circumstance of having first started his inoculations with matter from an outbreak of a very mild Small Pox, and the mild character of this variety was, for a time, successfully propagated from arm to arm. Adams[1] obtained still more striking results, which I will relate in his own words.

" By continuing with great caution to inoculate at the hospital from pearl Small Pox, and afterwards by selecting those arms which had the most appearance of Cow Pox, we at last succeeded in procuring a succession of arms so nearly resembling the vaccine, that an universal suspicion prevailed among the parents, that

[1] Adams, *loc. cit.*, p. 27.

VIII.th day.

VII.th day.

XII.th day.

XX.th day.

COW POX.   SMALL POX.

(BALLHORN AND STROMEYER).

they were deceived by the substitution of one for the other. This
will be readily understood by the following register :

" REGISTER I.

"August 14th, 1805, William Croft was inoculated, with several
others, from a subject who had casual Small Pox. Croft had
diarrhœa three days after he was inoculated, a circumstance in
children often favourable for the future disease.

" On the 3rd day, the insertion appeared elevated.

" 6th, a vesicle.

" 8th, the vesicle spread.

" 10th, has a vaccine appearance with fever.

" 13th, one hundred and fifty pustules appeared which passed
regularly through their stages, somewhat shortened, as often
happens in inoculation.

" Rogers was inoculated 26th August, from Croft, in two places.
Only one took effect, which was perfectly vaccine in all its stages.
The child had been previously ill, so that it was difficult to
ascertain whether any or what degree of constitutional disorder
was produced by the inoculation.

" Mary Ann Dobins, having been previously inoculated from
Croft without effect, was,

"September 2nd, inoculated from Rogers. The arm proved
vaccine in all its stages.

" On the same day, were inoculated from Rogers—

" I. Richard Jude. His arm was vaccine in every stage.

" On the 13th day, as the arm was drying, appeared one hundred
and fifty variolous pustules.

" II. Eleanor Watts. Arm vaccine.

" Pustules appeared on the 11th day.

" On the 13th, five hundred were counted; all maturated, but
dried early.

" III. Elizabeth Gray. Her arm regularly vaccine to the 8th
day.

" On the 10th, appeared stationary, in consequence of which
inoculation was repeated from Edward Christian's arm, who had
been inoculated twelve days.

" 12th day, the arm first inoculated retains its vaccine appearance, though somewhat jagged with elevations round the vesicle. She had fever the day before, and pustules first appeared on the body.

" 13th, the arm retains its circumscription, but is yellow. The fever considerable all night.

" 14th, the first inoculation dry; the second contains a yellow crystalline lymph with areola. Has upwards of sixty small circumscribed pustules.

" 15th, arms drying, pustules suppurating.

" 19th, pustules drying.

" 22nd, scabbed.

" IV. Thomas Dyson. His arm was perfectly vaccine in all its stages.

" 10th day, a few pustules appeared ; had been sick on the 9th evening.

" 12th day, the arm drying.

" From Dobins, seven were inoculated ; of these

" Five had no eruption ; the arms were vaccine in all the stages, and in the appearance of the scab.

" One had a perfectly vaccine appearance on the arm, areola, and brown scab, with one hundred variolous pustules, which appeared on the 12th day, and began to dry on the 16th ; but the desiccation was not completed till the 29th, when the appearance was horny.

" The other had a vaccine arm somewhat irregular, with fever, but no pustules.

" From the last, were inoculated four.

" Of these, two had vaccine arms, perfect in all their stages, and without pustules.

" One had the vaccine vesicle regular, excepting that the edges sloped in such a manner, that the base was broader than the apex. The top was, however, flat, and the whole appearance such as occasionally occurs in the genuine vaccine.

" The other had small pustules, which dried, as well as the place of insertion, by the 15th.

" Elizabeth Gray, we have observed, had pustules. Two were inoculated from her arm, and two from her pustules.

" The two from the arm had the legitimate vaccine appearance.

" One, from the pustules, had fever with general efflorescence.

"The other had all the symptoms of vaccination, with the areola; but the contents of the vesicle became yellow before it dried.

"It is unnecessary, in this place, to pursue this register any further. Suffice it to say that the enemies to vaccination, about this time, excited so great a clamour that every mother was suspicious lest her child should be clandestinely inoculated with the Cow Pox; and even those who saw matter taken from secondary pustules, and applied to the arm, were scarcely satisfied unless their own children had unequivocal symptoms of Small Pox. Reflecting, therefore, that an event of this kind must either occur again, or be unsatisfactory from being unsupported, we contented ourselves with the record preserved in the register, waiting till it should be explained by subsequent occurrences.

"This is not the only time that we have been interrupted in our attempt to perpetuate a favourable Small Pox. For though it was urged to the parents, that before the discovery of Cow Pox, the inoculation of the Small Pox was sometimes only followed by a pustule at the arm, with the attendant fever; yet the suspicions of many were equal to their prejudices : nothing less than secondary pustules would satisfy them, and some even expressed their doubts, if the eruption was scanty or disappeared early."

It was not until many years afterwards, that Guillon[1] also, found that a vesicle, with the physical characters of the vaccine vesicle, could be raised from Small Pox by cultivation.

Dr. Thiele, of Kasan, in 1839, succeeded in the following manner. Lymph from human Small Pox was allowed to remain, for ten days between slips of glass fastened together with wax. The

---

[1] *The London Medical Repository and Review*, p. 426. 1827.

virus was then diluted with warm cow's milk, and inoculated like ordinary vaccine lymph. Large vesicles resulted. There were febrile symptoms from the third to the fourth day, and a secondary onset of fever, much more pronounced, between the eleventh and the fourteenth days. The areola was strongly marked, and not confined to the inoculated place which was occasionally surrounded by minute secondary vesicles. The scar was larger and deeper than usual, and the edges occasionally sharply defined.

If watched through ten removes, the vesicles were found gradually to assume all the classical characters of the vaccine vesicle. As soon as the secondary fever ceased to occur, inoculation from arm to arm was practised without diluting the lymph with cow's milk.

This variety of vaccine lymph was, later, designated *lacto-varioline*. That a " vaccine vesicle " could be produced direct from human Small Pox, without, that is to say, the intervention of the cow, was regarded as an extraordinary and novel fact. But the results were precisely the same as those obtained by Adams and by Guillon, which, so far as I am aware, had been entirely overlooked. The production of a " vaccine vesicle " from a mixture of variolous lymph and milk was not vaccination in the strict meaning of that term, but simply *variolation* in an extremely mild form.

Precisely similar results were obtained by Gassner

in 1801, who succeeded in reducing the effects of Small
Pox virus to the production of " vaccine vesicles " on
one out of eleven cows which had been inoculated.

The ordinary phenomena of vaccination were observed in four children inoculated from this cow,
and similar results followed in seventeen children
inoculated from them.

In 1828, Dr. McMichael reported to the Royal
College of Physicians that several physicians in Egypt,
had succeeded in raising " vaccine lymph " by inoculation of cows with Small Pox, and that children were
successfully " vaccinated."

In 1830, Dr. Sonderland, of Barmen, claimed to
have produced vaccine in cows by infection from
human Small Pox. An account of these experiments
was published in the *Medical Repository*, with the
following introduction :—

"The author of the paper which we shall here translate
almost without abridgement, if his experiment be correct, has
at length succeeded in establishing what physicians have long
laboured to discover, a satisfactory and simple explanation of
the protective power of Cow Pox against Small Pox, and, as
announced, we will venture to say, the most important discovery
which has been made in the pathology of these diseases since
vaccination was first introduced, by showing that they are
modifications of one another, and that Cow Pox in the cows
is simply Small Pox in man, and may be produced in that
animal at will by the variolous contagion. Of the authenticity
of his facts we don't pretend to judge ; all we can say is that
the author, if we judge from the language of Boufleu towards
him, is a respectable practitioner, and a public medical officer."

" 'The simplest and surest mode of producing Cow Pox in the cow, and thus proving indisputably the identity between the contagion of Cow Pox and that of human Small Pox, is to follow the procedure here laid down. Take a woollen bedcover which has lain on the bed of a Small Pox patient who has died during the suppurating stage, or is suffering from the disease in a considerable degree, and is lying in a small imperfectly-ventilated apartment; and, when it is well penetrated by the contagion, roll it up immediately after death or the fourteenth day of the disease; wrap it in a linen cloth, and then spread for twenty-four hours on the back of a quey in such manner that it cannot be thrown off by the animal, then place it for twenty-four hours on the backs of each of three other queys, and afterwards hang in such manner in their stalls that its exhalation may rise upwards and be inhaled by them. In a few days the animal will fall sick and be seized with fever; and on the fourth or fifth day, the udders, and other parts covered with hard skin, will present an eruption of pustules which assume the well-known appearance of Cow Pox, and become filled with lymph. This lymph, which exactly resembles the lymph of genuine Cow Pox, if used for inoculating the human subject, will induce the vaccine or protective pock. The only precaution which it is necessary to observe is that the person about to be inoculated should not be exposed in any manner to the contagious effluvia of the cow-house, either directly or during the intervention of the experimentalist's clothes, otherwise he may have natural Small Pox. A bedcover, impregnated with the variolous contagion, if firmly rolled up and wrapped in linen, and afterwards in paper, and then properly packed in a bucket, will retain the contagion for at least two years, so as to infect the cow with Cow Pox, provided it can be kept in a cool shady place, where the temperature does not fall under thirty-two, or above fifty-two, degrees.

" 'My present occupations prevent me at this particular period from giving a full and scientific exposition of the consequences which must follow from this discovery, but I may state them shortly in the aphoristic form :—

" ' 1. This discovery is new; for, although many have suspected the identity of Small Pox in man and Cow Pox in the cow, and have in consequence performed inoculation with the matter of both, yet no one has previously ascertained the possibility of transmitting the contagion to the cow in the gaseous form so as to decide the question beyond all doubt.

" ' 2. The desire of physicians and governments to discover Cow Pox in cows, in order to revive the vaccine lymph is more than fulfilled by the discovery of a simple method of engendering Cow Pox into the cow at will.

" ' 3. Jenner's discovery of the protective power of vaccination hitherto imperfect, is now perfected, because the previously unknown nature and origin of Cow Pox are laid open.

" ' 4. All previous uncertainty regarding the quality of vaccine matter, its degeneration, the loss of its protective property, and the like, must now cease, because we have obtained a clear insight into the nature of Cow Pox, and can lay down a substantial theory of its operation.

" ' 5. This discovery must tend to widen the boundaries of physiology, pathology, and therapeutics, since it shows how the subtle contagion of Small Pox was hostile to the nervous system of man; may be conveyed in the aeriform state from him to the cow, and excite in that animal a similar disease; but in doing so, be changed by the special constitution of this class of animal into a permanent contagion of a different kind.

" ' 6. An instructive lesson may be drawn from this discovery, how the poison of diseases in the gaseous form may be communicated to the lower animals, and according to the difference in their constitution, engender diversified products which may then be used as protective means against the diseases from which they originated. Such, for example, may be subsequently proved of scarlet fever, measles, yellow fever, and plague.

" ' 7. It is now clear why, in recent times, Cow Pox has been seldom or never seen in the cow; for the Cow Pox of the cow arises merely from infection by the variolous exhalations from men recently affected with Small Pox and coming in contact with the cow. As epidemics of Small Pox have been rare during the last thirty years, cows could seldom be exposed to infection, and have therefore seldom exhibited the disease.' "

Although attempts to confirm Dr. Sonderland's experiments failed in the hands of Ceely in England, and Macpherson and Lamb in India, and at Alfort, Berlin, Weimar, Bergen, Dresden, Kasan, Utrecht, and Stockholm on the Continent; nevertheless, his aphorisms were accepted in support of the theory, the popular doctrine of the present day, that Cow Pox is Small Pox, modified by transmission through the cow. Had Dr. Sonderland and his followers been acquainted with the characters of the *natural* Cow Pox, and had they appreciated the fact that a vesicle with the physical characters of the vaccine vesicle, could be produced on the human subject, by management of variolous lymph without the intervention of the cow, they could hardly have come to such a conclusion. But this doctrine, owing to the explanation it afforded of the alleged protective power of Cow Pox against Small Pox, was a most seductive one. It was very widely accepted, and led to a complete misinterpretation of the successful variolation experiments which followed.

Dr. Thiele made a number of attempts to inoculate *cows* with variolous virus, and, at last, succeeded in producing a vesicle with the physical characters of the vaccine vesicle. From this he raised a stock of lymph, which at the time of his publication had passed through seventy-five generations, and had been used for the " vaccination " of over three thousand individuals. Thiele succeeded in confirming his first results. He insisted upon the necessity of selecting the animals. Cows from four to six years old, which had recently calved, and those with delicate pink skins, were preferred. The udder was shaved, and variolous *lymph* was alone employed, and the animals were exposed to a proper temperature (15° R.).

Before Dr. Thiele's experiments were published in this country, Mr. Ceely of Aylesbury, impressed with Dr. Sonderland's seventh aphorism, and *influenced by the strong presumptive evidence of Baron* that Small Pox had been common to men and brutes, determined to test the validity of Dr. Sonderland's experiments.

Attempts to infect cows by enveloping them with the sheets and blankets of Small Pox patients were without result. Ceely nevertheless persevered, and proceeded to try the effect of variolous *inoculation*.

In order to avoid all sources of error, Ceely himself took the Small Pox virus in the presence of his assistant, Mr. Taylor, on points that could never have been used before, as they were the teeth of a large comb cut for the purpose. Lymph was also collected in *new* capillary tubes. This lymph was inoculated on one side of the vulva of a heifer, and Cow Pox lymph on the other. One of the variolous punctures developed into an enormous vesicle, very unlike an ordinary vaccine vesicle. There can be no doubt that Ceely succeeded in raising a *variolous* vesicle. But it is

very commonly supposed to have had a vaccinal
origin, from the lancets having been mixed, or th
vaccine transferred to the opposite side by the anim
tail.

The variolous character of this vesicle was
borne out by the result of the accidental ino
of his assistant.

"My assistant, Mr. Taylor, to whom I had entrusted
used in opening the variolous vesicle in the first exp(
the tenth day, while I was engaged in the tedious
charging points thereform, punctured the skin of his
between the thumb and forefinger, with the instrun
moist with lymph, a circumstance with which at the time I ..
unacquainted. On the fourth day afterwards, he directed my
attention to a hard, deep red, papular elevation on the spot,
stating the cause, and at the same time assuring me that he had
been vaccinated in infancy, and had subsequently had modified
Small Pox. On the fifth day, there was a papulo-vesicular elevation, surrounded with a dark red areola, and much uneasiness
in the part. In the evening, headache and other febrile symptoms
appeared, with roseola and fiery red papulæ on the face and
other parts. On the sixth day, a more diffused and lighter areola
surrounded the less abrupt elevation, which was now more perfectly vesicular ; the constitutional symptoms increased, and the
papulæ, on the face, neck, trunk, and limbs, exhibited ash-coloured
summits, and, through a lens, appeared to have slight central
depressions. On the seventh day, it was manifest that the
disease had reach its acme on the previous day. The areola
was diminished, the vesicle was more apparent, some of the
papulæ presented straw-coloured summits, and the roseola was
declining, with an abatement of the febrile symptoms, a diminution of the tenderness of the axilla. On the eighth day, all these
changes were more obvious, although he was not free from headache ; the papulæ were more yellow and some were desiccating ;

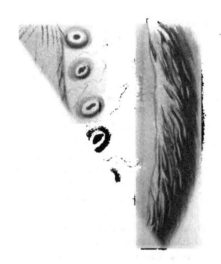

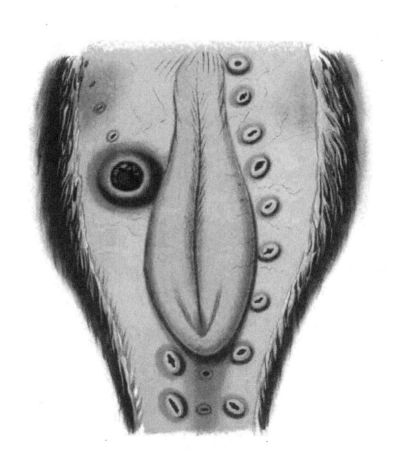

VARIOLATION OF THE COW (CEELY).

the vesicles were larger but less active, and the areola was comparatively pale."

Chauveau, also, is of opinion that Mr. Taylor had an attack of Small Pox, and no doubt this is the true interpretation of what occurred. But Ceely's eyes were blinded by Sonderland's seventh aphorism. He looked upon this giant vesicle as the experimental confirmation of the doctrine that Cow Pox is modified Small Pox, and hence the opinion he expressed of Mr. Taylor's case, "this was evidently modified vaccine in a sanguine habit, with roseola and vesicular or vaccine lichen."

Points charged with lymph from the variolous vesicle were used on children. " Vaccine vesicles " were produced with the primary constitutional symptoms slight, and the secondary, proportioned to the extent and character of the areola. One child who suffered severely, had vomiting and delirium and extensive roseola, but no eruption was observed in any other case.

In December, 1840, Mr. Badcock,[1] of Brighton, quite independently of Ceely, succeeded in variolating a cow. He was led to undertake the experiment from having suffered from a dangerous attack of Small Pox in 1836, which impressed his mind with the view " that the old vaccine had lost its protective influence by passing through so many constitutions." After making inquiries with a view to raising a

[1] Vol. ii., p. 513 *et seq.*

fresh stock of vaccine from the cow, he came to the conclusion that the only satisfactory way would be to inoculate a cow with Small Pox matter. In the month of December 1840, he inoculated a fine young cow, on the teats and on the external labium, with Small Pox virus. No details of the operation have been recorded, but the result was successful. There was one well-developed vesicle on the external labium, and the lymph from it was employed by Badcock for " vaccinating " his son. The case excited considerable interest, and more than thirty members of the profession examined the boy. In four years, Badcock was able to repeat this experiment upon upwards of ninety cows, and, from occasional successful cases, to raise fresh supplies of " vaccine." According to the testimonials published by Badcock, there were slight differences observed, by several physicians, on comparing the vesicles with those produced by the current vaccine lymph. Badcock ultimately successfully variolated 37 out of 200 cows experimented upon. The vesicles were only perfect in 33, and these cases furnished lymph for 400 practitioners. In 1857, it was estimated that 14,000 people had been " vaccinated " with Badcock's lymph, and subsequently it was stated that Badcock himself had " vaccinated " upwards of 20,000 individuals.

It is quite a mistake to speak of this operation as *vaccination.* This method was simply a modification

of the Suttonian system of Small Pox inoculation,
in which, in the first remove, the cow was substituted
for the human subject. I repeat, that all those who
have been inoculated with Ceely's or Badcock's
" variola-vaccine " lymph have not, in the true sense
of the word, been *vaccinated; they have not been Cow
Poxed, but they have been variolated.* This is amply
verified by the results which have followed in the
hands of others who have variolated cows, and used
the products for " vaccination."

In 1836, Dr. Martin, of Attleborough, Mass., inoculated the cow's udder with variolous lymph, and by
inoculating children from the variolated cow, produced
an epidemic of Small Pox with fatal cases.

In 1839, Reiter, of Munich, after fifty unsuccessful
attempts, succeeded in producing a vesicle with all
the characters of the vaccine vesicle. The variolous
lymph which had been employed in that case, when
inoculated into another cow, gave rise to results
similar to those obtained by Chauveau. A child inoculated from the *successful* vesicle, contracted Small
Pox.

In 1847, variolation of the cow was successfully
performed at Berlin, but the products inoculated in
the human subject resulted in retro-variolisation, and
one of the experimental children died of confluent
Small Pox.

In 1864, the Lyons Commission encountered similar

disasters. Chauveau, in his classical experiments, made in the name of the Lyons Commission, 1863 — 1865, inoculated seventeen animals with virulent variolous lymph (*en pleine activité*). He obtained very small papules, which became insignificant in the second remove. The contents of these papules inoculated into children always produced Small Pox, which recalled, in its course, the results obtained by the early inoculators of Small Pox. One of the children transmitted Small Pox to another child, who communicated it to the mother. Some of the children died. In 1871, Chauveau produced precisely similar results. He inoculated Small Pox and Cow Pox on the same animal. The Small Pox virus still produced Small Pox, and the Cow Pox virus produced Cow Pox. The two viruses mixed and inoculated in bovines engendered Cow Pox only ; and a similar result was obtained in children after six successive transmissions through the cow. Chauveau therefore believes in the autonomy of Cow Pox ; in other words, in the impossibility of transforming Small Pox into Cow Pox.

More recently, Voit, at the vaccination station at Hamburg, succeeded in producing " variola-vaccine." He inoculated a calf with Small Pox lymph and Cow Pox lymph, on parts of the body far distant from each other. The variolous lymph had been collected on the fourth day. The Cow Pox took feebly ; the punctures, for the most part, were abortive, but those which

developed, took the ordinary course. Of five inoculations with variolous lymph, four failed entirely, the
fifth was transformed into a large, round, greyish
vesicle, flattened, but not umbilicated. On the sixth
day, it measured six millimetres. The areola was
indistinct. It was excised on the sixth day, and the
contents inoculated on the scrotum of a calf, three
months old, and very fine vesicles, with the characters
of vaccine vesicles, resulted. After successive cultivation on calves through twenty generations, the only
difference in this virus from ordinary vaccine lymph
was its slightly greater activity. But lymph taken from
the second remove produced, in a child, marked fever
after the sixth day, and acute eczema on the left
knee ; on the ninth day, swollen glands in the axilla,
and on the twelfth and sixteenth, eruptions (*petites
nodosités disseminés*), which indicated its true variolous
character.

The lymph from the third remove of calves, inoculated on four children, produced in three, serious
complications, erysipelas, angina, and pneumonia. With
lymph of the eighth remove, accidents continued to
follow, but happily no deaths occurred. Voit was of
opinion that the pustulous eruptions (*pustules de
variola-vaccine*) which resulted on inoculation of the
variolous virus in a cow, was true Small Pox of the
cow, and that the nodular exanthem described by
Chauveau was to be considered as an abortive form.

From the mere resemblance which existed between late removes of "variola-vaccine" and ordinary vaccine, Voit believed that he had succeeded in transforming Small Pox into Cow Pox. Voit was misled by appearances, in precisely the same way as Ceely, and others who have succeeded in reducing Small Pox to the appearances of a vaccine vesicle. The true variolous character of the "variola-vaccine" lymph, and the tendency, in less early removes, to produce Small Pox, is probably the reason why Voit has abandoned its use, in favour, as I am informed by M. Layet, of the ordinary spontaneous Cow Pox lymph, from the vaccination station at Rotterdam.

The doctrine that Cow Pox is modified Small Pox was adhered to with extraordinary tenacity, and it became the official dogma that, as Small Pox protected against Small Pox, so Cow Pox, being modified Small Pox, must of necessity protect against Small Pox. Even distinguished pathologists and scientists were misled, and the doctrine was all the more acceptable in that it met a host of objections. It is interesting now to look back and see the reception meted out to Chauveau's opposite conclusions. Dr. Seaton, for example, in his *Handbook of Vaccination*, 1865, thus speaks of M. Chauveau's experiments :—

"With serosity taken from one of the cows and one of the horses, local vesicles, followed by general varioliform eruption, were in fact produced on three children, and from these children other variolous inoculations were performed. These results are regarded by the experimenters as showing that the inoculation of variola on horses and cows produces a true variolous infection, and that the organism of these animals is therefore incapable of transforming variola into vaccine. But they do not appear to me to lead at all necessarily to the conclusions thus drawn. The local effects produced by these inoculations were not in any respect greater than those produced by Ceely in cases which he regarded as failures, nor than the results which followed some variolous inoculations of horses (two) performed in 1863 by MM. Le Blanc and De Paul, which were regarded by them 'as unsuccessful. And it is not in the least improbable that if Mr. Ceely, or MM. Le Blanc and De Paul had, in the cases they describe, dealt with the tumid papules that arose as M. Chauveau and his colleagues did, they might have got from them the same stuff (*sic*) they had put in—stuff which had undergone no sort of transformation whatever, but which had lain where it was put as in a pouch, quite inert, giving rise only to local irritation, without inducing any sort of general affection or disease."

But Chauveau was perfectly correct. The eruption which follows inoculation of bovines with Small Pox, whether papular or vesicular, is still variolous. Ceely, Badcock, Chauveau, Voit, and others succeeded in *ingrafting* Small Pox on the cow, and when suitable lymph and suitable subjects were employed, a more or less benign vesicle resulted. And they ought to have known that similar results had been obtained on the human subject by Sutton and Dimsdale, and identical results by Adams, without transmission through the cow.

I, therefore, agree with Chauveau, with the exception of his statement that the persons so variolated must necessarily convey infection. This is only partly true; it is not necessarily the case, as is amply borne out by the experience with Badcock's lymph. In this case, there has been no tendency for the inoculated to spread variola by infection, proving that a strain of benign variolous lymph can be cultivated by judicious selection, and completely deprived of any infectious properties.

CHAPTER X.

CATTLE PLAGUE AS A SOURCE OF "VACCINE LYMPH."

BARON states in reference to the affinities alleged to exist between Cow Pox and Small Pox, that in no former instance did historical evidence and remarkable pathological phenomena so singularly and beneficially throw light on each other.

In this chapter, I propose to inquire into the historical evidence collected by Baron, and to ascertain whether his literary researches justified his opinion, and in what way they affected the practice of vaccination.

Jenner always considered that Small Pox and Cow Pox were modifications of the same distemper ; and Baron, in an elaborate dissertation, not only endeavours to justify, but to fully establish, the doctrine of *variolæ vaccinæ*. I have already pointed out the train of thought which led Jenner to speak of Cow Pox as variolæ vaccinæ. From the similarity of the inoculated Cow Pox to the inoculated Small Pox, he concluded that these two diseases were derived from a source in common. He believed that "grease," by successive transmission through the human subject, became Small Pox, but, transmitted through the cow, it manifested itself in the form of Cow Pox. Cow Pox might, therefore, in this sense be regarded as Small Pox of the cow.

Baron took an entirely different ground for the establishment of this doctrine. He reasoned in this way. Eruptive diseases affecting man and the lower animals, had been known at different times, and in different countries. Just as there were numerous writers on Small Pox in man, so there were also many who had described an eruptive, pestilential disease existing among animals, especially cattle, to which they applied the name VARIOLA. The question then was whether the variolæ of men and of the lower animals were essentially and originally the same.

In order to elucidate this question, Baron[1] made an elaborate investigation into the history of this cattle disease. He quotes Lancisi, who asserted in his treatise, *De Bovilla Peste*, that this disease among horned cattle was epidemic in the Papal Territory in 1713 and 1714, and was similar to the outbreak which occurred in Italy nearly two centuries before, of which Frascatorius had given a description. In 1690, Ramazzini described this disease, and gave the following account of an outbreak in Italy in 1711 :—

---

[1] Baron, *loc. cit.*

" The kind of affection which seemed to have declared exterminating war on the whole race of oxen, was evidently a
malignant, destructive, and (if you will) a pestilential fever
commencing with chills, rigor, horripilatio, succeeded quickly by
pungent, violent heat diffused over the whole body, with frequency
of pulse, and accompanied by great anxiety and heavy panting,
together with stertor, and, in the commencement of the fever, with
stupor and a kind of lethargy ; a continual flow of stinking matter
from the mouth and nostrils ; a most fœtid discharge from the
bowels, and this at times bloody ; loss of appetite and rumination
was altogether destroyed ; on the fifth, or sixth day, pustules
broke out over the whole body of the animal, and tubercles
resembling *variolæ* in kind and appearance ; death common to
all, and in the same manner, about the fifth or seventh day ; a
very few escaped, and these rather by chance than the efficacy
of any remedies."

Baron also quotes from the account published by
Dr. Layard in the *Philosophical Transactions for* 1780.

" The disease among horned cattle is an eruptive fever of the
variolous kind : it bears all the characteristic symptoms, crisis
and event of the *Small Pox;* and whether received by contagion,
or by inoculation, has the same appearance, stages, and determination, except more favourable by inoculation, and with this
distinctive and decisive property, that a beast once having had
the sickness, naturally or artificially, never has it a second time.

" According to the several prejudices of different countries,
various opinions have arisen of the nature of this sickness. Such
as are averse to inoculation, have obstinately refused to acknowledge it was similar to the Small Pox in the human body, and
have very idly asserted, that the only intention of declaring this
contagion to be a species of Small Pox, was purposely, and with
no other view than to promote inoculation for the Small Pox.
Others have as positively declared it to be a pestilential putrid
fever, owing to a corrupted atmosphere, and arising from infected
pastures. But unfortunately for the supporters of this opinion,
while the contagious distemper raged with the utmost violence

on the coasts of Friesland, North and South Holland, Zealand, and Flanders there was not the least appearance of it on the English coast, from the North Foreland to the Humber, although the coast and climate are the same."

This destructive disease, so graphically described by Dr. Layard, appears to have been first noticed in England in the year 1745, and it was said to have been imported from Holland. I may continue Baron's argument in his own words.

"When Dr. Layard wrote, it was of less importance than it is now, to illustrate the connection between the diseases of man and the inferior animals; no trials, therefore, were made to ascertain whether the *variolæ* of man could be communicated to the brute, or *vice versâ.* The discovery of the Variolæ Vaccinæ has fully established the latter point; and although attempts to demonstrate the former have failed in the hands of some, other investigators have been more successful. . . . It was quite unlooked for, and at first almost an incredible thing that a disorder immediately derived from one of our domestic animals should exert an influence so powerful and so beneficial on the human frame. But if it should appear that the disease incident to man and to beasts, had one common origin, and that an analogy, close and well-defined, may be traced in their subsequent history and progress, we shall have obtained evidence to explain pathological facts which are of the utmost value to mankind.

"From what has been adduced, it is clear that a fatal, pestilential, eruptive disease, common to man and the inferior animals, has been known from the earliest period of authentic history; that the same, or at least a disease somewhat similar, continues to exist in various regions of the earth, often attended with great mortality. That it appears to have undergone various modifications in respect to virulence, and to be susceptible, by artificial communication, of still greater modifications.

"Should it appear that the views which I have attempted to illustrate rest upon a solid foundation, they will tend, I would

hope, to give a stability to the practice of vaccine inoculation
which was not formerly experienced. They will also explain
how sheep and horses or any other animals may be subject to
the disease as well as cows or oxen; that it is not a poison
peculiar only to one variety, but may be found and propagated
among many. It will not, therefore, excite surprise, that *matter*
capable of producing the genuine pustules should be found in
the horse, as it unquestionably has been in this country and
elsewhere; or that the disease should make its appearance among
sheep, as it is reported to do in Persia, and in goats in other
countries. . . .

"As the existence of the Variolæ Vaccinæ in the dairies of
England would seem not to have been of very long duration,
I think there is good ground for believing that the disease, as
originally noticed by Dr. Jenner in Gloucestershire, was the
endemic or local remains of the more general or epizootic disease
which prevailed in many parts of the island at the period when
Dr. Layard wrote."

Baron was Chairman of the Vaccination Committee
of the British Association, and in its report these
views are again brought forward, and there was no
hesitation in speaking of Cow Pox as *Cow Small Pox*.

In order to make this account agree, to some
extent, with Jenner's belief in the origin of Cow Pox
from the horse's heel, Baron says that he regarded
this doctrine as substantially true. He considered that
it had been established by unquestionable evidence
that matter from the horse produced a vesicle similar
in appearance to the vaccine vesicle; but, that this
fact, though it proved in his opinion the identity of
the diseases, did not establish the fact of their both
originating in the horse.

" It seems certain that there are, at least, four animals—the horse, the cow, the sheep, and the goat—which are affected with a disorder communicable to man, and capable of securing him from a malignant form of the same disease."

The disease which Baron was describing was not Cow Pox but cattle-plague, and the totally erroneous views into which he had drifted, arose from that initial nosological error committed by Jenner, who branded Cow Pox as *Variolæ Vaccinæ*, or Small Pox of the Cow. That cattle-plague has a close affinity with human Small Pox is perfectly true, but it has no relation or connection whatever with Cow Pox. I shall give a brief history of the disease referred to by Baron, and then I shall pass on to describe the disastrous results which followed the reception of the *variolæ vaccinæ* theory in India.

The outbreak of cattle-plague, described by Dr. Layard, commenced in England in 1745, and died out at the end of twelve years; it did not reappear until the summer of 1765. In 1769, the disease was again so prevalent and fatal as to be referred to by George III. in his speech at the opening of Parliament, in January 1770.

The resemblance of cattle-plague to human Small Pox had long been recognised, and this view was endorsed in more recent times by Murchison,[1] who regarded the analogy as very close. He pointed out that Small . Pox is the only acute contagious disease

---

[1] *Report* of the Commissioners appointed to inquire into the Origin and Nature, etc., of Cattle Plague, 1866, p. 74, *et seq*.

in man that assumes a pustular form. The eruption
in rinderpest also, consists of pustules and scabs, while
such differences as exist, may be explained by the
differences in the skin of man and cattle, and are not
greater than the differences which exist between varieties
of human Small Pox. Murchison continues :—

"In both, the eruption extends from the skin to the interior
of the mouth and nostrils; in both, the pustules and the scabs
are preceded or accompanied by patches of roseola; in both,
they are occasionally interspersed with petechiæ; and in both,
they sometimes leave behind pitted scars and discolorations on
the cutis. . . . The other prominent symptoms of rinderpest are
also those of Small Pox, viz., pyrexia, lumbar pain, saliva-
tion, and running from the nostrils; alvine flux, albuminuria,
hæmaturia, and 'the typhoid state.' The anatomical lesions
of the internal organs in rinderpest and unmodified Small
Pox are identical, viz., congestion or inflammation of the
mucous membranes of the air passages and digestive canal,
patches of ecchymosis and even gangrene of the stomachs, and
other mucous surfaces, and dark coloured blood. . . . In both
rinderpest and Small Pox, the duration of the pyrexial stage is on
an average about eight days. In both diseases, a peculiarly of-
fensive odour is exhaled from the body before and after death.
The perspiration and other secretions of healthy cattle smell very
differently from those of man, so that we can readily understand how the same disease may generate very different odours
in the two animals. It may be mentioned that a medical
correspondent in the country compared the smell of rinderpest
to that of human variola weeks before he was aware of the
intimate resemblance of the two maladies. . . . The two diseases
resemble one another in their extreme contagiousness, and in
the facility with which the poison is transmitted by fomites.
Both diseases can be easily propagated by inoculation, and in
both cases the inoculated disease is milder and less fatal than
that resulting from infection. In both diseases, there is a

period of incubation which is shorter when the poison has been introduced by inoculation than when it has been received by infection.   Vaccinated persons are constantly exposed to Small Pox poison with impunity; and with regard to rinderpest, there are numerous instances in which individual cattle or entire herds have appeared to lead charmed lives in the midst of surrounding pestilence.   This last fact has never been explained, but it would be readily accounted for on the supposition that rinderpest was the equivalent of Small Pox, and that the cattle who have enjoyed the immunity from it had previously suffered from ordinary Cow Pock."

Murchison admitted, that the theory that rinderpest was simply bovine Small Pox might be objected to, on the ground that there was no proof that it had communicated Small Pox to the human subject, and that, in fact, human Small Pox was far less prevalent in 1866, than it was a few years previously, when there was no rinderpest.   Ceely, however, like Baron, maintained that cattle-plague was simply malignant Cow Pox; and he did so principally from the fact that in the accidental transmission of rinderpest to the human subject, a vesicle was produced presenting the appearances, and running the ordinary course, of inoculated Cow Pox.   The following is the case as reported by Ceely[1]:—

"On the 3rd December, 1865, Mr. Henry Hancock, veterinary inspector, Uxbridge, was engaged in superintending the autopsy of a bullock, recently dead of cattle plague.   His assistant,

---

[1] *Notes of the History of the Case of Mr. Henry Hancock, Veterinary Surgeon and Inspector, Uxbridge,* drawn up by Robert Ceely, Esq.   [*Report* of the Commissioners, *loc cit*, p. 79.]

who was performing the operation, while occupied in removing the skin from the scrotum, accidentally punctured the back of Mr. Hancock's hand with the point of the knife. The puncture being slight, was disregarded at the time, but was washed as soon as practicable, and thought of no more. On the 8th, five days afterwards, a small, slightly elevated, hard pimple was felt and seen on the site of the puncture. This gradually advanced till the 9th day of the puncture, the 4th from papulation, when the enlargement became distinctly vesicular. At that time there were but slight constitutional symptoms. On the next day, the 10th from the receipt of the puncture, the 5th from papulation, and the 2nd from vesiculation, he called upon his friend Mr. Rayner, of Uxbridge, who, on seeing the hand, inquired if the patient had been handling the udder of a cow, for that he could recognise a Cow Pock vesicle of the 9th day. The vesicle was then distended with limpid lymph, its margin elevated and rather brown, centre depressed and rather brown, and was surrounded with a large bright red areola. There was then considerable tumefaction extending from the knuckles above the wrist. The absorbent vessels were considerably inflamed. They, and the axillary glands, were tender and painful ; the pulse, naturally slow, was accelerated ; there was much pain in the back and limbs, severe distracting headache, etc. ; all of which symptoms continued to increase during the two following days. At the end of that time the diffused areola had extended as far as the elbow. On the 18th December, fifteen days after the puncture, and ten days after papulation, the patient was seen in London by Drs. Klein and Murchison, and Professors Spooner and Simmonds. The local inflammation and the constitutional symptoms had partially subsided. The vesicle contained a rather turbid brownish fluid, and there were present all the indications of a declining vaccine vesicle. The above particulars were detailed to me by Mr. Hancock and Mr. Rayner on my visit to them at Uxbridge on the 20th December, and on my exhibiting the different phases of the vaccine vesicle on the hand of the milker (depicted in Plates III., IV., and V., in *Further Observations on the Variolæ Vaccinæ, Transactions of the Provincial*

Medical and Surgical Association, vol. x.),[1] Mr. Hancock immediately recognised there the exact correspondence with
those which occurred on his hand. On this day, December 20th,
being the 18th of the puncturation and the 13th of papulation,
I observed manifest declining œdema on the back of the
hand, as far as the elbow, with some patches here and there
of declining redness near it. The vesicle, which had been
many days poulticed, was depressed in the centre, puckered at
its margin, but still raised on a palpably firm basis. It
certainly exhibited the appearances I have often seen at a corresponding stage of the loose vascular skin on the back of the
hand of milkers affected with casual Cow Pox. A similar
vesicle I have depicted (Plate V., fig. 2)[2] in the work above
referred to. The conclusion drawn from the appearance of
the vesicle at this time was fortified by a consideration of the
history of its development. The late appearance after the
puncture, the tardy and gradual papulation and vesiculation,
the period of the advent of the areola, its progress, extent and
period of decline, all corresponding to those phenomena
resulting from the casual inoculation of the milker by the cow
affected with vaccinia. I could not, however, but regret that
lymph was not abstracted at the proper time with a view to
excluding all doubt as to its actual character."

Murchison, in describing this case, gives practically
the same account, with a few additional details. The
appearances, as well as the entire history, were very
different from the results of an ordinary poisoned
wound, but coincided with those observed after
vaccination. Murchison observed that Mr. Hancock
had been vaccinated in infancy, and had one good
vaccination mark upon his arm. In commenting
further upon the case, Murchison pointed out that

---

[1] *Vide* Plates XIII., XIV.   [2] Plate XIV., fig. 1.

there was no evidence of cattle-plague, or Cow Small
Pox, being transmitted by *infection* to man, but he
attributed this to a difficulty in transferring the disease from one species to another, and he considered
that it was, therefore, not surprising, on the supposition that rinderpest is a form of Small Pox, that
human beings have not suffered from it; but he adds,
it is not unreasonable to expect that inoculation of
human beings with the virus of rinderpest, unprotected
by vaccination, or by a previous attack of Small Pox,
may, now and then, produce results similar to those
obtained in India by Messrs. Macpherson, Brown, and
Furnell, and those recently observed in this country
in the case of Mr. Hancock, just as Small Pox in
man is transmitted with great difficulty back to cows.
Murchison concluded by pointing out that these
remarks were adduced not to prove the identity of
rinderpest and variola, or even that they were pathological equivalents, but to establish the very close
analogy between the two diseases.

It was not unnatural that Murchison should have
recommended vaccination as a prophylactic measure.
In a supplementary report we read :—

" Successful vaccination seemed to confer temporary immunity
from the cattle plague, for in certain herds the vaccinated cattle,
and they alone, escaped the disease. Further experience, however, has proved that this immunity, if real, is very transient.
Cattle that have been successfully vaccinated, and in which
the vaccination has run its course, when brought in contact

with animals suffering from cattle plague, or when inoculated with
the virus of cattle plague, have contracted the disease and died
of it. The obvious inference is, that notwithstanding the close
analogy between the cattle plague and human Small Pox, the
former disease, like the so-called Small Pox of sheep, is unin-
fluenced by ordinary vaccinia, and, like it therefore, is in all
probability a distinct species of disease from human Small Pox."

I will now pass on to describe the consequences in
India, of Jenner and Baron's teaching that the terms
Cow Pox and Cow Small Pox are interchangeable.

The cattle in Bengal were long subject to a malignant disease, which the natives designated by the same
term as human variola—viz., *Bussunt*, *Mhata* or *Gotee*.

When the medical men in India heard that the
source of vaccine lymph was a disease of cows with
an eruption on the udder, called Cow *Small* Pox,
it is not to be wondered at, that in order to raise
a stock of lymph they resorted to a disease which
had pustules on the udder, and was called Cow Small
Pox by the natives of India.

In 1832, a series of inoculations was performed by
Mr. Macpherson [1] in Bengal. I will give his account
in extenso, from the report which he furnished as
superintendent of vaccination at Moorshedabad.

"Small Pox raged with the most destructive virulence in
the city and vicinity during the months of May, June, July,
and August last; and soon after receiving the Board's instructions, I made many attempts to introduce the disease in cows

---

[1] *Transactions of the Medical and Physical Society of Calcutta*,
p. 169. 1883.

by exposing them to variolous contagion, covering them with the blankets of patients labouring under the disease, and by inoculation ; but all to no purpose, although, in these instances, the animals had very marked feverish symptoms, and in one those symptoms were followed by a few small ulcers on the abdomen, from which two cows were inoculated on the udder and teats; but no local or constitutional effects followed the operation or experiment.

" Finding I could not thus introduce variola I had two young cows inoculated with vaccine virus taken from the arm of a fine healthy child on the eighth day. Both cows had slight fever, and local inflammation on the third day. In one a vesicle formed on the fifth day, from which two children were inoculated, and in both instances the operation was followed by local and slight constitutional effects; but the pustules were elevated and opaque, they had no areola, and ran their course in five days, evidently spurious, consequently no attempt was made to carry this experiment farther. On inquiry among the natives, I learned that the cows in Bengal are subject to a disease which usually makes its appearance about the latter end of August or early in September, to which the same names are given as to variola in the human subject—viz., Bussunt, Mhata or Gotee, and on the 24th August, I was informed that several cows belonging to a native of Moidapore were affected. I consequently determined on again attempting to regenerate the vaccine virus from the original source. The animals which were first affected, amounting in one shed to eighteen or twenty, had been, for a day or two previously, dull and stupid ; they were always seized with distressing cough, and much phlegm collected in the mouth and fauces. The animals had apparently at this time no inclination for food, or, at all events, they were unable to satisfy their hunger. Their sufferings seemed to be greatest on the fifth and sixth days, when there was considerable fever, and pustules made their appearance all over the body, especially on the abdomen, which terminated in ulceration, the hair falling off wherever a pustule had run its course. The mouth and fauces appeared to be the principal seat of the disease, being in some instances one mass of ulceration, which in all probability extended to the stomach and alimentary canal. In those cases where the mouth was very much affected the animals died apparently from inanition; whereas those cases in which the power of mastication, or even of swallowing, was retained, recovered much more rapidly than might have been expected from the previous severe sufferings and reduced state of the animals. The mortality may be calculated at from 15 to 20 per cent. From the above description of the disease, the Board will immediately observe that it assumes a much more serious complexion in this country than we have been taught to believe it does at home. I say taught, because I presume it has fallen to the lot of few to witness the disease in England ; and it must be inferred from Dr. Jenner's and other medical writings on the subject that the animal not only continued to secrete milk, but that the milk was used; while in this country the little that is secreted is never made use of, and perhaps owing to this very circumstance the Guallahs or milkers in India are not affected with Cow Pox, as is the case with this description of persons in Gloucestershire and other counties in England where the disease is most prevalent. It is an extraordinary fact, and worthy of remark, that while the cows were thus affected no case of variola amongst the natives in the village presented itself, and although the people were ordinarily averse from handling or going much amongst the cattle at the time of disease, still they all scouted the idea of infection, stating they never heard of any one contracting disease from the cow, consequently they were under no alarm on that score. In consequence of the extreme jealousy with which all my inquiries on this subject were watched by the Hindoos, coupled with my own anxiety to conceal the object in view, I should have found very great difficulty in prosecuting my investigations had not the disease assumed the character of an epidemic, all the cattle in the neighbourhood becoming affected, and amongst others two belonging to one of my own vaccinators. I had them covered with blankets, leaving merely the udder and teats exposed to the air. On the seventh day two small pustules made their appearance on the teats of one, which dried·up on the tenth, and the crusts were removed on the twelfth day ; from those crusts eleven native children were inoculated. No effects whatsoever were produced on six of this number. Two had very slight inflammation on the arms on the third and fifth days ; two had considerable local inflammation and slight heat of surface on the fifth, sixth, and seventh days, but no vesicle formed, although there was marked induration round the puncture. The remaining child's arm was slightly inflamed on the fourth morning, and a vesicle was apparent the next day, which continued to increase till the ninth day, when I was much gratified to find that it assumed all the characteristics of true vaccine. The poor little child, the subject of this experiment, was about five months old, and suffered much from fever for four days, by which he was greatly reduced, but very soon recovered.

" Two children were vaccinated from this patient with the most complete success, but the symptomatic fever was more severe than I have ever observed it in former instances. Five children were vaccinated from those just mentioned, and the result was equally successful, after which no difficulty was experienced in disseminating the disease. With the view, however, of satisfying myself that true Cow Pox was introduced, I had two children who had been vaccinated with the fresh virus inoculated with Small Pox, and both were happily found to be secure. Another instance of the preservative powers of the new lymph deserves mention. Five children in the Gorah Bazaar at Berampore were vaccinated, and shortly afterwards were accidentally exposed to the variolous contagion by residing in the same huts where the disease was raging very dreadfully, but not one of those vaccinated was in the slightest degree affected by variola. Many children belonging to His Majesty's 49th Regiment and others in the families of residents, both civil and military, at this station and its vicinity, had been vaccinated with the regenerated virus. My friend Dr. French, who invariably has recourse to Bryce's test; Mr. Skipton, the superintendent surgeon, and several other medical men, have expressed themselves completely satisfied with the result. It is a gratifying fact that since the introduction of the new lymph the symptomatic fever has been more marked, and the natives have much greater confidence in the efficacy of the operation; in proof of which I need merely mention that the number presented for vaccination within the last three months has much exceeded that of any similar period for the previous two years. Variola has been more or less prevalent in this neighbourhood for the last seven months, and is now committing dreadful ravages in several parts of the city. Many instances are daily presenting themselves of the disease attacking those who have been previously affected, either naturally or by inoculation, and I am credibly informed that several of the latter have fallen victims to this dreadful scourge. It is melancholy to reflect that a city of ignorant and mercenary beings, such as the Tikadars in this country, are permitted annually to regenerate the disease, and thereby keep up a continual source of contagion, by which thousands of lives are sacrificed. Accompanying I have the pleasure to send some vaccine crusts, and ivory points armed with virus taken two days since, from which, I entertain no doubt, the disease will be readily introduced in Calcutta, and should more be required it shall be immediately supplied."

According to Dr. Duncan Stewart[1] this lymph was distributed throughout India.

Mr. Macpherson's example was followed by Mr. Furnell,[2] in Assam, in 1834. He wrote as follows :—

"Being very anxious to obtain a constant supply of vaccine virus, that which I got from Decca at various times having been followed by eruptions all over the body, and often with much fever, I was much interested by the account in the Transactions of the Medical Society detailing Mr. Macpherson's success in procuring vaccine lymph from the original source, the cow. I, therefore, in September last endeavoured to procure it in the same way, and having heard that several cows in the neighbourhood of Silhet were affected with the disease called Mhata or Gotee, I succeeded in getting one that was recovering, but it had a number of dried scabs over its body ; from those

---

[1] Duncan Stewart. *Report on Small Pox in Calcutta.* p. 146.
[2] *Transactions of the Medical and Physical Society of Calcutta*, p. 453. 1835.

scabs I vaccinated four children without effect. My health being very bad at the time I was recommended to try Chirra for change of air, and left Silhet, requesting Mr. Brown, who kindly undertook my duty, to follow up the trial, at the same time offering a reward to any person who would bring a cow having the disease. Ere I returned to Silhet, Mr. Brown vaccinated several children, the first four, direct from the cow, and afterwards continued vaccinating from these children in succession. In the first four, the vaccine vesicle appeared most favourable on the eighth day, and in those who were vaccinated from them, the disease also appeared well marked on the eighth day. On my return, I found all in a fair train, as I thought, and continued vaccinating until the middle of November, when I was again obliged to go to Chirra for the benefit of my health. During my absence, Mr. Brown vaccinated Major Orchard's child on the 23rd of that month. On my return on the 30th, I found that the vesicle did not appear in so forward a state as it should have been, but from its appearance, I thought that it had only been retarded in its progress, as at the time the babe was vaccinated she had a slight teething rash. On the 1st December, it looked much better, and on the evening of that day, the eighth of the vaccination, she had slight fever, and got in the evening a grain of calomel, and in the morning following, some castor oil, which affected her bowels slightly. On the evening of the second, the dose of calomel was repeated, and followed by oil next morning; the fever continued but slight. On the 3rd day, from the commencement of the fever, an eruption similar to that preceding Small Pox appeared, and in four days from that, she was completely covered with an eruption resembling the Small Pox at its confluent point, which ran through the same course as natural Small Pox. She was quite well on the 18th December, with a few pocky scabs scaling off. Before the above-mentioned eruption made its appearance three native children that were vaccinated on the same day as Mrs. Orchard's child, and from the same source, were brought to me, and the vesicles having a most favourable appearance, I vaccinated my own baby from one of them. On the 1st December, being much alarmed on

seeing the eruption on Mrs. Orchard's little girl, I sent for the
boy from whom she was vaccinated, and found that he had
had very little fever, but he had a few scabs, about twenty
on his entire body. I also had the three children, who were
brought to me on the day my little one was vaccinated, with me
daily; none of them had fever for more than one day; in two
of them a slight eruption, and on the third child there was not
an eruption of any kind, and the vaccine vesicle in all of them
went through its regular course. Notwitstanding this I took
every precaution, and on the eighth day of vaccination, slight
fever having come on, my little one had a little calomel and
on the following morning some oil; yet the fever increased,
and the dose was repeated on the following evening and the
oil next morning with the desired effect. On the third day of
the fever, a very thick eruption appeared on the face, and
followed the course of Small Pox in its worst form. On the
seventh day, from the commencement of the eruption her
mouth and throat became so sore that she was unable to take
the breast or any other food: it was very necessary to try
to support her by a nourishing injection, notwithstanding which
she sank on the 20th. The above report, it is hardly necessary
to say, is given with great pain; but I feel that it is right to
do it, and to warn my brethren of the danger that sometimes
occurs after taking the virus from the cow in this climate.
Mhata in the cow of this country is decidedly a much more
serious disease than the vaccine diseases in the animal in
Europe. And it will be seen from the above statement that
the inoculation from it is, in the human subject, followed by a
most dreadful disease, but I will refrain from further remarks;
but I think it is necessary to state that such precautions were
taken in this trial that it was almost impossible that any
admixture of the variolous disease could have been made, as
all the children mentioned were vaccinated direct from the cow.[1]
Two native vaccinators were deputed to vaccinate at the
houses of the natives, and the third, in whom I had great

---

[1] "The first four from the cow; in the remainder the lymph was propagated from the first four children by Mr. Brown or myself."

confidence, was employed about the station, and brought weekly three or four healthy subjects to be vaccinated from those vaccinated by myself or Mr. Brown. Neither should we have known that the vaccination had been followed by any serious result had it not been for the above melancholy case, as, on the strictest inquiry, I cannot learn that any of the native children vaccinated, suffered from illness, not one having got any medicine ; not the slightest pitting followed in either, as the eruption left no pits on Major Orchard's child. I have been so ill since the 22nd of last month that I have been obliged to leave Silhet, or I should have given this report earlier. I have within a few days learned that Captain Fisher's suffered also from a severe eruptive fever after vaccination from virus sent from Silhet.

" In answer to your question I mentioned yesterday that I had heard from Silhet that young Mr. Tereneau was suffering under an affection of the kind.

"I give you the words of my correspondent. 'In my letter yesterday I mentioned that young Tereneau had an eruption which I took for one of the patches of roseola. To-day, however, it has singularly enough been assuming the identical appearance which came out on your baby.' He was twice vaccinated, first in India, and afterwards in Scotland, and all right. I can only suppose that he caught the infection from Mrs. Fisher's child. I heard of several cases of Small Pox in Silhet about the time my little one was vaccinated. The native vaccinator, designated the third in the report, was taken ill about the 24th of December. His case was mentioned as a case of Small Pox ; however, if it was, it was a very slight eruption. He did not keep his bed after it appeared. He was inoculated when a child."

According to Dr. Duncan Stewart, Mr. Brown made use of the scabs taken from the back or abdomen of the diseased cattle. These were reduced to a pulp with water, and employed for inoculating the four children mentioned above.

"'In all four, vesicles in every respect resembling in their progress and when mature genuine vaccinia, made their appearance, and went the same regular course, the constitutional disturbance on the eighth day only being more severe than I have usually seen it in the latter.[1]'"

"From these many other native children were inoculated, and no doubts of the genuineness of the lymph were excited until two English children were punctured from one of them, and it was then found that Small Pox supervened in both of these cases, and this was more than suspected to have happened in many of the native children, who had generally dispersed a few days after the operation, and were not afterwards heard of. One of the English children unhappily died."[2]

According to Baron, in 1837, another series of inoculations was performed by Mr. Macpherson in Bengal with virus from diseased cows, "on which occasion an eruptive complaint of the true variolous nature was produced;" and similar phenomena were observed at Gowalpara by Mr. Wood in 1838.

"In several of his cases the symptoms were so severe as to excite apprehension that the disease would terminate fatally. He was so strongly impressed with this fact, that he thought it would be better to take human Small Pox rather than Cow Small Pox for inoculation, when the latter assumes its dangerous and fatal form."

From all these independent observations, if we accept them as correct, there would seem to be no doubt that cattle-plague virus inoculated in the human subject will produce a vesicle with the physical characters

<hr />

[1] _Quarterly Journal, Calcutta Medical Society_, April 1837
[2] _Report on Small Pox in Calcutta_, p. 148, by Duncan Stewart, M.D. 1844.

of the vaccine vesicle, and succeeded occasionally by an eruption which appears to have the characters of the eruption of cattle-plague. That cattle-plague is not infectious to man in the ordinary sense affords no proof that the disease may not be cultivated in the human subject by inoculation.

But these occurrences had to be explained away, for such circumstances were incompatible with the Small Pox theory of Cow Pox. We have only to turn again to Dr. Seaton's *Handbook of Vaccination* to find that ingenious explanations were forthcoming.

First of all, with regard to Dr. Macpherson's cases, Seaton admitted that the " vaccinations " were genuine, and that a stock of " vaccine " was established and was afterwards regularly continued. But he adds :—

" From these facts it is not to be doubted that a case of Cow Pox in the cow had been met with ; but what is to be doubted is that the Gotee—the malignant disease above referred to—was the source of this infection."

It was evidently impossible for Seaton to admit that a vaccine vesicle could be produced *by " management " of cattle-plague.* But having admitted that a vaccine vesicle had somehow resulted, the only way out of the difficulty was to suppose that in some extraordinary way a case of Cow Pox had cropped up amidst the epidemic of cattle-plague. Nor does the fact that these experiments were repeated by Furnell in another part of India, appear in the least to have shaken his opinion. But while Seaton throws doubt upon the Gotee as the source of the lymph, he admits that the cows had "a generalised eruption of some kind or another," and he explains the pustular eruption in the inoculated children as the result of an accidental admixture of either inoculated or casual human Small Pox. If we are to accept Seaton's view, we must, in some similar fashion, explain away the independent experience of Mr. Wood, of Gowalpara, and reject Ceely's and Murchison's accounts of inoculated cattle-plague on the hand of Mr. Hancock.

CHAPTER XI.

SHEEP Pox, or *variola ovina*, is a common disease in some parts of Europe. In France, the disease is called *la clavelée*, and in Italy, *vaccuolo*. It has been introduced on several occasions into this country, but has been effectually stamped out. As in human Small Pox, there are varieties; the benign and the malignant; the discrete and the confluent. It is an acute febrile disease accompanied by a general vesiculo-pustular eruption, highly infectious, and capable of being propagated by inoculation or *clavelisation*.

It is very closely analogous to human Small Pox, and as another result of the misleading theory of Cow Pox being Cow *Small* Pox, not only was vaccination employed to protect sheep from Sheep Pox, but "vaccine lymph" was raised from Sheep Pox to protect human beings from Small Pox. These experiments were first performed in Italy, and have been described in detail by Sacco.[1]

"In 1802, Dr. Marchelli communicated to the *Società di*

---

[1] Sacco. *Trattato di Vaccinazione.* p. 144. 1809.

Emulazione of Genoa, to which I have also the honour to belong, the fact, that Small Pox of sheep might be substituted for Cow Pox; but as he had then made only a very few experiments, with a view of ascertaining if it were efficacious or harmful when transmitted to man, he undertook to continue his researches, and then to publish the results. However, as he has recently informed me, he has not been able to do so in consequence of a long and severe illness from which he has been suffering; it is this which has retarded the publication of these valuable observations which would have led to important results, and would have thrown light on this branch of science.

" Since I published my practical observations, I have suggested the vaccination of sheep in order to protect them from the malady to which they are subject. I had indeed vaccinated more than seventy; but never having had the opportunity of seeing the Small Pox of these animals in our midst, I have not been able, for many years past, to ascertain whether by means of this inoculation they have been really protected. During the many journeys which I made with a view to extending vaccination in the kingdom, I redoubled my efforts in vain; I only succeeded in meeting with it in the State of Naples, at Capua. Passing through it in 1804, I saw a peasant who was driving a flock of seven sheep to the butcher's; as I was obliged to stop in this town, I endeavoured to profit by the opportunity and to gain information on the subject.

" Having noticed the miserable and dejected appearance of these sheep I stopped; and after putting various questions to the peasant, and examining the nature and character of the eruption and of the symptoms which accompanied it, I felt sure that the malady was the true Small Pox of sheep. The peasant told me that the malady was common in the neighbourhood, that fifty-four sheep had already been slaughtered, and that they would continue this method if the malady should develop in others, because treatment, besides being costly and difficult, was often useless, and exposed the rest of the flock to the contagion of the illness. I, with great care, collected matter from the finest vesicles, in small tubes, with the intention of testing it at the first opportunity.

"On returning to my own province on Christmas Day of the same year, I went as soon as I had reached *La Cattolica*, which was then the last place on the frontier of the kingdom of Italy, in search of Dr. Legni. I informed him of my design, and my desire to make experiments with the matter obtained from the sheep, at Capua; he kindly seconded my project. He procured me six children, who were all inoculated with the matter, which was still fluid; I also inoculated two other infants with true vaccine, in order to institute a comparison. I then left the neighbourhood, entrusting the examination of the inoculated children to the above-named physician, who was to inform me of the results. A month later he sent me an exact account of all he had observed, the substance of which was, that the inoculations advanced at the different stages in the way which is usual with the vesicles of Cow Pox, and that he had failed 'to see any appreciable difference. He continued to vaccinate with the same matter for several years, and always with the same success.[1]

"I had no sooner arrived at Milan than I put to the test the remains of the matter which I had brought with me. I at once inoculated four infants with it, but was greatly surprised to find that it produced no effect upon them; for want of fresh *virus* from the sheep I was then obliged to suspend further experiments.

"In the month of October, 1806, I visited the Apennines

---

[1] Extract from the letter of Dr. Mauro Legni, of June 29th, 1808 :—
"Having pointed out its characters, I will now endeavour to sum up all that I have already written on the Small Pox of sheep; it has substantially a course in every way analogous to Cow Pox; although the vesicles produced by the first insertions of the original matter appear to have had but little vigour; they were otherwise well formed. I have used this matter for two years, and I have inoculated more than three hundred infants with it, of whom one hundred were at Pesaro, where Small Pox has since reigned for three consecutive years; and where, in spite of such a prolonged and fatal epidemic, all those inoculated with the sheep *virus* have been preserved from this fatal distemper, although they were in very close communication with those who were attacked by Small Pox."

with the object of helping the different districts by rendering the practice of vaccination general, and I then found means of verifying my theory. In many places I had the opportunity of observing this epidemic disease of sheep and of following it in all its stages.

"I recommenced my researches in the neighbourhood of Montemiscoso, by inoculating the same malady in other sheep, and I ascertained that its course was only a little milder and more rapid, and that it acted precisely in the same way as inoculated Small Pox does in man. But, as this inoculation, although producing a milder disease, was still accompanied by the inconvenience of spreading the contagion and further diffusing it in the flock, I determined to vaccinate several sheep, with the object also of trying upon them the subsequent effects of Sheep Pox. The vaccination ran its proper course, and the experiment was successful, for the Sheep Pox no longer appeared, although the sheep associated with others which were infected. I had, therefore, assured myself by this experiment, that vaccination had rendered these sheep insusceptible of a similar malady.

"As the ovine virus, inoculated in sheep, gave rise to a disease with symptoms which were regular, constant, and benign, I was induced to inoculate three infants with *virus* taken from a lamb which did not appear to be very ill : two others were inoculated in one arm with the ovine virus, and in the other with vaccine. I had on this occasion the satisfaction of seeing that all that Dr. Legni had written to me, from La Cattolica some years before, of the results of the inoculation which I had made with Sheep Pox, whilst passing through that place, was fully confirmed. Of the first three children inoculated with the sheep *virus*, two had one vesicle each ; of the second children, one had only one vesicle on each arm, and the other had two, but only of the Cow Pox. The vesicles which had developed were so similar, that if I had not made a mark to remind myself on which arms I had inoculated the Cow Pox, and on which the Sheep Pox, I could not have distinguished one from the other. A few days after desiccation I inoculated with human Small Pox, the two children in whom the virus of the sheep had been completely successful, but no effects, either general or local, resulted.

"Continuing my journey by Fosdinovo and Aulla, I had the opportunity of seeing the same sheep disease in various places, and of continuing my observations.

"I inoculated several persons at Fosdinovo, amongst others the sons of Cancelliere Uccelli; others were made in Barbarasco near Aulla, where I also inoculated a cow with the same matter. I observed the course of those made at Fosdinovo, and in all, the ordinary vesicle was similar to that of Cow Pox. I left the Barbarasco cases to be observed by Dr. Magnani, an accomplished surgeon at Aulla, who sent me, eventually, an exact account of them.[1]

"Proceeding to Lucca, I used the same *virus* to inoculate various people, and continued to vaccinate also in other places, always renewing the matter which had been originally taken from

---

[1] Account sent by Doctor Antonio Magnani of Aulla, to Professor Luigi Sacco, Director-General of Vaccination, at the request of the latter conveyed in a memorandum of December 9th, 1806 :—

"1. On 8th and 11th of the month, I went to Barbarasco to see the four children whom you had inoculated with virus from the sheep, and designated in your list as Nos. 13, 14, 15, and 16, I saw only two of them, who had contracted the malady, namely, the brothers Gioacchino and Domenico Biondi; the former had two very beautiful vesicles on each arm, and the latter had only a single one on the right arm. After a very careful examination, I found that the vesicles on both boys were like those of true Cow Pox, surrounded by a red circle; I further observed that the matter in both cases was different to that of true Cow Pox, that is to say that on the eighth day it was of a yellowish colour; and on this same day I noticed, moreover, that the vesicles already began to form a crust, and this was of a colour which tended to yellow.

"2. On my first visit to these boys I took the virus from their vesicles, and found it to be serous, of a yellowish colour, and not at all limpid. With this matter I inoculated two other persons; in both cases two vesicles on each arm appeared on the seventh day, filled with limpid matter, and I afterwards observed that these vesicles ran their course in the same manner as those of vaccinated persons.

"3. However, the matter from these vesicles having been taken on the seventh day, I wished to inoculate three more persons in the commune of Tendola; I found on visiting them on the eighth day, that they all

Sheep Pox, its course being always very regular, and its effect constant, as if it had been derived from a genuine Cow Pox."

In more recent times, extensive experiments were carried out in England to test the protective power of vaccination against Sheep Pox. According to Marson and Simmonds, it was very difficult to get Cow Pox to take on sheep, and when an effect was produced, the resulting affection, even when developed to its fullest extent, was very unlike the same disease in the human subject. In the sheep, it seldom produced anything more than a small papule, which occasionally resulted in the formation of a minute vesicle, or more commonly, a pustule, which was sometimes, although very rarely, surrounded by a slight areola. Generally, however, neither vesication nor pustulation followed ; but a small scab was produced, which soon fell from the site of the puncture, leaving no trace behind. The disease passed quickly,

---

had two vesicles on each arm ; and I remarked besides that the humour which they contained was limpid and crystalline.

"4. On inspection of the cow which you inoculated at several points with the same matter, I found on the udder a single vesicle, from which I took matter, which was yellowish in colour and not limpid, and used it to inoculate two other boys ; the first had two vesicles on each arm, and on the second I found only one, on the left arm ; in other respects the *virus* contained in the two vesicles was exactly similar to that of true Cow Pox. I have vaccinated with this matter other persons, and from these again I inoculated others, whom I visited soon after, hoping that they would succeed equally well ; the result was, and still is, most successful.

"AULLA, *January 29th*, 1807."

and irregularly through its several stages, and terminated by the eighth or ninth day, and not unfrequently even before that time. Lymph was but rarely obtainable, and then only in the smallest quantity, and this on the fifth or sixth day succeeding the vaccination. The effects were only local, and the animal's health was not impaired.

Sheep were found to be just as susceptible of the Cow Pox virus on subsequent repetition of the inoculation as they were in the first instance, and hence the conclusion that Cow Pox was utterly worthless as a protective against Sheep Pox.

According to Depaul, however, Cow Pox takes characteristically on sheep, and Sheep Pox lymph inoculated on cows produces a perfect " vaccine." It is impossible to say whether these conflicting results depended upon the employment in the experiments of different breeds of sheep, or different stocks of vaccine lymph.

But the experiments of Marson and Simmonds, which have just been referred to, were not the only ones made in this country. Marson succeeded in raising on the *human subject*, a vesicle with the physical characters of the vaccine vesicle, and thus confirmed Sacco's " vaccinations."

" When Small Pox appeared in this country in the sheep in 1847, we tried to communicate it, by inoculation, to the human subject, and thought we had succeeded in doing so, and the virus was carried on from one to another for several weeks in succession. The pock produced was very like Cow Pox, having only, as we thought, a bluer tinge, and was protective against Small Pox, as we ascertained by inoculating the patient afterwards with the lymph of human variola ; but we had unfortunately used for the original *ovination* the same lancet instead of having a new one, as we ought to have had, that we had previously used for vaccinating ; and although it was, as we believe, perfectly clean and free from vaccine lymph, nevertheless, as the disease could not be produced again in the human subject, either by Mr. Ceely of Aylesbury, who made repeated trials with the lymph of Sheep Pox, or by ourselves, the experiment was never brought before the profession."

The failures in subsequent attempts do not invalidate the successful experiment, just as the numerous failures to raise a " vaccine vesicle " by variolation of cows, in no way disprove the results of more fortunate experimenters. In both cases, the effects depend upon the nature and " management " of the lymph.

CHAPTER XII.

GOAT POX AS A SOURCE OF "VACCINE LYMPH."

GOATS are subject to an eruptive disease, which is alleged to be similar to Small Pox in man.

Dr. Valentine and others proved that it was possible to vaccinate the goat and to retro-vaccinate the human subject; and Professor Heydeck, at Madrid, meeting with an outbreak of an eruptive disease of goats known as Goat Small Pox, and influenced, no doubt, by the doctrine that vaccine lymph was derived from Cow *Small* Pox, proposed to employ the lymph from this source to afford human beings protection from Small Pox. A friend of Mr. Dunning received the following letter briefly referring to these experiments :[1]—

"MADRID, *March 9th,* 1804.

"I am not able to send you, at present, our observation on the Goat Pock subsequent to the 8th of June last, because it is not finished yet; for the king ordered in September last that all the children in the Foundling-house, and those who are in the Desamparados should be inoculated with the Goat Pock, which did its effects; we are now employed in the contra-proofs, and after everything is finished, shall send the whole process to you for the

---

[1] Baron, *loc. cit.*

inspection of your medical friends and Dr. Jenner; and as I am
at present on another discovery, not less useful than the Goat Pock,
I shall give also an account of its results in my next letter."

His friend replied :—

" I wrote to the Professor about three weeks ago, told him that
his discovery had excited very much the attention of the medical
world in England, and more immediately Dr. Jenner's, and urged
him to forward his further observations with all the expedition in
his power, and that I would transmit them to you."

Mr. Dunning published an account of these experiments, but Jenner discountenanced the idea. In a
letter to Mr. Dunning, he wrote :—

" I believe we have had no correspondence since your *Spanish
paper* appeared in the *Medical and Philosophical Journal.* To be
plain with you, and use the familiarity of a friend, I do not like it.
The paper is not now before me ; but if I recollect right, it went
only to prove that goats are subject to spontaneous pustules upon
their nipples ; that the matter of these pustules was inserted into
the arms of human subjects; and that it produced local effects. Is
there any quadruped that is not subject to diseased nipples? Even
the human animal, we know from sad experience, is not exempted.
The cow, like other animals, is subject to a spontaneous pock upon
its teats, the fluid of which, when brought in contact with the
denuded living fibre, is capable of exciting disease ; but I positively assert, this is not one grand preventive. When you hear
again from Madrid, do not fail to tell me what the Spaniards say
about it. I have already anticipated."

And in a postscript he added :—

" Do not fail to write soon. I want to know your further sentiments of the Goat Pox."

I have not been able to ascertain whether any

further experiments were made at the time, or what became of the stock of goat lymph "which did its effects." Nor have I been able to obtain the history of similar experiments with any diseases of the goat, in more recent times.

CHAPTER XIII.

THE description given by Jenner in the *Inquiry*, was the first published account of Cow Pox. He described the disease in the cow as consisting of irregular pustules on the teats, of a palish blue colour, surrounded by an erysipelatous inflammation, and characterised by a tendency to degenerate into phagedenic ulcers. The animals were indisposed, and the secretion of milk lessened.

This description is not so complete as that given, a few months afterwards, by Clayton,[1] a veterinary surgeon in Gloucester, and published by Mr. Cooke.

"The Cow Pox begins with white specks upon the cow's teats, which, in process of time, ulcerate, and if not stopped, extend over the whole surface of the teats, giving the cow excruciating pain :—that if this disease is suffered to continue for some time, it degenerates into ulcers, exuding a malignant and highly corrosive matter; but this generally arises from neglect in the incipient stage of the disease, or from some other cause he cannot explain :—that this disease has not a regular process of commencing and terminating without a remedy, because, if not attended to, it would end in a mortification

---

[1] Cooke. *Contributions to Physical and Medical Knowledge, collected by Thomas Beddoes*, p. 392. 1799.

of the teats, and probably death of the animal:—that this disease may arise from any cause irritating or excoriating the teats, but the teats are often chapped without the Cow Pox succeeding. In chaps of the teats, they generally swell; in the Cow Pox, the teats seldom swell at all, but are gradually destroyed by ulceration:—that **this disease first breaks out upon one cow, and is communicated by the milkers to the whole herd, but if one person was confined to strip the cow having this disease, it would go no farther**:—that the Cow Pox is a local disease, and is invariably cured by local remedies:—that he never knew this disease extend itself in the slightest degree to the udder, unless mortification had ensued, and that he can at all times cure the Cow Pox in eight or nine days, by his usual local remedies:—that he is conversant with the diseases of the horse, and extensively employed, particularly in curing the Grease:—that he cannot recollect ever to have had horses with the Grease and cows with the Cow Pox, under cure at the same time, and at the same farm:—that he is very certain he has frequently had cows with the Cow Pox, where no horses whatever have been kept:—that he considers the Grease as a name, having great latitude in the diseases of horses, because sometimes it may be cured merely by topical remedies, and at other times it is only to be completed by internal remedies:—that he does not consider the Grease an infectious disease amongst horses, since greasy horses and horses in perfect health frequently stand in stables together indiscriminately, without infecting each other; and although it is probable, if the discharge of Grease was to be applied in its most acrid state to the heels of a sound horse, it would inflame and excoriate them, yet it would not produce the Grease:—that Grease is most prevalent in winter, at which time he has never known the Cow Pox to occur, and therefore cannot think it at all probable that the Grease can have the least influence in producing the Cow Pox."

Mr. John Sims,[1] in a letter dated February 13th, 1799, corroborated the account given by Clayton.

---

[1] Sims, *Medical and Physical Journal.* 1799.

"There is a gentleman of eminence in the law, now living at
Bristol, who has had the Cow Pox thrice, and being afterwards
inoculated for the Small Pox, had it in so great abundance that his
life for some time was despaired of. He describes the Cow Pox
as the most loathsome of diseases, and adds that his right arm
was in a state of eruption both the first and the second time from
one extremity to the other; the pain was excessive, and his fingers
so stiff he could scarcely move them. The gentleman alluded
to was the son of a farmer who kept seventy cows, of which
he, being then a lad, milked eighteen himself; they were all of
them infected with this disorder at one time; he caught it, and
such was the abhorrence it created in the family that they made
no use of the milk as long as it lasted. He never heard, nor does
he believe, that this complaint originates, as supposed by Dr.
Jenner, from any communication with that acrid humour called
the grease in horses."

Dr. Bradley, one of the editors of the *Medical and
Physical Journal*, commenting on this case, says :—

"What this gentleman remarks of the loathsomeness of the
disease, although a circumstance overlooked in Dr. Jenner's
account, appears to be in itself a formidable objection, should it
be found to answer the purpose for which it has been recommended."

Dr. Bradley, in the same paper, briefly referred to
the outbreak of Cow Pox which occurred in London in
February 1799, and gave a coloured plate of the
disease on the arm and fingers of a milker. The
Cow Pox, he adds, in this instance, "appears to have
been very mild, for no loss was experienced by the
farmers from the deficiency of milk as usually happens."

This early description was supplemented by an

account of Cow Pox [1] by Mr. Lawrence, author of *A Philosophical and Practical Treatise on Horses and on the Moral Duties of Man towards the Brute Creation.* This article on Cow Pox not only affords further evidence of this disease being known to those who had the care of cattle, before Jenner's paper was published, but it shows that it had also been made the subject of practical observation and study, by veterinary surgeons.

Lawrence was of opinion that the disease had no connection with grease, and thus relates his experience :—

"Concerning the real ætiology of the disease, I have, for many years, been without any uncertainty in my opinion. Too sudden repletion and thickening of the fluids, after the fatigue of long driving and inanition is an auxiliary and accelerating cause of Pox upon the teats, accompanied by low fever, considerable debility, and a diminution both of the quantity and quality of the milk. This hypothesis, I think, will at least not be condemned as irrational, when it is considered that the disease is nearly or altogether unknown, except in the dairy counties, and in large towns where the animals which are its victims are congregated in such great numbers and stowed so close.

"That it is often taken in so slight a way as to have no preventive effect of the Small Pox, I apprehend pretty numerous proofs might be obtained.

"The Pox among cows I always supposed to arise from the contagion of their own atmosphere ; a cause fully adequate to the effect produced ; and this effect ceases with the cause or from the influence of some casual and unknown cause, and is reproduced indefinitely with the recurrence of the original cause.

---

[1] *Med. and Phys. Journ.*, vol. ii., p. 113. April 1799.

" Whatever may be the fate of Cow Pox inoculation it has and will give further occasion to a pretty large and open discussion, which is always beneficial, as having a tendency to produce discovery and promote improvement, and when the public ardour for the present topic shall have become a little cool and satisfied, I hope it will be turned by enlightened men towards another, perhaps of nearly as great consequence, namely, the prevention of the original malady in the animals themselves. Those who had witnessed it and only reflected upon the excessive filth and nastiness which must unavoidably mix with the milk in an infected dairy of cows, and the corrupt and unsalubrious state of their produce in consequence, will surely join me in that sentiment."

Lawrence was almost a century before his time. Cow Pox was not again brought forward in this light until 1887–88, when I reported the " filth and nastiness" at a Wiltshire Farm, and advocated the advisability of placing this disease under the Contagious Diseases (Animals) Act.

CHARACTERS OF THE DISEASE IN THE COW.

The numerous details, wanting in the early accounts of Cow Pox, have been supplied by the painstaking and laborious researches of Robert Ceely.[1] From his classical papers in the *Transactions of the Provincial Medical Journal*, we have a complete picture of the features of the natural disease in the cow.

In Ceely's experience in the Vale of Aylesbury, outbreaks occurred at irregular intervals, most commonly appearing about the beginning or end of the spring; rarely during the height of summer. There were outbreaks at all periods, from August to May and the beginning of June; cases also being met with even in autumn and the middle of winter, after a dry summer. The

---

[1] *Vide* vol. ii., p. 363, *et seq.*

disease was occasionally epizootic, or occurring at times in several farms at no great distance from each other, but more commonly sporadic or nearly solitary. It was to be seen sometimes at several contiguous farms; at other times, at one or two farms. Many years might elapse before it occurred at a given farm or vicinity, although all the animals might have been changed in the meantime. Cow Pox had broken out twice in five years in a particular vicinity, and at two contiguous farms, while at a third adjoining dairy, in all respects similar in local and other circumstances, it had not been known to exist for forty years. It was sometimes introduced into a dairy by recently purchased cows. Twice it had been known to be so introduced by milch heifers. It was considered that the disease was peculiar to the milch cow; it came primarily while the animal was in that condition, and it was casually propagated to others by the hands of the milkers. Sturks, dry heifers, dry cows, and milch cows milked by other hands, grazing in the same pastures, feeding in the same sheds, and at contiguous stalls, remained exempt from the disease.

For many years past, however, the spontaneous origin of Cow Pox had not been doubted in the Vale of Aylesbury. In all the cases that Ceely had noticed he never could discover the probability of any other source.

Condition of Animals primarily affected.—There was much difficulty in determining with precision at all times, whether this disease arose primarily in one or more individuals in the same dairy. Most commonly, however, it appeared to be solitary. The milkers believed that they were able to point out the infecting individual. In two instances, there could be very little doubt on this point. In August 1838 three cows were affected with the disease. The first was attacked two months after calving and seven weeks after weaning. This animal was considered to be in good health, but it looked out of condition. She had heat and tenderness of teats and udder as the first noticed signs. The other two were affected in about ten days. In December 1838, in a large dairy, a milch cow slipped her calf, had heat and induration of the udder and teats, with vaccine eruption, and subsequently leucorrhœa and greatly impaired health; the whole dairy, consisting of forty cows, and some of the milkers, became subsequently affected. In another dairy, at the same time, it first appeared in a heifer soon after weaning, and in about ten or twelve days, extended to five other heifers and one cow, milked in the same shed, and it also affected the milkers. In another dairy, at the same time, thirty cows were severely affected, and also one of the milkers. It appeared to arise in a cow two months after calving. The only symptoms noticed were that the udder and teats were tumid, tender, and hot, just before the disease appeared.

Condition of Animals casually affected.—In some animals the attack was less severe than in others, depending on the state and condition of the skin of the parts affected, and the constitution and habits of the animal. It was sometimes observed to diminish the secretion of milk, and in most cases it commonly did affect the amount obtained artificially; with this exception, and the temporary trouble and accidents to the milk and the milkers, little else was observed; the animal continued to feed and graze apparently as well as before. The topical effects varied very much in different individuals, the mildness or severity being greatly influenced by temperament and condition of the animal, and especially by the state of the teats and udder, and the texture and vascularity of the skin of the parts affected. Where the udder was short, compact, and hairy, and the skin of the teats thick, smooth, tense, and entire, or scarcely at all chapped, cracked, or fissured, the animal often escaped with a mild affection, sometimes with only a single vesicle. But where the udder was voluminous, flabby, pendulous, and naked, and the teats long and loose, and the skin corrugated, thin, fissured, rough, and unequal, then the animal scarcely ever escaped a copious eruption. Hence, in general, heifers suffered least and cows most from the milkers' inoculations and manipulations.

Progress of the Disease.—Cow Pox, once arising or introduced, and the necessary precautions not being adopted in time, appeared in ten or twelve days, on many more, in succession, so that among twenty-five cows perhaps by the third week nearly all would be affected; but five or six weeks or more were required to see the teats perfectly free from the disease.

Propagation by the Hand of the Milker.—Ceely was able to confirm the way in which the disease was said to spread. In December 1838, on a large dairy farm, where there were three milking-sheds, Cow Pox broke out in the home or lower shed. The cows in this shed being troublesome, the milker from the upper shed, after milking his own cows, came to assist in this for several days, morning and evening, when, in about a week some of his own cows began to exhibit the disease. It appears that, having chapped hands, he neglected washing them for three or four days at a time, and thus seemed to convey the disease from one shed to another. During the progress of the disease through this shed, one of the affected cows, which had been attacked by the other cows, was removed to the middle shed, where all the animals were perfectly well. This cow, being in an advanced stage of the disease, and of course difficult to milk and dangerous to the milk pail, was milked first by a juvenile milker for three or four days only, when, becoming unmanageable by him, her former milker was called in to attend exclusively to her. In less than a week all the animals of this shed showed symptoms of the disease, though in a much milder degree than it had appeared in the other sheds, fewer manipulations having been performed by an infected hand.

Topical Symptoms of the Natural Disease.—For these, Ceely was almost always, in the early stage, compelled to depend on the observations and statements of the milkers. They stated that for three or four days, without any apparent indisposition, they noticed heat and tenderness of the teats and udder, followed by irregularity and pimply hardness of these parts, especially about the bases of the teats, and adjoining the vicinity of the udder; that these pimples on skins not very dark were of a red colour, and generally as large as a vetch or a pea, and quite hard, though in three or four days many of these increased to the size of a horse-bean. Milking was generally very painful to the animal; the tumours rapidly increased in size, and some appeared to run into vesication on the teats, and were soon broken by the hands. Milking now becomes a troublesome and occasionally a dangerous process. Ceely adds :—" It is very seldom that any person competent to judge of the nature of the ailment has access to the animal before the appearance of the disease on others of the herd, when the cow first affected, presents on the teats **acuminated, ovoid,** or **globular vesications,** some entire, others broken, not infrequently two or three interfluent ; those broken have evidently a central depression with marginal induration ; those entire, being punctured, diffuse a more or less viscid amber-coloured fluid, collapse, and at once indicate the same kind of central and marginal character. They appear of various sizes, from that of a pin's head, evidently of later date, either acuminated or depressed, to that of an almond or a filbert, or even larger. **Dark brown** or **black solid uniform crusts,** especially on the udder near the base of the teats, are visible at the same time, some, much larger, are observed on the teats ; these, however, are less regular in form and less perfect. **Some are nearly detached, others quite removed, exhibiting a raw surface with a slight central slough.** On the teats, the crusts are circular, oval, oblong, or irregular ; some flatter, others elevated ; some thin and more translucent, being obviously secondary. The appearance of the disease in different stages, or at least, the formation of a few vesicles at different periods, seems very evident. The swollen, raw, and encrusted teats seem to produce uneasiness to the animal only while subjected to the tractions of the milkers, which it would appear are often nearly as effectual as usual." Referring again to the character of the vesicles, Ceely says that those "fortunate enough to have an opportunity of watching the disease in its progress may observe that when closely examined they present the following characters :—In animals of dark skin, at this period, the finger detects the intumescent indurations often better than the eye, but when closely examined, the tumours present, at their margins and towards their centres, a glistening metallic lustre or leaden hue ; but this is not always the case, for occasionally they exhibit a yellowish or yellowish-white appearance."

In describing more fully the crust, Ceely said that "**large black solid crusts, often more than an inch or two in length, are to be seen in different parts of these organs, some firmly adherent to a raw elevated base, others partially detached from a raw, red, and bleeding surface ; many denuded, florid, red, ulcerated surfaces, with small**

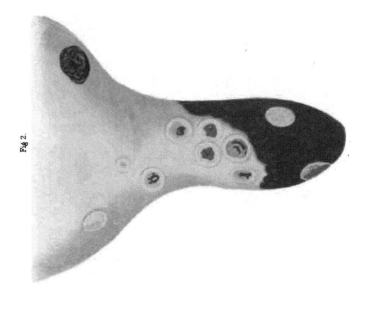

Fig 2.

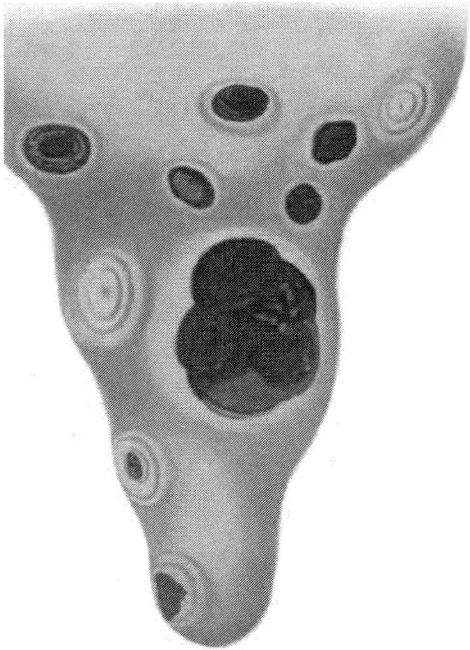

Fig 1.

NATURAL COW POX (CEELY).

central sloughs secreting pus and exuding blood, the teats exceedingly tender, hot, and swollen. . . . In some animals, under some circumstances, this state continues little altered till the third or fourth week, rendering the process of milking painful to the animal, and difficult and dangerous to the milker." [1]

" In many, however, little uneasiness seems to exist. The parts gradually heal; the crusts, although often partially or entirely renewed and renewed, ultimately separate, leaving apparently but few deep irregular cicatrices, some communicating with the tubuli lactiferi, the greater part being regular, smoothly-depressed, circular, or oval."

With regard to papulæ, " the milkers seldom notice the first period of papulation. Nor is this to be wondered at. It is, in truth, very difficult for an experienced observer, at all times, to escape error in this latter particular, and oversights will occur to the most vigilant from various causes, especially from peculiarity of colour, vascularity and texture of skin, as well as temperament of the individual."

With regard to central depression of the vesicles, Ceely found that " in three or four days from their first appearance the papulæ acquire their vesicular character, and have more or less of central depression, continuing gradually to increase. In three or four days more, they arrive at their fullest degree of development, and sometimes are surrounded with an areola, and always embedded in a circumscribed induration of the adjacent skin and subjacent cellular tissue."

If we carefully analyse this description of Cow Pox, we find that we have a most faithful account of the disease, as it actually occurred under Ceely's eyes. But, here and there, we see an attempt to harmonise these observations with the classical description of the inoculated disease. In ordinary vaccination, we recognise the stages of the papule, the vesicle with its central depression, the scab, and the scar. And Ceely, it will

---

[1] Compare Plate X.

be observed, describes the natural Cow Pox under
each of these headings.   But when describing the
vesicles, he practically admits that the classical character
of umbilication is absent, for he says that *those broken*
had evidently a central depression ; and again, that
vesicles, three or four days after the appearance of
papules, have *more or less* of a central depression.

There can be little doubt that in the use of these
ambiguous expressions, Ceely was probably misled by
constantly having in his mind the effects of ordinary vaccination.   And the appearances depicted in the elaborate
pictures of Cow Pox on the cow's teats, which illustrate
his classical memoir, can therefore be explained.   The
second plate is a faithful picture of the disease on the
teats as it is ordinarily met with.   [Plate IX.]   The first
plate is apparently a composite picture, representing the
eruption as ordinarily observed in the cow, and a number
of depressed vesicles as they appear after artificial inoculation.   The outline of this drawing is, I am of opinion,
distinctly *after* Sacco.   It is, however, an improvement on
the latter, which can only be described as an imaginary
diagram, representing the udder and teats of a cow,
covered with an eruption purporting to be that of the
natural Cow Pox.   Jenner had described the vesicles
in natural Cow Pox, as possessing a bluish tint, and
Sacco deliberately represents the natural disease by a
drawing of clusters of vesicles of inoculated Cow Pox,
coloured bright blue, and with a silvery lustre.   Ceely

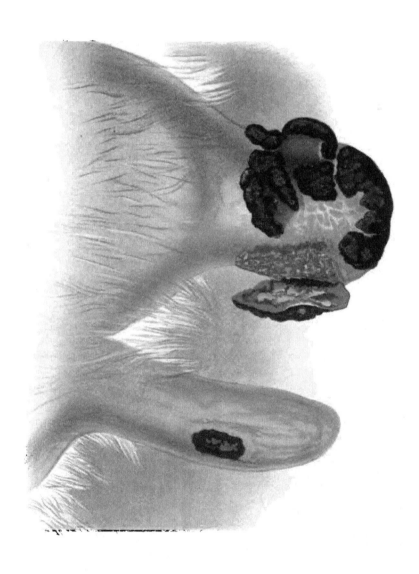

has outlined his drawing from Sacco's, but he has represented the crusts and scabs on the teats as he really saw them, though he has unfortunately added the vesicular stage, as he always wished to see it. I say unfortunately, for while Sacco's plate was accepted as a genuine representation of the natural disease in the cow for the first half of this century, Ceely's plate has been accepted (particularly in this country) for the latter half. It has, to my knowledge, been used in a veterinary school to represent what Cow Pox would be like, if it were ever again discovered!

Hering has given a coloured plate of the natural Cow Pox, and it will be noticed that it is totally different from either Sacco's or Ceely's drawing. On the teats are a number of oval or circular bullous vesicles and crusts. More recently, Layet has pointed out the same character in the Cow Pox discovered at Cérons in 1883. The characters of the inoculated disease were wanting, particularly the central depression of the vesicle. In Wiltshire I could only distinguish on the cow's teats, globular and broken vesicles, thick prominent crusts and ulcers; appearances which had very little in common with the characters of the inoculated disease.

CASUAL COW POX ON THE HANDS OF MILKERS.

The early accounts of the "loathsome" character of the disease will appear by no means exaggerated

to those, who have had an opportunity of studying
its effects on the hands of milkers, or indeed to those
who have made themselves familiar with the descriptions given by Jenner and others. To illustrate this, I
will briefly refer to some of Jenner's cases :—

" JOSEPH MERRET had several **sores** on his hands : swelling and
stiffness in each axilla, and much indisposition for several days.

" MRS. H. had **sores** upon her hands, which were communicated to
her nose, which became inflamed and very much swollen.

" SARAH WYNNE had Cow Pox in such a violent degree that she
was confined to her bed, and unable to do any work for ten days.

" WILLIAM RODWAY was so affected by the severity of the disease
that he was confined to his bed.

" WILLIAM SMITH had several **ulcerated sores** on his hands, and
the usual constitutional symptoms, and was affected, equally
severely, a second and a third time.

" WILLIAM STINCHCOMB had his hand very severely affected with
several corroding ulcers, and a considerable tumour in the axilla.

" SARAH NELMES had **a large pustulous sore** on the hand and the
usual symptoms.

" A GIRL had an **ulceration on the lip** from frequently holding her
finger to her mouth to cool the **raging** of a Cow Pox **sore** by blow-
ing upon it.

" A YOUNG WOMAN had Cow Pox to a great extent, **several sores**
which maturated having appeared on the hands and wrists.

" A YOUNG WOMAN had **several large suppurations** from Cow Pox
on the hands."

Pearson met with similar experiences in his investigations, and was informed of others.

" THOMAS EDINBURGH was so lame from the eruption of Cow
Pox on the palm of the hand, as to necessitate his being for some
time in hospital. For three days he had suffered from pain in the

armpits, which were swollen and sore to the touch. He described the disease as **uncommonly painful**, and of long continuance.

" A SERVANT at a farm informed Pearson that in Wiltshire and Gloucestershire, the milkers were sometimes so ill as to lie **in bed for several days**.

" MR. FRANCIS said that Cow Pox was very apt to produce **painful sores** on the hands of milkers.

" A SERVANT of Mr. Francis said that Cow Pox affected the hands and arms of the milkers, with **painful sores as large as a sixpence**.

" MR. DOLLING described the disease as a swelling under the arm, chilly fits, etc., not different from the breeding of the Small Pox. After the usual time of sickening, namely, two or three days, there is **a large ulcer** not unlike a carbuncle, which discharges matter.

" DR. PULTENEY described the disease as causing 'a soreness and swelling of the axillary glands as under inoculation for the Small Pox, then chilliness and rigors and fevers, as in the Small Pox.' Two or three days afterwards, **abscesses, not unlike carbuncles**, appear generally on the hands and arms, which ulcerate and discharge much matter.

" MR. BIRD wrote a short account of Cow Pox, 'It appears with red spots on the hands, which enlarge, become roundish, and suppurate, tumours take place in the armpit, the pulse grows quick, the **head aches**, pains are felt in the back and limbs, with sometimes **vomiting and delirium**.'

"ANNIE FRANCIS had pustules on her hands from milking cows. These pustules soon became scabs, which, falling off, discovered **ulcerating and very painful sores**, which were long in healing. Some milk from one of the diseased cows, having spurted on the cheek of her sister and on the breast of her mistress, produced, on these parts of both persons, pustules and sores similar to her own on her hands."

Pearson classified the cases of which he had received information into :—

1. Those in which the patients are inflicted with so

much painful inflammation as to be confined to their beds for several days, and have painful phagedenic sores for several months.

2. Those cases which are so slight that the patients are not confined at all, but get well in a week or ten days.

I will now proceed to point out that, in more recent times, these descriptions have been confirmed.

In 1836, Cow Pox was discovered at Passy, near Paris, and was investigated by Bousquet.[1] A cow had Cow Pox six weeks after calving. Bousquet had no opportunity of seeing the eruption in the early stage, but at the time of his examination, he found reddish-brown crusts on the teats, which later gave place to puckered scars.   The milk-woman, Fleury, who had had Small Pox, nevertheless contracted the disease from the cow. She had several vesico-pustules on the right hand and on her lips.   A vesico-pustule on her hand, when opened with a lancet, *discharged like an abscess.*

Ceely,[2] in 1840-42, very fully described the casual disease in milkers :—

"As in the cow so in man, it does not appear always necessary that the skin should be visibly fissured or abraded to insure infection, although very often we find those conditions in existence. A thin and vascular skin seems capable of absorbing lymph, if copiously applied and long enough retained. The parts upon which the disease is commonly observed are the back of the hands, particularly between the thumb and fore-

---

[1] *Vide* vol. ii., p. 312.
[2] Ceely, *loc. cit.*

finger, about the flexures of the joints and on the palmar, dorsal, and lateral aspects of the fingers. The forehead, eyebrows, nose, lips, ears, and beard, are often implicated from incautious rubbing with the hands, during or soon after milking. In women, the wrists and lower parts of the naked forearm coming in contact with the teats are apt to be affected. If the skin of the hands be very thin and florid, especially if chaps and fissures abound, the individual often suffers severely, having, soon after the decline of the disease, **abscesses and sinuses** of the subcutaneous cellular tissue and often considerable **swelling and inflammation of the absorbents and the axillary glands.** The inflamed spots or papulæ which announce the disease are more circumscribed, better defined, harder, deeper, and more acuminate, than the papulæ produced by some of the other contagious eruptions of the cow. They vary in colour from a deep rose to a dark damask or purple hue, according to the vascularity and texture of the parts affected. If the papulæ be small, there is often no perceptible central depression in the early period of their change to the vesicular state; but they exhibit an ash-coloured or bluish, rather acuminated apex, which gradually becomes relatively flatter as the base enlarges and elevates, when the central depression is more obvious and exhibits a yellowish tinge.

" Larger vesicles, especially on the back of the hand and sides of the fingers, have a well-marked central depression in the early stage, and often a livid or irregularly ecchymosed appearance similar to what is observed on the cow; when fully developed, they present a bluish or slate-coloured hue, which increases in depth, and is more conspicuous towards their decline. This bluish colour, though very common, is often absent, even in some of the vesicles on the same hand. It evidently depends upon and is influenced by the vascularity of the part, the greater or less translucency of the epidermis, the quantity of lymph, the depth and extent of the vesicle. When the epidermis is stripped off from such vesicles, the zone-like adventitious membrane appears diaphanous, and has a bluish or livid hue, derived, doubtless, from the highly congested state of its vessels; here and there, are often seen spots of actual ecchymosis. Where the epidermis is thick, the vesicles are generally well defined, circular, or oval, if the parts will admit, and have only a slight slate-coloured tint in the centre, but more frequently this colour is superseded by an opaque white or a dusky yellowish hue. Where the skin is loose, thin, dark, or dusky, the vesicles are jagged, irregular and puffed at their margins, and, saving the central depression, very much resemble a scald. In size they vary from that of a vetch to a fourpenny-piece, sometimes larger, especially when depending on a wound or extensive fissure. The vesicles are frequently broken, or, when the epidermis is thin, spontaneously burst, causing deep **sloughing of the skin** and cellular tissue and **ulcerations, which slowly heal.** There is often, consequently, much attendant local irritation and considerable symptomatic fever.

"**Papular, vesicular, and bullous eruptions** are occasionally seen attendant on casual Cow Pox, especially in young persons of sanguine temperament and florid complexion, at the height or after the decline of the disease. They are generally of the same character as those known to attend the inoculated disease; but now and then we are told by the patients that these eruptions, either solitary or in clusters, resemble the vaccine vesicles.

"Although the casual Cow Pox in man is mostly found in those who have not previously gone through variola or the vaccine, it is by no means rare to meet with it on persons who have passed through the latter and a few who have had the former disease."

To illustrate this account of casual Cow Pox in man, I will give the particulars of cases observed by Ceely, in October, 1840.

"I. MR. POLLARD, æt. fifty-six. When first observed, the vesicles on the hand and finger had burst, the secondary constitutional symptoms were declining, and the centres of the vesicles, as usual, were in **a sloughing state**. About ten days after the discovery of the disease on the cows, the patient observed two itching small pimples on the site of the present **ulcers**, which, according to his account, ran the normal course of the vaccine vesicle; as soon as the areolæ commenced, having felt scarcely any indisposition before, pain and tenderness of the axillary glands, with the usual constitutional symptoms, arose, and gradually increased for four or five days, but were never severe enough to confine him to the house. When seen later the topical inflammation was rapidly departing, the vesicles were quite broken up, and a **blackish-brown slough** adhered to their centres, their base being surrounded with an elevated induration of a hard red colour.

"II. JOSEPH BROOKS, æt. seventeen, felt the glands and lymphatics of his neck stiff and tender; and noticed a pimple on the temporo-frontal region, which he could not resist scratching. He also observed a red pimple on his finger, of the size of a pin's head, and one very small one on the thumb. In neither situation was there to his knowledge any visible wound or abrasion of the cuticle.

"On the 21st, he had headache, general uneasiness, and pains of the back and limbs, with **tenderness and pain** in the course **of the** corresponding **lymphatic vessels** and **absorbent glands**, particularly of the axilla, which increased till the 23rd, when **nausea** and **vomiting** took place. His right eyelids became swollen, and were closed on that day; but after this period he became better in all respects, never having been confined to the house, although disabled from work. The engravings [Plates XI., XII.] represent the vesicles as they appeared on the 23rd, when the constitutional and local symptoms were subsiding. The vesicle on the temporal region had a well marked central depression, with a slight crust, a general glistening appearance, and was of a bright rose or flesh colour, with a receding areola; and there was an inflamed, tumid, and completely closed state of the corresponding eyelids.

"On the finger, the vesicle was small and flat, with a slightly depressed centre, containing a minute crust. It had a beautiful pearly hue, and was seated on a bright rose-coloured slightly elevated base. On the thumb, the vesicle was also flat and broad, but visibly depressed towards the centre, where there appeared a transverse linear-shaped crust, corresponding, doubtless, with a fissure in the fold of the cuticle. The vesicle was of a dirty yellowish 'hue, and visibly raised on an inflamed circumscribed base. Lymph was obtained from the vesicle on the temple, in small quantity, by carefully removing the central crust, and patiently waiting its slow exudation. In this, as in most other respects, it strikingly resembled the vesicle on the cow, and appeared as solid and compact. The lymph was perfectly limpid, and *very* adhesive. No lymph was taken from the vesicles on the finger and thumb, with a view to avoid any interruption of their natural course.

. "On the 26th and 27th, when the redness and elevation of the base of the vesicles had materially diminished, the vesicles themselves had become greatly enlarged. On the thumb and finger, they were loosely spread out at the circumference, each having **a dark and deep central slough.** On the temple, the margin of the vesicle (as on the cow) was firm and fleshy, its diameter being nearly ten lines, and its centre filled with **a dark brown firmly adherent slough.** In about seven or eight days, with the aid of poultices, the sloughs separated, and the **deep ulcers** healed, leaving cicatrices like variola, deep, puckered, and uneven, which were seen on the 25th of November. The scar on the temple was nearly as large on the 5th of December as the vesicle represented in the engraving:

"JOSEPH WHITE, æt. eighteen ; fair complexion, thin skin. Had never before had variola or vaccine. He had not been long engaged in milking at Dorton before he received the infection ; he first noticed the pimples on the thumb and dorsum of the left hand on the 25th of May. On the 30th, the sixth day of papulation,[1] he first felt the mild constitutional symptoms and the axillary swelling and tenderness. The next day these symptoms increased ; but on the following day, the eighth of papulation, they abated ; yet as his hand was more painful, and he found himself incapable of work, he called on Mr. Knight for advice. Lymph was then abstracted and used by that gentleman ; the areolæ were just commencing. On the 2nd of June, the ninth

---

From our inability to determine the precise period of infection, we are obliged to reckon from the earliest period of recognised papulation.

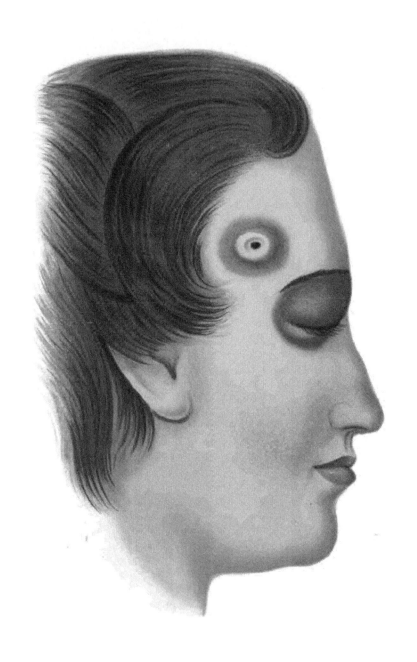

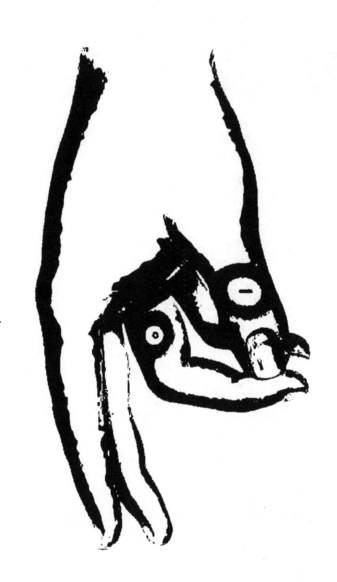

day of papulation, he came to Aylesbury, when the following appearances were observed. On the side of the thumb [Plate XIII.]. between the root of the nail and above the last articulation, was a flat vesicle of a dirty white hue, with a slight central *discolouration* rather than *depression*, and a pale red areola extended around the vesicle and beyond the last joint of the thumb. On the back of the hand there was a smaller vesicle, of a different colour and character; it was visibly raised, overlapping at the outer margin, and depressed in the centre, on a less circumscribed but obvious base. The vesicle was of a light flesh colour; its central crust dark brown, and a moderate light rose-coloured areola, and some tumefaction surrounded and raised the whole. A small red imperfectly vesiculated pimple was seen on the left cheek—noticed by the patient now for the first time. The axillary glands and absorbent vessels were very tender; and though early in the morning the patient felt generally better, in the evening there was increase of all the symptoms.

"*June 3rd, tenth day of papulation.* — To-day worse in all respects; both vesicles considerably enlarged, and the areolæ much increased. There was considerable tumefaction of the thumb and the back of the hand; and the **absorbent vessels, highly inflamed,** could be traced by the eye into the axilla.

"*June 4th, eleventh day of papulation.*—The vesicles enlarging ; areolæ rapidly subsiding; constitutional symptoms less in the morning, but in the evening augmented ; the areolæ then quite gone, but much puffiness of integuments remaining ; and some red absorbents still visible on the arm. The vesicle on the face now contains a light amber crust.

"*June 5th, twelfth day of papulation.*—Better in all respects; less tumefaction of the hand, etc.; vesicles expanding. That on the thumb was of a dull dirty white horn-colour, and it had still a dull red areola around the raised and tumid base ; the centre of the vesicle, scarcely depressed, was of a dirty yellowish-brown colour. On the hand the vesicle was of a dull pearly hue, though rather more glistening than before ; it was much puckered at the centre and the margin : the centre was deeply depressed, and contained a small dirty yellowish-brown crust. The areola was dull, and brighter than that on the thumb.

"*June 8th, fifteenth day of papulation.*—The vesicle on the thumb [Plate XIV.] was still characteristic, though it had acquired a vesicated margin. The vesicle on the hand [Plate XIV.] was also characteristic, though puffed exceedingly at its circumference. The vesicle on the face was now capped with a hard light brown crust [Plate XIV.].

"*June 12th, nineteenth day of papulation.*—The **stage of ulceration** was **fully developed** [Plate XIV:], and the extent of topical disorganisation was now sufficiently manifest.

" In about a fortnight, the ulcers were perfectly healed, leaving scars like those succeeding variolæ or any other disease attended with entire destruction of the corium."

In a letter to Mr. Badcock, dated April 3rd, 1845, Ceely, referring to a new stock of lymph raised from a milker's hand, wrote :—

" In the enclosed lymph I see nothing unusually severe, except on very thin skins, although the milker's hand exhibits now **rough ulcers**, one on the hand **deep enough to encase a bean**."

After Ceely's cases in 1840-41, no cases of casual Cow Pox on the hands of milkers, in this country, were recognised as such and recorded for nearly fifty years. In December 1887, Cow Pox broke out on farms near Cricklade in Wiltshire, and the disease was communicated to nearly all the milkers.

JOHN RAWLINS, milker, informed me that he was the first to catch the eruption from the cows. He states that it came as a hard, painful spot, which formed "matter" and then a "big scab." He had been inoculated about seven weeks ago. He pointed to the scar which remained on his right hand. This scar presented the characters of an irregular cicatrix, indicating considerable loss of substance. He states that he had also two places on his back, where he supposes he had inoculated himself

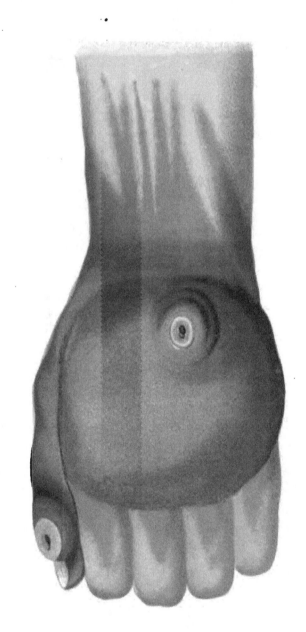

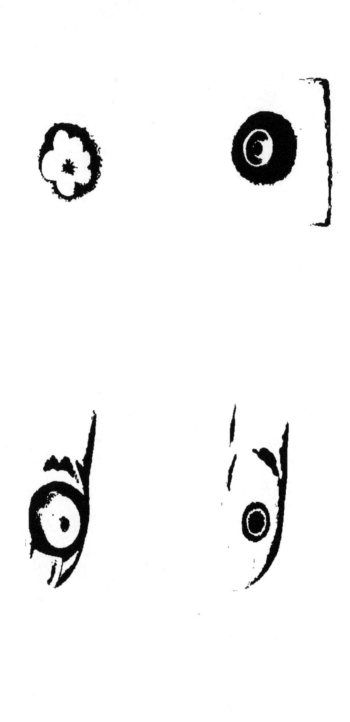

by scratching. He had continued milking ever since, but had had no "fresh places."

WILLIAM HIBBERT, milker. He states that he was inoculated from the cows about the same time as J. R. They were the two milkers of the herd in which the Cow Pox first made its appearance. The eruption appeared in one place on each hand. He pointed to two irregular scars as the remains of the eruption.

JOSEPH LANFEAR, milker, states that he also caught the disease from the cows. On his right hand, "a spot appeared which formed a blister, then discharged matter, and produced a bad sore." Lumps formed at the bend of his elbow and in his armpit. He lost his appetite, felt very poorly, and was obliged to leave off work for two or three days, and stay at home.

He states that about a fortnight or three weeks afterwards, while milking a very bad case, a sore on his left hand, resulting from a wound with a rusty nail, became inflamed, and another place broke out at the tip of one of his fingers, but he was not poorly, nor did lumps appear in his left armpit.

WILLIAM KING works on the farms, but was put on as a milker to take the place of one of the others with bad hands. After his fifth or sixth milking, that is to say about three days after first milking the cows, pimples appeared on his hands, which became "blistered and then ran on to bad sores." He pointed to three irregular scars on the first and third fingers and palm of the right hand. Lumps appeared in his elbow and in his armpit, but he did not feel very poorly in consequence.

JAMES FEBRY, milker, states that about a month ago he noticed spots which appeared on both hands. His fingers swelled and were painful. He says it came first like a pimple and felt hard. Then it "weeped out" water, in four or five days. There were red marks creeping up to his arm. There was a sort of throbbing pain, and he could not sleep at night.

When I saw him, I found on the right hand a scar, but on the left hand, there was an ulcer about the size of a shilling covered with a thick black crust. The crust was partially detached and exposed a granulating ulcer. It was, in this stage, the exact counterpart of the ulcers on the cow's teats.

WILLIAM HIBBERT, JUN., milker, states that he had both hands bad about a month ago. First the index finger of the left hand, and then the knuckle on the right hand and between the first and second fingers.

He says that it came up like a hard pimple, and the finger became swollen and red. After a few days it "weeped out" water and then matter came away. Both his arms were swollen, but his left arm was the worst.

About a fortnight after, he noticed kernels in his armpits, which were painful and kept him awake at night. His arms became worse, he could not raise them, and he had to give up milking. He also had had a "bad place" on the lower lip.

On examination, I found that the axillary glands were still enlarged and tender. He volunteered the statement that the places were just like the sore teats. [Plate XVII., Fig. 4.]

JOHN HARDING, the bailiff's son, also milked the cows. He had a sore on the upper lid of his right eye and on his left hand. In both cases, he had been previously scratched by a cat, and the scratches were inoculated from the cow's teats. The right hand also had been inoculated. The eruption broke out a fortnight ago. His hands were swollen, red, and hot. He felt very poorly and went to bed. Little spots like white blisters appeared on the back of his right hand. His mother remarked that they "rose up exactly as in vaccination." Thick dark brown scabs formed. He was very ill for two or three days, but did not send for a doctor. He had painful lumps at the bend of his arm and in the armpit. He gave up milking and had not taken to it since.

On examining him, the thick crusts on his right hand were identical with the stage of scabbing in ordinary vaccinia. [Plate XV.]. The scabs fell off in about three weeks to a month and left permanent depressed scars.

WILLIAM PLOWMAN, milker. He had taken the place of one of the other milkers who had vesicles on his fingers and had been obliged to give up milking. After the seventh time of milking, he noticed a small pimple on his right cheek (Nov. 27th). The pimple became larger and, as he expressed it, "rose up like a blister."

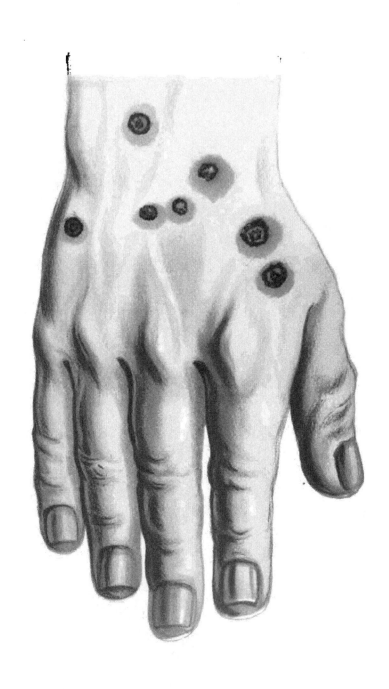

On December 2nd, the date of my visit, there was a depressed vesicle with a small central, yellowish crust and a tumid margin, the whole being surrounded by a well-marked areola and considerable surrounding induration. [Plate XVI., Fig. 1.]

After puncturing the tumid margin and collecting clear lymph in a number of capillary tubes, I raised this central incrustation and observed a crater-like excavation, from which lymph welled up and trickled down the boy's cheek.

On the following day, the crust had re-formed and was studded with coagulated lymph. The areola had become more marked, and on pricking the margin of the vesicle the contents were slightly turbid.

From this day, the surrounding infiltration increased enormously, the whole cheek was inflamed, and the eyelids so œdematous that the eye was almost closed. There was enlargement of the neighbouring lymphatic glands. The crust, which had re-formed, thickened day by day, and on Dec. 9th, there was a thick reddish-brown crust, still bearing the character of central depression, situated on a reddened, raised, and indurated base. [Plate XVI., Fig. 2.]

From this date, the surrounding induration gradually diminished. The crust changed in colour from dark-brown to black, and finally fell off on Dec. 15th, leaving an irregular depressed scar. This scar, when seen several months afterwards was found to be a permanent disfigurement.

A vesicle also formed on the thumb of the left hand. Two days after the pimple appeared on his cheek, the lad says that he noticed a pimple on his thumb, and this, on my visit on Dec. 2nd, presented a greyish flattened vesicle, about the size of a sixpence. On the following day, its vesicular character was much more marked, and a little central crust had commenced to form. [Plate XVII., Fig. 1.] On Dec. 4th, especially towards the evening, the margins became very tumid, giving it a marked appearance of central depression. On Dec. 5th, I punctured the vesicle at its margin with a clean needle, and I filled a number of capillary tubes from the beads of lymph which exuded.

On Dec. 7th, suppuration had commenced; the vesicle

contained a turbid fluid, and the areola was well marked. [Plate XVII., Fig. 2.] On Dec. 9th the crust had assumed a peculiar slate-coloured hue, and, on pressing it, pus welled up through a central fissure. [Plate XVII., Fig. 3.] The areola had increased, and there was considerable inflammatory thickening. The lymphatic glands in the armpit were enlarged and painful. Though there was deep ulceration, which left a permanent scar, the ulceration did not assume quite so severe a character as in some· of the other milkers. Possibly this may be accounted for to some extent by the fact that the pock was covered with a simple dressing, instead of being subjected to the irritation and injury incidental to working on the farm.

There were in all eight milkers, varying in age from seventeen to fifty-five, who contracted the disease from milking the cows. Seven had been vaccinated in infancy, but not since ; one had been revaccinated on entering the navy at fifteen. They were all vaccinated after complete recovery from the casual Cow Pox (that is to say, from three to four months afterwards), and were all completely protected. On the other hand, two milkers who had not had the casual Cow Pox were vaccinated, with the result in one of typical revaccination, in the other of very considerable local irritation.

Effects of Inoculation of Virulent Cow Pox Lymph.

Severe symptoms are not limited to milkers casually infected from the cow. Occasionally, intentional inoculation of fresh virus from the cow reproduces the disease without any mitigation. Thus in Jenner's cases[1] :—

"JAMES PHIPPS. The incisions assumed, at their edges, rather a darker hue than in variolous inoculation, and the efflorescence around them took on more of an erysipelatous look. They terminated in scabs and subsequent eschars.

---

[1] *Vide* vol. ii., p. 172.

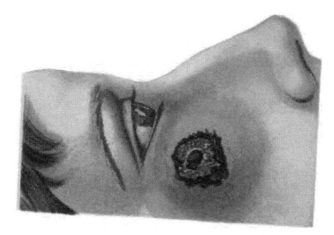

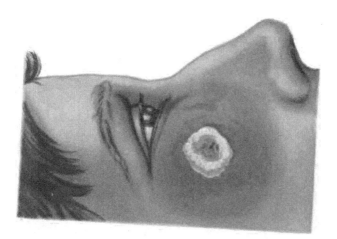

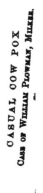

CASUAL COW POX
CASE OF WILLIAM PLOWMAN, MILKER.

M. Gauci lith. ad nat. Ara.

PLATE XVI.

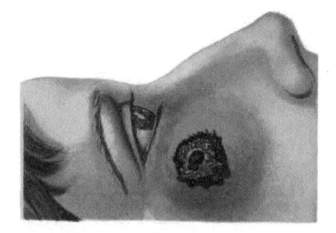

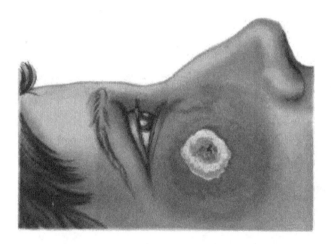

CASUAL COW POX
CASE OF WILLIAM PLOWMAN, MILKER.

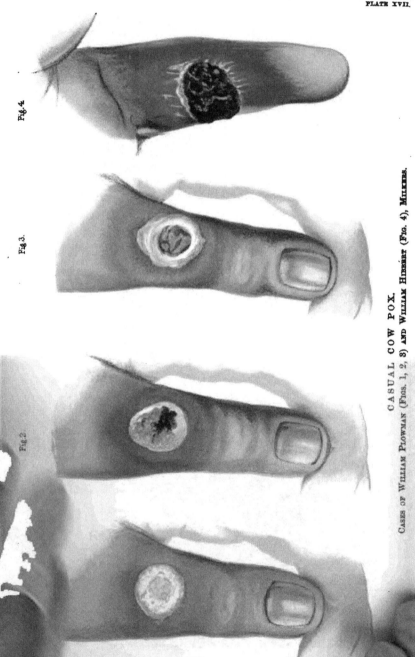

Fig. 4.

Fig. 3.

Fig. 2.

CASUAL COW POX.

CASES OF WILLIAM PLOWMAN (FIGS. 1, 2, 3) AND WILLIAM HERBERT (FIG. 4), MILKERS.

"SUSAN PHIPPS was inoculated from the cow, by inserting matter into a superficial scratch, on Dec. 2nd.

"6th. Appearances stationary.

"7th. The inflammation began to advance.

"8th. A vesication perceptible on the edges, forming . . . an appearance not unlike a grain of wheat with the cleft or indention in the centre.

"9th. Pain in the axilla.

"10th. A little headache; pulse 110; tongue not discoloured; countenance in health.

"11th—12th. No perceptible illness; pulse about 100.

"13th. The pustule was now surrounded by an efflorescence interspersed with very minute pustules, to the extent of about an inch. Some of the pustules advanced in size and maturated. . . The child's arm now showed a disposition to scab, and remained nearly stationary for two or three days, when it began to run into an **ulcerous state,** and then commenced a febrile indisposition, accompanied with an increase of axillary tumour. **The ulcer continued spreading nearly a week, during which time the child continued ill, when it increased to a size nearly as large as a shilling.** It began now to discharge pus; granulations sprung up and it healed.

"MARY HEARN, inoculated from the arm of Susan Phipps.

"6th day. A pustule beginning to appear, slight pain in the axilla.

"7th. A distinct vesicle formed.

"8th. The vesicle increasing; edges very red.

"9th. No indisposition; pustule advancing.

"10th. The patient felt this evening a slight febrile attack.

"11th. Free from indisposition.

"12th and 13th. The same.

"14th. An efflorescence of a faint red colour extending several inches round the arm. The pustule, beginning to show **a disposition to spread,** was dressed with an ointment composed of *hydrarg. nit. rub.* and *ung. cerae.* The efflorescence itself was covered with a plaster of *ung. hydr. fort.* In six hours it was examined, when it was 'found that the efflorescence had totally disappeared.' The application of the ointment of *hydr. nit.*

rub. was made use of for three days, when the state of the pustule remaining stationary, it was exchanged for the *ung. hydr. nit.* This appeared to have a more active effect than the former, and in two or three days, the virus seemed to be subdued, when a simple dressing was made use of; but the sore again showing a disposition to inflame, the *ung. hydrarg. nit.* was again applied, and soon answered the intended purpose effectually."

Jenner's lymph was employed by Mr. Cline with similar results.

"The child sickened on the seventh day, and the fever which was moderate subsided on the eleventh. . . . The ulcer was not large enough to contain a pea."

But the lymph raised by Pearson and Woodville from the "mild" outbreak of Cow Pox in London produced a correspondingly mild effect. This was the result, for example, in the very first case inoculated by Woodville [1] from the cow.

"MARY PAYNE, 3rd day. The inoculated part elevated and slightly inflamed.

"6th day. The local tumour extended to about one-third of an inch in diameter, and was nearly of a circular form, with its edges more elevated than its centre, and with the surrounding inflammation not greater than is usual in cases of inoculated Small Pox. The vesicle upon the middle of the tumour was now very large and distended with a limpid fluid.

"8th day. The redness surrounding the tumour seems returning, and the thirst and. other febrile symptoms are much abated.

"9th day. She is perfectly free from complaint; the inoculated part is scabbing, but surrounded with a hard tumefaction of a bright red colour."

---

[1] *Vide* vol. ii., p. 100.

Consequently Woodville, after describing two hundred cases of inoculated Cow Pox, wrote :—

" We have been told that the Cow Pox tumour has frequently produced erysipelatous inflammation, and phagedenic ulceration, but the inoculated part has not ulcerated in any of the cases which have been under my care, nor have I observed inflammation to occasion any inconvenience except in one instance, when it was soon subdued by the application of aqua lithargyri acetati."

Similar experiences have been encountered since, in the early removes of fresh stocks of virulent lymph. Bousquet,[1] in 1836, in the first trials with his new lymph, made three punctures, but he had soon to abandon this practice, because the intensity of the inflammation was sometimes so great that it spread over the arm and into the axilla. In one case, the vesicles were enormous, and the inflammation so violent that baths, poultices, fomentations, and antiphlogistic diet scarcely sufficed to reduce it. The crusts when they fell off, left *ulcerations* which were very slow to undergo cicatrization.

In some cases, the vesicles which resulted hollowed out the skin so deeply that they left *regular holes*.[2]

It was then that Bousquet appreciated Jenner's fears (*les frayeurs de Jenner*) and understood his anxiety to suppress the vesicle by every means in his power, including cauterisation.

The following year, Estlin,[3] in England, started a

---

[1] *Vide* vol. ii., p. 311.
[2] Compare p. 426.
[3] *Vide* vol. ii., p. 323.

stock of fresh vaccine virus from the cow, and soon
found that the new lymph was extremely active.

"JANE, inoculated from the hand of a milker, had three large
fine prominent circular vesicles, and subsequently Estlin learnt
that the child became 'very poorly.' SARAH OWENS was inoculated with lymph from Jane.

"Each vesicle was perfect, rising abruptly from the arm, its
upper part almost overhanging the base; its surface was much
flattened, and it yielded freely limpid fluid, when punctured before
the areola appeared. On the thirteenth day, the child's body and
extremities were covered with a rash in patches much elevated
from the skin, and she was constitutionally indisposed. On the
fifteenth day, the surface of the vesicle was becoming brown,
and the areola, rash, and general indisposition had disappeared."

In contrasting this new lymph with the current
lymph, Estlin said :—

"The depth in the cellular membrane to which the vesicle
extends is a marked feature in the new lymph. In some cases
under my care, when during the third week the scab has been
rubbed off, there have been deep, though not wide, circular
cavities, that would have contained the whole of a pea-nut
of the smallest size."

Estlin's lymph was employed on sixty-eight children
by Messrs. Michell and Prankard, of Langport in
Somersetshire, and the results which they reported to
Estlin were :—

In 52 the disease was regular.
   1 Severe erysipelas.
   4 Erythematous eruptions of a violent character.
   2 Highly inflamed ulcerated arms.
   1 No effect after twice vaccinating.
   8 Result unknown ; supposed to have been favourable.

In one of the patients, two months old, erythema appeared on the back, and gradually extended to the feet. The child had much dyspnœa, with croupy cough, and died on the 21st. Mr. Estlin's correspondent wrote :—

"I do not attribute its death to vaccination, nor does the mother wholly, as she lost an infant previously with a similar affection of the air passages, but her neighbours set it down to vaccination entirely."

The case of erysipelas, and two more cases of erythema were serious. The attacks occurred during the first week, two of them on the day following vaccination.

The alarm caused by these violent symptoms was so great that Messrs. Michell and Prankard suspended the use of the new lymph.

Estlin supplied some of his lymph to the National Vaccine Establishment. Trials were made, but details were suppressed from publication, from which we may perhaps conclude that in some instances similar results to those experienced by the Langport practitioners were met with. The lymph was condemned, the practice of going back to the cow was discountenanced, and the Report insinuated (without mentioning his name) that Mr. Estlin was disseminating "spurious" Cow Pox.

"We are sorry to hear an anxiety expressed that a recurrence should often be made to the disease of the cow which first supplied the genuine protective matter; for in the first

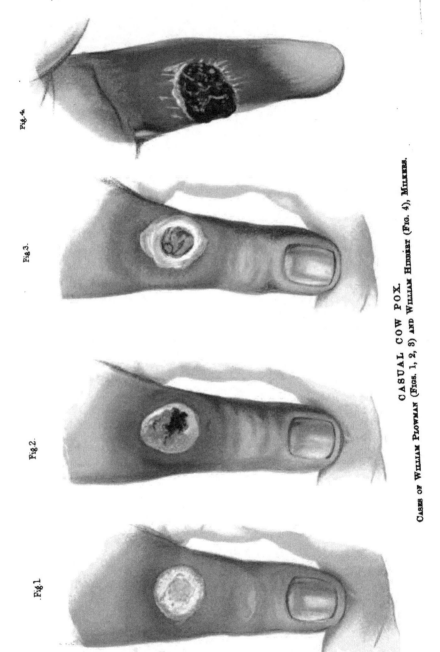

Fig. 4.

Fig. 3.

Fig. 2.

Fig. 1.

CASUAL COW POX.

CASES OF WILLIAM PLOWMAN (FIGS. 1, 2, 3) AND WILLIAM HIRBERT (FIG. 4), MILKERS.

CHAPTER XIV.

JENNER included all spontaneous eruptions on the teats in the term "spurious Cow Pox." None of them were capable of yielding the "grand preventive." True Cow Pox, as he designated the source of his "vaccine lymph," was the eruption on the cow's teat which, according to a prevalent belief among farmers, originated from the grease. This disease was thus briefly described in Jenner's *Inquiry*.[1]

"There is a disease to which the Horse from his state of domestication is frequently subject. The Farriers have termed it *the Grease*. It is an inflammation and swelling in the heel, accompanied at its commencement with small cracks and fissures, from which issues matter possessing properties of a very peculiar kind."

If the men who dressed the horses' heels were called upon to milk cows, they communicated to them the malady known as the Cow Pox.

In support of these statements several cases were given.

Case 1. Several horses belonging to a farm began to have *sore-heels*, which a man named Merret attended to. He milked

---

[1] *Vide* vol. ii., p. 7.

the cows. They soon became affected with Cow Pox, and several sores appeared on his hands.

Case 2. One of the horses on a farm had *sore-heels*, and it fell to the lot of William Smith to attend to the animal. By these means the infection was carried to the cows, and from the cows it was communicated to Smith. On one of his hands were several ulcerated sores, and he was affected with such symptoms as have been before described.

Case 3. Simon Nicholls was employed in applying dressings to the *sore-heels* of one of his master's horses, and at the same time milked his master's cows. The cows became affected in consequence, though not until several weeks after he had begun to dress the horse.

Case 4. A mare, the property of a dairy farmer, began to have *sore-heels*, which were occasionally washed by the servant men of the farm,—Thomas Virgoe, William Wherret, and William Haynes. They contracted "sores on their hands, followed by inflamed lymphatic glands in the arms and axillæ, shiverings succeeded by heat, lassitude and general pains in the limbs ;" and the disease was also communicated to the cows.

From another case in his experience, Jenner thought it highly probable that not only the heels of the horse, but other parts of the body of that animal, were capable of yielding the virus which produces Cow Pox.

" ' An extensive inflammation of the erysipelatous kind appeared without any cause upon the upper part of the thigh of a sucking colt. . . . The inflammation continued several weeks, and at length terminated in the formation of three or four small abscesses.' Dressings were applied to the colt by those who milked the cows, and all of them had Cow Pox."

When Woodville discovered Cow Pox, and raised a stock of " vaccine lymph," it was the ordinary "spontaneous" Cow Pox, arising quite independently of any disease of the horse's heels. Jenner nevertheless pronounced the vaccine to be genuine, and abandoned for a while, the horse-grease theory. In *An Account of the Origin of the Vaccine Inoculation*,[1] and in his evidence before the Committee of the House of Commons, he omitted any reference whatever to this malady.

Thus when Jenner had published his famous *Inquiry*, he found that grease, transmitted direct to man, was not protective against Small Pox. In one case, Small Pox was produced by inoculation, and in another, by infection, after an attack of grease. To explain this, Jenner assumed that the virus from the horse's heel must be modified by passage through the cow in order to acquire the peculiar properties which converted it into a protective against Small Pox. Later he abandoned horse grease altogether and advocated " spontaneous " Cow Pox, but still later he reverted to grease, and formally adopted it as the "true life-preserving fluid."[2]

Jenner recognised tha this vaccinogenic "grease" was not limited to the heels of the horse. The fullest description which he wrote of the disease was the following :—

"The skin of the horse is subject to an eruptive disease of a vesicular character, which vesicle contains a limpid fluid, showing itself most commonly in the heels. The legs first become œdematous; and *then* fissures are observed. The skin contiguous to these fissures, when accurately examined, is seen

---

[1] *Vide* vol. ii., p. 271.   [2] p. 393.

studded with small vesicles surrounded by an areola. These
vesicles contain the specific fluid. It is the ill management
of the horse in the stable that occasions the malady to appear
more frequently in the heel than in other parts ; I have detected
it connected with a sore on the neck of the horse, and on the
thigh of a colt."

According to Baron, Jenner had observed a case of
transmission of grease to sheep :—

" Dr. Jenner, in like manner, had ascertained that the cow
was not the only animal capable of receiving the infection of
the *grease*. A sheep that had three lambs, of which two
perished, being incommoded by the superabundance of milk,
was drawn by a servant who, at the same time, dressed the
greasy heels of a horse. Pustules, similar to those of the
Vaccine, appeared on the teats of the sheep : the same person
who milked the sheep immediately afterwards milked two cows,
and communicated the disease to them. From the cows thus
infected a servant of the house received the Cow Pox."

Jenner summed up his reasons for attributing Cow
Pox to grease as follows :—

" First. I conceived this was its source, from observing that
where the Cow Pox had appeared among the dairies here (unless
it could be traced to the introduction of an infected cow or
servant) it had been preceded at the farm by a horse diseased
in the manner already described, which horse had been attended
by some of the milkers.

" Secondly. From its being **a popular opinion** throughout
this great dairy country, and from its being **insisted on by
those who here attend sick cattle.**

" Thirdly. From the total absence of the disease in those
countries, where the men servants are not employed in the dairies.

" Fourthly. From having observed that morbid matter
generated by the horse frequently communicates, in a casual
way, a disease to the human subject so like the Cow Pox, that

in many cases it would be difficult to make the distinction between one and the other.

"Fifthly. From being induced to suppose, from experiments, that some of those who had been thus affected from the horse resisted the Small Pox.

"Sixthly. From the progress and general appearance of the pustule on the arm of the boy whom I inoculated with matter taken from the hand of a man infected by a horse; and from the similarity to the Cow Pox of the general constitutional symptoms which followed."

Baron has published Jenner's reasons from MS. notes, which contain several important additional details.

"1st. From its being the fixed opinion of those who have been in the habit of attending to cows infected with this disease for a great number of years.

"2ndly. From its being a popular opinion in this great dairy-country, and from the cautions the farmer observes when he has a horse with a sore heel.

"3rdly. From observing, in almost every instance, that the appearance of the Cow Pox at a farm was preceded by some disease of a horse at the same farm, which produced the discharge of some fluid from the skin.

"4thly. From having attempted, in vain, to give the Small Pox to the son of a *farrier* who had had sores and a fever, from dressing a diseased horse.

"And 5thly. From the peculiar appearance of the pustule, and its disposition to run into an ulcer in the arm of the boy who was inoculated with matter taken from the hand of a man who received the infection from dressing a slight spontaneous sore on a horse's heel."

In testimony of its being a popular opinion, Jenner published a letter on this subject from the Rev. Mr. Moore, of Chalford Hill :[1]—

---

[1] *Vide* vol. ii., p. 169.

" In the month of November, 1797, my horse had diseased heels, which was certainly what is termed the grease; and at a short subsequent period my cow was also affected with what a neighbouring farmer (who was conversant with the complaints of cattle) pronounced to be the Cow Pox, which he at the same time observed my servant would be infected with: and this proved to be the case; for he had **eruptions on his hands, face, and many parts of the body, the pustules appearing large, and not much unlike the Small Pox, for which he had been inoculated a year and a half before, and had then a very heavy burthen.** The pustules on the face might arise from contact with his hands, as he had a habit of rubbing his forehead, where the sores were the largest and thickest.

" The boy associated with the farmer's sons during the continuance of the disease, neither of whom had had the Small Pox, but they felt no ill effects whatever. He was not much indisposed, as the disease did not prevent him from following his occupations as usual. No other person attended the horse or milked the cow, but the lad above mentioned. I am firmly of opinion that the disease in the heels of the horse, which was a **virulent grease**, was the origin of the servant's and the cow's malady."

Jenner remarks :—

" From the similarity of symptoms, both constitutional and local, between the Cow Pox and the disease received from morbid matter generated by a horse, the common people in this neighbourhood, when infected with this disease, through a strange perversion of terms, frequently called the Cow Pox. Let us suppose then such a malady to appear among some of the servants at a farm, and at the same time that the Cow Pox were to break out among the cattle; and let us suppose too that some of the servants were infected in this way, and that others received the infection from the cows. It would be recorded at the farm, and among the servants themselves, wherever they might afterwards be dispersed, that they had all had the Cow Pox. But it is clear that an individual thus infected from the horse would neither be for a certainty secure himself, nor would he impart security to others, were they inoculated by virus thus .generated. He still would be in danger of taking the Small Pox. Yet were this to happen before the nature of the Cow Pox be more maturely considered by the public, my evidence on the subject might be depreciated unjustly."

Jenner also received the following account[1] from Mr. Fewster, of Thornbury, "a gentleman perfectly well acquainted with the appearances of the Cow Pox on the human subject:"—

"WILLIAM MORRIS, aged thirty-two, servant to Mr. Cox of Almonsbury, in this county, applied to me the 2nd of April, 1798. He told me, that four days before he found a stiffness and swelling in both his hands, which were so painful, it was with difficulty he continued his work; that he had been seized with pain in his head, small of the back, and limbs, and with frequent chilly fits succeeded by fever. On examination I found him still affected with these symptoms, and that there was a great prostration of strength. Many parts of his hands on the inside were chapped, and on the middle joint of the thumb of the right hand there was a small phagedenic ulcer, about the size of a large pea, discharging an ichorous fluid. On the middle finger of the same hand there was another ulcer of a similar kind. These sores were of a *circular* form, and he described their first appearance as being somewhat like blisters arising from a burn. He complained of **excessive pain**, which extended up his arm into the axilla. These symptoms and appearances of the sores were so exactly like the Cow Pox, that I pronounced he had taken the distemper from milking cows. He assured me he had not milked a cow for more than half a year, and that his master's cows had nothing the matter with them. I then asked him if his master had a *greasy* horse? which he answered in the affirmative;

---

[1] *Vide* vol. ii., p. 170.

and further said, that he had constantly dressed him twice
a day for the last three weeks or more, and remarked that the
smell of his hands was much like that of the horse's heels.
On the 5th of April, I again saw him, and found him still
complaining of pain in both his hands, nor were his febrile
symptoms at all relieved. The ulcers had now spread to the
size of a seven-shilling gold coin, and another ulcer, which I had
not noticed before, appeared on the first joint of the forefinger of the left hand, equally painful with that on the right.
I ordered him to bathe his hands in warm bran and water,
applied escharotics to the ulcers, and wrapped his hands up
in a soft cataplasm. The next day he was much relieved, and
in something more than a fortnight got well. He lost his nails
from the thumb and fingers that were ulcerated."

Mr. Tanner was the first to succeed in experimentally transmitting grease to the cow by inoculating
some of the liquid matter from the heel of a horse.
The result was the production of a " vaccinal vesicle,"
and he wrote :—

"From handling the cow's teats, I became infected myself,
and had two pustules on my hand, which brought on inflammation
and made me unwell for several days. The matter from the
cow and from my own hand proved efficacious in infecting
both human subjects and cattle."

Jenner received some of Tanner's equine virus while
he was in London, in April 1800, and some of it, he
passed on to Mr. Wachsel of the Small Pox Hospital.

In the same month some observations tending to
confirm Jenner's opinion were made by Mr. Lupton,
a surgeon of Thame, Oxfordshire, which were communicated to Jenner by Sir Christopher Pegge, and
published in the *Medical and Physical Journal.*

In the year 1801, Dr. Loy published his experiments in a work entitled *Some Observations on the Origin of Cow Pox*.[1] Coleman, Woodville, and Simmons had negative results when they experimented on cows, with grease, but Dr. John Loy met with very different experience. Mr. Loy, surgeon at Pickering, had undertaken experiments from having met with the following cases :—

"I. A farrier applied to him with an eruption on his hands, composed of distinct pustules, containing a thin fluid, and surrounded by an inflamed ring. The vesicle had an appearance similar to that arising from a burn. They were all regularly circumscribed, and a small dark speck could be discovered in the middle of each. The patient had been dressing a horse affected with the grease. He had had Small Pox.

"II. A young man, a butcher, at Middleton, near Pickering, was affected with painful sores on both his hands, particularly about the roots of the nails. These sores in a few days became inflamed, and a vesicle formed upon each. Soon after the appearance of the vesicles, a number of red painful lines, which appeared to be inflamed lymphatics extended from the pustules to the arm-pit, where a tumor formed; he had also a pustule, of the same appearance as those on his hands, upon one eyebrow, which, he said, had been affected with an itching, inducing him frequently to scratch it; and the pustule had no doubt been communicated in that manner from his fingers. He had a considerable degree of fever, which continued obstinate till the absorption from the pustules was prevented by destroying them with caustic, when the tumor in the axilla also dispersed. This patient, like the former, had been for some time employed in applying remedies to the heels of a horse affected with the grease, and was continuing to do so at the time he begun to be indisposed. He had never undergone the Small Pox."

[1] *Vide* vol. ii., p. 279.

Mr. Loy, being curious to ascertain whether this disease could be communicated by inoculation, took a quantity of matter from the pustules of this patient and inserted it into the arm of his brother, with the following results :—

"In a few days, some degree of inflammation appeared, and on the eighth day, a vesicle formed ; my patient had now some slight feverish symptoms, which continued a day or two.

"This disease had exactly the appearances of the genuine Cow Pox, and I intended to have tried the effect of the Small Pox virus, had not the fears of the boy's parents prevented me."

At the same time that Mr. Loy performed this experiment, Dr. John Loy inoculated the udder of a cow with matter from the pustule of the same patient. When the animal was inspected on the ninth day, there was a vesicle with a "rose-coloured rim." Matter was taken and inserted into the arm of a child. The inflammation, vesication, and scabbing which followed corresponded with Cow Pox. On the sixth day of the disease, the child was inoculated with Small Pox. The wound "seemed to be rather inflamed on the third day, but in a few days more it healed."

Dr. Loy then inoculated another child, with matter taken direct from Mr. Loy's patient. The results were similar to the effects of Cow Pox, and subsequent inoculation of Small Pox produced no effect. The next experiment was with another case of grease. A cow was inoculated, and in a few days, a vesicle formed containing a large quantity of watery fluid, and of a purple tinge. A quantity of the limpid water was inserted into the arm of a child. A vesicle formed on the ninth day, and the same day, the child was inoculated with Small Pox without effect.

Dr. John Loy then inoculated a child direct from a horse suffering from grease.

"On the third day, a small degree of inflammation surrounded the wound. On the fourth, the inoculated place was much elevated, and a vesicle, of a purple colour, was formed on the fifth day : on the sixth and seventh, the vesicle increased, and the inflammation extended, and became of a deeper colour ; on the same day, a chilliness came on, attended with nausea and some vomiting. These were soon succeeded by increased heat, pain in the head, and a frequency of breathing ; the pulse was very frequent, and the tongue was covered with a white crust. When in bed, the child was much disposed to sweat. By the use of some medicines, and exposure to cool air, the feverish symptoms soon abated, and disappeared entirely on the ninth day. On the sixth day, Small Pox matter was inserted into the same arm in which the matter of Grease had been placed, but at a considerable distance from it. On the fourth and fifth days of the Small Pox inoculation, some redness appeared about the wound, and on the sixth a small vesicle. The inflammation now decreased, and on the ninth day, the vesicle was converted into a scab."

On the sixth day of the inoculation, four other children were inoculated with matter from this child. On the tenth day, an extensive erysipelatous efflorescence surrounded the vesicles. On the same day, they were all inoculated for the Small Pox, in the arms free from the former inoculation. Nothing appeared except a very small degree of inflammation. It is not stated whether the lymph stock was carried on.

PEDIGREE OF THE FIRST STOCK OF DIRECT EQUINE LYMPH.

HORSE
|
A Child
|
Five Children

Loy had made a number of experiments with grease, but only in certain cases did he succeed in getting positive results, for which he gave the following reason :—

"This fact induces me to suspect, that two kinds of Grease exist, differing from each other in the power of giving disease to the human or brute animal ; and there is another circumstance which renders this supposition probable. The horses that communicated the infection to their dressers were affected with a general, as well as a topical disease. The animals, at the commencement of their disease, were evidently in a feverish state, from which they were relieved as soon as the complaint appeared at their heels, and an eruption upon the skin. The horse, too, from whom the infectious matter was procured for inoculation, had a considerable indisposition, previous to the disease at his heels, which was attended, as in the others, **with an eruption over the greatest part of his body** ; but those that did not communicate the disease at all, had a local affection only. From this, perhaps, may be explained, the want of success attending the experiments of the gentlemen I have mentioned."

Loy also observed that the grease appeared to act with greater mildness after having been cultivated on the cow, or the human subject. Thus after direct inoculation from the horse, a purple tinge was observed, but this did not appear with lymph which had been passed either through the medium of the cow or the human subject.

With regard to the application of the variolous test, all Loy's experiments were deprived of any value. No conclusions could be drawn when the inoculation was performed at or near the height of the disease, which had been produced by insertion of the virus of grease. Loy ought to have been fully aware that under such circumstances, inoculation would prove abortive.

Jenner was the first to perform arm-to-arm indirect, and Loy was the first to perform arm-to-arm direct equination.

Jenner sent a copy of Loy's work to the Duke of Clarence with a letter, in which he made the following remarks :—

" In obedience to the wish your Royal Highness expressed to me at Lord Grantley's, I have done myself the honour of sending you Dr. Loy's pamphlet on the Origin of the Cow Pox, which decisively proves my early assertions upon that subject. This discovery is the more curious and interesting as it places in a new point of view the traditionary account handed down to us by the Arabian physicians that the Small Pox was originally derived from the camel. The whole opens to the physiologist a new field of inquiry, and I sincerely hope it may be so cul-tivated that human nature may reap from it the most essential benefit."

Dr. Loy also corresponded with Jenner on this subject.

DR. LOY TO DR. JENNER.

"SIR,—I have not yet had an opportunity of making any further experiments respecting the origin of the Cow Pox, on account of the disease of grease having been of late remarkably rare in this country. From the evidence, however, I have had of the truth of your opinion, and from some observations which have been made on my experiments by my worthy preceptor, Dr. Duncan, of Edinburgh, I consider myself in some degree called upon to pay more attention to this curious subject, and you may, Sir, be assured that you shall be informed of my success.

"I have the satisfaction to mention that the subject inoculated with the grease matter on Experiment VI. has withstood the action of the Small Pox, by way of repeated exposure to the natural disease. Several of those also who were inoculated with vaccine virus, generated by inoculation with the equine, have been exposed more than once to the natural infection of the Small Pox, but without the least effect. Dr. Duncan seems to conjecture that the persons on whom the experiments were performed might have previously had the small Pox; but any foundation for such a supposition is perfectly groundless. Most of the persons who were subjected to the experiments had never been within several miles of the Small Pox till inoculated. And that the small Pox matter I made use of was good is proved by the same virus giving readily the disease to others.

"There is not the least doubt but the experiments will remain successful; and that they were fairly performed many respectable gentlemen in this neighbourhood can testify. One gentleman at my request saw me inoculate one of his cows from the greased heels of his horse, with a lancet which he himself supplied me at the time of experiment. This trial was successful. . . .

"Give me, Sir, the honour to subscribe myself,

"Your faithful friend and servant,

"John Glover Loy.

"Whitby, *December 26th*, 1802."

Experiments with grease were also made, about this time, on the Continent. Dr. De Carro appears to have been the first to communicate to Jenner the result of some experiments conducted by Sacco.

"If you have felt so much pleasure in hearing that your discovery is known and practised in India, I hope that my late intelligence of the true Cow Pox, produced at Milan with the *giardoni* on Dr. Sacco's own horse and that of one of his neighbours, has not been less agreeable to you."

And in a reply to his letter Jenner makes some observations on this subject.

DR. JENNER TO DR. DE CARRO.

" *March 28th*, 1803.

"Since the commencement of our correspondence, great as my satisfaction has been in the perusal of your letters, I do not recollect when you have favoured me with one that has afforded me pleasure equal to the last. The regret I have experienced, at finding that every endeavour to send the vaccine virus to India in perfection, again and again failed, is scarcely to be described to you ; judge, then, what pleasure you convey in assuring me that my wishes are accomplished. I am confident that had not the opponents, in this country, to my ideas of the origin of the disease been so absurdly clamorous (particularly the *par nobile fratrum*) the Asiatics would long since have enjoyed the blessings of vaccination, and many a victim been rescued from an untimely grave. The decisive experiments of Dr. Loy on this subject have silenced the tongue of these gentlemen for ever.

" I am happy to see this interesting work translated by you, and hope it will travel the world over.

" It is very extraordinary, but certainly a fact, that the plate which I gave in my first publication of the equine pustule (although its origin was detailed) was by almost every reader considered as the *vaccine*. There are probably some varieties in the pustules which arise among horses. You will observe, by a reference to my publication, that the virus in the instance I now allude to, was so very active that it infected every person who dressed the horse.

" I am happy to find an opinion taken up by me, and mentioned in my first publication, has so able a supporter as yourself. I thought it highly probable that the Small Pox might be a *malignant variety* of the Cow Pox. But this idea was scouted by my countrymen, particularly P. and W. . . ."

In a subsequent letter, De Carro gave an account of some important experiments by Dr. La Font.

DE CARRO TO DR. JENNER.

"VIENNA, *21st June*, 1803.

"MY DEAR SIR,—My friend Dr. Marcet wrote to me lately that the accounts I have sent to you of Dr. Sacco's experiments have afforded you great satisfaction. The motive which induces me to write to you to-day is another confirmation of your theory which has taken place in a country where you scarcely expect it from, the more so that it is accompanied with veterinary observations which appear to me very nice and curious.

"Monsieur La Font, a French physician established at Salonica in Macedonia, has been one of the most active vaccinators I know on the continent . . . Some time afterwards, I sent him a translation of Dr. Loy's experiments, and desired him to make as many veterinary observations and experiments as he could. He has some reason to suppose that the Cow Pox reigns in that country, according to the report of several Albanese peasants. As to the *grease* (which he calls javart), he says that the farriers at Salonica know it very well. Dr. La Font began his experiments with the kind of grease which the Macedonian farriers call the *variolous*. He found a horse which had been attacked with feverish symptoms, that ceased as soon as the eruption appeared. The fore legs were much swelled; the left had four ulcers, one upon the heel, a second some inches higher, a third on the articulation, a fourth near the breast. The eruption on the legs was, he says, very like the Small Pox, but none was to be seen on the other parts of the body. He took matter from the upper ulcer, which was of twelve days' standing. The matter was limpid, but a little yellowish and *filamentous* (thready); first, a cow was submitted to this inoculation, but without success; secondly, a girl twelve years old, without effect; but this girl

had been vaccinated some months before without success, and
was suspected to have had the Small Pox; thirdly, two boys,
one six, the other five, years old, were inoculated with the same
equine matter; and in both, a pustule appeared, which followed
the regular course of a vaccine pustule. The colour was less
white, and more purple than usual. Those two children had
a pretty strong fever, for which some cooling medicines were
administered. Those inoculated with matter from them underwent the disease in its usual mild way.

"These particulars, I hope, will silence all those who still
doubt of the truth of your doctrine. These observations enhance
the merit of your discovery. The *means* of making it were
everywhere; yet nobody before you had the least idea of that
singular connection between the grease, the Cow Pox, and the
Small Pox."

On March 25th, 1803, Sacco communicated to
Jenner the details of his experiments.

"I have for a long time been making experiments with grease
in order to confirm your opinion of the origin of vaccine. Until
the beginning of this year, I have had only negative results.
Studying Mr. Loy's little book encouraged me to make another
attempt. In the winter of this year grease could not have been
more common than it was, in consequence of the quantity of
water which there was and the mud which resulted on the roads;
thus nearly all the horses suffered from grease, my servant
was attacked by it on both forearms, having five vesicles from
dressing one of my horses suffering from grease. He only
informed me of it when the vesicles were beginning to dry up.
This encouraged me to continue my experiments. I inoculated
several children and several cows with the virus which came
from grease at different stages, but always without effect. A
coachman came to the hospital to be examined with an eruption
which he had on his hands; it was at once recognised that
it was vaccine taken while treating horses, which in fact he had
dressed. He was taken to the foundling hospital, where some
inoculations were made. He came to me the same day, and

I made nine inoculations on as many children, and I inoculated the teat of a cow as well. Three of these children had an eruption exactly like Cow Pox. Nothing happened in the cow. I made other inoculations with matter taken from these children, and I have already reached the fourth remove, which reproduces itself with the same effect as vaccine. I have already inoculated several of these individuals with Small Pox, but without any effect. It is therefore very certain that the grease is the cause of Cow Pox, and the name may at once be changed to *equine* or into anything which you think better. I have also at last obtained, with the virus of grease inoculated with six more children, two vesicles exactly like those of vaccine. I am construing my observations. Everything points to the conclusion that we shall procure from grease a virus for protection against Small Pox without the *intermedium* of the cow.

" I hope that this new proof will remove the doubts which still existed about the origin of Cow Pox. I will publish the results of these experiments in a work on vaccination, to which I will add a coloured plate of *grease*."

Jenner replied to Sacco, expressing his confidence in his original theory.

" Accept my best acknowledgments for your very kind attention. I am extremely gratified by your goodness in sending me your pamphlet on Vaccine Inoculation, your obliging letter, and above all the virus from the plains of Lombardy. I am confident that wherever the horse and the cow are domesticated together, and the same human being that attends the one, under a peculiar malady of the foot, milks the cow also, that there the disease called the Cow Pox may arise."

In Paris, according to Baron, equination was practised in 1812.

" A coachman who had not had Small Pox, and who dressed a horse affected with the *grease*, had a crop of pustules on his hands, which resembled the vaccine. Two children were inoculated from these pustules, and the genuine vaccine was excited in both : from this stock many successive inoculations were effected, all possessing the proper character. A similar series of inoculations took place from another infant who was infected from one of the scabs taken from the pustules on the hand of the coachman."

In spite of these results the theory was still discredited in London, and Jenner wrote to Moore, July 23rd, 1813, giving information of a fresh stock of equine virus which he had been using for months.

"In one of your letters you seemed not perfectly satisfied that the fact respecting the origin of the vaccine was clearly made out. For my part, I should think that Loy's experiments, independently of my own observations, were sufficient to establish it, to say nothing of Sacco's and others' on the Continent. However, I have now fresh evidence, partly foreign and partly domestic. The latter comes from a Mr. Melon, a surgeon of repute at Lichfield. He has sent me some of his **equine virus, which I have been using from arm to arm for these two months past,** without observing the smallest deviation in the progress and appearance of the pustules from those produced by the vaccine. I have at length found the French document I formerly alluded to, which, with Melon's, shall be sent to you in the course of the ensuing week."

Jenner wrote, again, on the same subject, August 1st, 1813.

To James Moore, Esq.

" Dear Moore,—My friend and neighbour, Mr. Hicks, will deliver to you the promised papers respecting equine virus. I **have been constantly equinating for some months,** and perceive not the smallest difference between the pustules thus produced and the vaccine. Both are alike, because they come from the same source."

And again, in a letter, dated October 27th, 1813 :—

" I am sorry you have not succeeded in infecting a cow. I have told you before that the matter which flows from the fissures in the heel will do nothing. It is contained in vesicles on the edges and the surrounding skin. Did I ever inform you of the curious result of vaccinating carters ? These people from their youth up have the care of the horses used for ploughing our corn lands. Great numbers of them in the course of my practice here have come to me from the hills to be vaccinated ; but the average number which resisted has been one half. On inquiry, many of them have recollected having sores on their hands and fingers from dressing horses affecteu with sore heels, and being so ill as to be disabled from following their work ; and on several of their hands, I have found the cicatrix as perfect and as characteristically marked as if it had arisen from my own vaccination."

Jenner now appears to have almost, if not entirely, abandoned vaccination for equination. On the 1st of April, 1817, he made the following memorandum :—

" Rise and progress of the **equine matter** from the farm of Allen, at Wansell. From a horse to Allen ; from Allen to two or three of his milch cows ; from the cows to James Cole, a young man who milked at the farm ; from James Cole to John Powell, by inoculation from a vesicle on the hand of Cole ; and to Anne Powell, an infant ; from Powell to Samuel Rudder ; from Rudder to Sophia Orpin, and to Henry Martin ; from H. Martin to Elizabeth Martin. All this went on with perfect regularity for eight months, when it became intermixed with other matter, so that no journal was kept afterwards. Proof was obtained of the patients being duly protected."

And among other entries to a similar effect, there was, on the 17th of May, the following :—

"Took matter from Jane King (**equine direct**), for the National Vaccine Establishment. The pustules beautifully correct."

This stock of equine lymph was widely diffused. Baron and many medical friends received supplies of it, and it was also introduced into Scotland.

Baron adopted equination, and made notes of cases of *grease*.

"It happened to me to see one case of this kind in the autumn of the year 1817. A young man in this neighbourhood, who had dressed a horse with the grease, had not less than fifty pustules on his hand and wrists. They exhibited the true character of the Variolæ Vaccinæ when taken in the casual way. The pustules were too far advanced to permit of any experiments being made with virus taken from them. I cannot refrain from remarking in this place, that as the disease, whether caught from the cow or the horse, is much more severe than when communicated by inoculation, so it likewise differs from the last in being sometimes what may be truly called an eruptive disease. Besides the case just specified, I know of instances where the disease, when it has been caught from cows in the dairy, has produced pustules more extensively diffused over the body than in the case above mentioned."

In the following year, Baron sent some fresh equine virus to Jenner. It was obtained from the hands of a boy who had been infected directly from a horse. The disease assumed a pustular form, and extended over both arms.

Jenner acknowledged the receipt of Baron's virus in the following letter:—

"Yesterday H. Shrapnell brought me the **equine virus** and your drawing, which conveys so good an idea of the disease that no one who has seen it can doubt that the vesicles contain **the true and genuine life-preserving fluid.** I have inserted some of it into a child's arm ; but I shall be vexed if you and some of your young men at the Infirmary have not done the same with the fluid fresh from the hand."

In 1818, Kahlert,[1] on the Continent, confirmed the experiments made by Loy and Sacco.

"In the month of May 1818, one of my friends remarked to me that two horses which he had just bought were not in their usual state of health ; that they quickly became fatigued, that their hind legs were stiff, and that they even went lame, and in fact he thought they were suffering from *javart* (*mauke*).

"These two horses were of the ordinary breed of the country (Bohemia), black, six years old, well nourished, and well cared for, but according to the groom they had for some time lost their spirit and appetite. . . . I at once noticed that the joint of the foot was swollen, that moisture exuded from it, and that the posterior part of the pastern was still slightly red and swollen. and hotter than the neighbouring parts. At the slightest touch, the animal showed signs of pain ; the hair was stuck together, and a clear yellowish fluid with a peculiar odour escaped. . . . I was not slow in recognising the *true equine preservative*. I collected the fluid on a lancet to inoculate cows and children."

The experiments on cows succeeded ; children were inoculated from the vesicles which resulted, and a lymph stock was started which was widely used.

In an appendix to the second volume of Jenner's *Biography*, published in 1837, Baron made the following remark :—

"I take this opportunity of expressing my regret that I have

---

[1] L'Almanach de Carlsbad. *Du javant preservatif trouvé en Bohême.* 1833. (Quoted by Auzias-Turenne.)

employed the word *grease* in alluding to the disease in the horse. *Variolæ Equinæ* is the proper designation. It has no necessary connexion with the grease, though the disorders frequently co-exist. This circumstance at first misled Dr. Jenner, and it has caused much misapprehension and confusion."

In 1840, Ceely remarked that there were farmers and others who had good reason for believing in the origin of Cow Pox from the equine vesicle, which he regarded as *eczema impetiginodes*.

Jenner's theory of the origin of Cow Pox has been discouraged, and completely replaced by the theory of Cow Small Pox, advocated so strongly by Baron, and supported by an erroneous interpretation of Ceely's and Badcock's variolation experiments; and thus the "Cow Pox" and the "grease" of the farmers were no longer of interest, while the hypothetical Cow *Small* Pox, which could never be discovered, has been credited with having become extinct, since the days of Jenner. At the present day the derivation of "vaccine lymph" from a disease of the horse is, almost, if not entirely, unknown to medical practitioners, and certainly vaccinogenic "grease" in this country is not differentiated by practical veterinarians of the present day, from the various diseases which it simulates. Like actinomycosis, it has been lost sight of under a variety of appellations. I would draw the attention of veterinarians to this, by giving a detailed account of the researches carried out by veterinary surgeons in France.

First Outbreak at Toulouse.

In 1860, the horses at Rieumes, near Toulouse, were attacked by an epizoötic malady. In less than three weeks, there were more than one hundred cases. According to the veterinary surgeon, M. Savrans, the animals suffered from slight fever, rapidly followed by local symptoms, the most marked of which were swelling of the hocks, and an eruption of small pustules on the surface of the swollen parts, which were at the same time hot and painful. After three to five days there was a discharge from the pastern, which continued for eight to ten days, during which the inflammation gradually diminished. The pustules dried up, and in about a fortnight the crusts with patches of hair fell off, leaving more or less marked scars.

The eruption appeared at the same time on different parts of the body, especially on the nostrils, lips, buttocks, and vulva. Savrans believed that the mares taken to the breeding establishment at Rieumes had been infected from the cords which had been used in tying up other affected animals and had become thereby infected with the virus of this disease.

One of the mares was taken by the owner, M. Corail, to the veterinary school, to be examined by M. Lafosse. About eight days after this visit, significant symptoms appeared: loss of appetite, lameness, stiffness of both pastern joints, and a hot, painful swelling of the left pastern joint.

The hair was staring, and there were vesicles on the skin, from which a liquid exuded having an ammoniacal odour, but less fœtid than the secretion in *eaux aux jambes*.

M. Lafosse regarded it as a case of acute grease, and this led him to inoculate a cow. This experiment, made on the 25th of April, a week after the eruption had first appeared on the mare, was completely successful. On the teats of the inoculated cow, at every puncture, there were large, flat, firm, round, umbilicated vesicles. They had all the characters of inoculated Cow Pox. Another cow inoculated with liquid from this first remove, manifested typical vesicles, which, transmitted to a child and to a horse, gave rise in both cases to a very fine "vaccinal" eruption. A child inoculated from the vesicle of this horse had also "vaccine vesicles." On making a comparative inoculation with current vaccine lymph on the same subject, the vesicles were found to be larger, finer, and slower in their development. When M. Lafosse detected the disseminated eruption on various parts of the body, especially around the lips and nostrils, he recognised that the disease was not an ordinary attack of grease.

The occurrences at Rieumes and Toulouse were communicated to the Academy of Medicine, in 1862,

by M. Bousquet; and M. Renault observed that the
original error in diagnosis, made after a cursory examination, by M. Lafosse, added greatly to the interest
of the inoculation experiment, because it might explain
the difference in the results obtained up to the present time by medical men and veterinary surgeons
who since Jenner had inoculated the grease. Renault
said :—" It may be possible that the few experimenters who assert that they have seen Cow Pox
result, under their hands and eyes, from accidental
or experimental inoculation of the matter of the grease,
were in reality dealing with the vesicular malady of
Toulouse, while the much larger number of them who
obtained no effect from their inoculations must have
employed the discharge from the true grease, which
was formerly so common."

Renault added :—" The occurrence at Toulouse is
of great importance in drawing attention to this
subject, which will lead to further discussion. It
will teach veterinary surgeons that there is an
affection, principally manifested on the horse's
heels, which appears up to this time to be readily
mistaken for the grease, from which, however, it can
be easily distinguished by attentive examination. It
will teach them how important it is to study at the
same time the characters of this disease, and the
effect of inoculation."

OUTBREAK AT ALFORT.

In 1863, the subject of Horse Pox again received
great attention in France. A student named Amyot
dressed a horse on which an operation had been performed. The leg which had been operated on (right
hind leg) became the seat of a very confluent eruption
of Horse Pox, which was followed by such an abundant flow of serosity that at first the nature of the
affection was mistaken, and it was thought to be a
complication of *eaux aux jambes*. Amyot had a
wound on the dorsal aspect of the first interphalangeal
joint of the little finger of his right hand ; in spite
of this, he continued to dress the horse entrusted to
his care. The sore on his finger was the seat
of an accidental inoculation with the virus which
flowed in such great abundance from the horse's
leg. The wound was made on the 3rd of August,
and the next day it was swollen and rather painful. On the 5th, Amyot suffered from *malaise* and
great weakness, on the 6th, 7th, and 8th, vesicles
appeared successively on the fingers of his left hand,
on his forehead, on a level with the root of his nose,
and between the two eyebrows. On the 9th, these
vesicles were fully developed ; those of the fingers
consisted of very large epidermic bullæ on a bluish-
red base. On opening them, a perfectly limpid fluid
escaped in such abundance that small test-tubes

might have been filled with it. The vesicle on the
forehead was surrounded by a bluish-red areola, within
which the epidermis of a leaden-grey hue was raised
and had a slight central depression. The liquid
which flowed from it when it was opened, and which
continued to ooze, was also very abundant and of
a deep citrine colour.

The vesicles which had developed on the dorsal
side of Amyot's fingers were extremely painful. The
incessant shooting pains, of which they were the seat,
prevented him from getting any rest for three days.
On the 10th, inflammation of the lymphatics followed ;
both arms were swollen and very painful, with red
lines indicating the course of the lymphatic vessels.
The glands of the axillæ were also enlarged.

The lymphatic glands behind the jaws were also
swollen and painful. Amyot's chief sufferings were
occasioned by the intense local pain caused by the
vesicles on the fingers, and by the inflammation of
the lymphatic vessels and glands, and they continued
in this state up to the 18th of August. It was only
at the end of the month that the vesicles were
completely cicatrized.

Bouley felt very great anxiety in the presence of
the grave symptoms which accompanied the eruption,
so closely did these symptoms resemble in their mode
of manifestation and their intensity the effects of an
inoculation much more alarming than those of the

virus of grease. The eruption on the forehead was, especially, a cause of great uneasiness, because glanders manifests itself in a similar way. But when, on the morning of the 9th, Amyot showed Bouley the pustules on his fingers and on his forehead fully developed, the latter was completely reassured, for he recognised without any hesitation, that they had the characters of " vaccine vesicles." This diagnosis was supported by Drs. Marchant, Auzias-Turenne, Bayer, Depaul, and Blot, who successively saw Amyot on the same day, and had only one opinion as to the nature of his malady. Amyot evidently had inoculated himself with the *grease* which Jenner and Loy had seen and described. They were of opinion, that Amyot's illness had been much more severe and had lasted for a longer time, than in others who had been victims, as he had been, of an accidental inoculation with Jennerian grease, or Loy's disease.

To complete the history of Amyot, and to demonstrate that the malady which he had contracted, while attending to the horse, was really Horse Pox, Bouley, on the 12th of August, inoculated the liquid taken from the vesicles on his fingers, in the scrotal region of a steer, and produced "magnificent Cow Pox," which, when inoculated on a child, was followed by a very fine vaccinal eruption.

This case of Amyot, so well circumstantiated and studied in all its details, was fresh evidence in favour of Loy's opinion that the equine virus is gifted with greater energy than that of the cow, and produces a much more marked effect on the human subject.

The outbreak at Alfort enabled exhaustive experiments to be made, by which it was definitely established that Horse Pox is never infectious, but, like Cow Pox, is transmitted solely by contact.

Not having been able to get any practical information on the subject of Horse Pox[1] in this country, I made it one of my principal objects during a visit to France to inquire into and, if possible, practically study this malady. It was, therefore, with great interest that I heard that Professor Peuch, of Toulouse, had not only investigated outbreaks of this disease, but also was in the possession of drawings illustrating its different manifestations. Professor Peuch described to me his experience, giving me the details of his observations, and allowed me to have copies made of his valuable drawings. I cannot, do full justice to M. Peuch's admirable researches unless I give the full details in his own words.

---

[1] The term *equine*, as a substitute for *vacciné*, was first employed by Sacco, in a letter to Jenner, in 1803 (p. 389); and both *equine* and *Horse Pox* were, independently, proposed by Mr. Brown of Musselburgh. *Vide An inquiry into the anti-variolous power of Vaccination*, p. 63. 1809.

Second Outbreak at Toulouse.

M. C. Baillet, Director of the National Veterinary School of Toulouse, having been informed that a contagious malady had developed in the mares which had been served by the stallions at the breeding establishment at Rieumes belonging to M. Mazères, delegated M. Peuch to inspect these animals in order to ascertain the nature of the illness with which they were affected, its mode of propagation, and the means of arresting it.

With this object in view, M. Peuch visited, on the 10th and 11th of May, 1880, at Bérat, Rieumes, and Labastide-Clermont, several mares which had been served by the stallions of M. Mazères, and also the stallions themselves.

M. Peuch reported the result of his investigations in the *Revue Vétérinaire de Toulouse*, the following July.

"At Bérat, I examined, in the presence of my colleague, M. Avéradère, three mares already attacked, and these I will speak of as Nos. 1, 2, and 3.

"No. 1. A mare (Isabel) eight years old, had been served on 25th, 27th, and 30th of April. This animal showed on the lips of the vulva a sort of cicatricial mark of a whitish colour, of an elongated form, with edges scalloped and slightly in relief, covered here and there by a few brownish crusts, and showing elsewhere, and principally in the neighbourhood of the folds of the vulval orifice, small reddish superficial ulcers. Towards the upper commissure of the vulva there were several round or oval scars, the size of a large lentil ; some obviously depressed in the centre, which was covered by a small crust ; others

were circular like little leprous marks. I did not observe any
pustule, or a trace of one on other parts of the body. There
was not any lesion on the nose, in the nostrils, on the internal
surface of the lips, or in the mouth. This mare, who was very
spirited, retained her full vigour, and it did not appear as if the
eruption had weakened her in any way.

"No. 2. A black mare, eight years old, had been served on the
26th and 28th of April. Several ulcerated, reddish, circular sores,
surrounded by a cicatricial zone, existed on the lips of the
vulva, notably towards their free edge. The majority had
attained the size of a twenty-centime piece. There was not
any eruption in the nostrils, the mouth, or the internal surface
of the lips ; no modification of the general condition ; no difficulty
in locomotion.

"No. 3. A bay mare, eight years old, had been served the
23rd, 25th, 27th, and 30th of April. At the circumference of
the vulva there were very numerous white, lenticular, slightly
elevated, isolated, or confluent marks, extending over the perinæum. These marks, which were only dried pustules, showed
at their centre, which was appreciably depressed, a blackish dry
and adherent crust, under which the skin had a bright red colour
when the central crust was raised. I also established the existence
of dried pustules, showing the same characters as the preceding,
on the under surface of the tail, where they were disseminated in
considerable numbers. I scraped off these crusts with the nail and
preserved them. On the lower part of the left flank a discoid
vesicle was discovered with a diameter of about a centimetre.
On raising the crust which covered it, a sero-sanguinolent
liquid oozed from the exposed surface. There was nothing to
remark on other parts of the body. The general state was
most satisfactory ; there was no lameness.

"Such were the symptoms which I observed at Bérat on the
10th of May. To what disease were they attributable ? Were
they to be considered as indications of the malady sometimes
known as syphilis, or the venereal disease of the horse (*maladie
vénérienne du cheval*) ? This is a very important question in the
interests of the breeder and the owner of stallions, which cannot
be too carefully investigated, for when an eruptive disease appears

after coition, in a locality abounding with breeding mares, the alarmed breeder thinks it must be a syphilitic malady, and it therefore remains for the veterinary surgeon to explain the true nature of the illness. But the symptoms which I have just described belonged obviously to an eruptive affection in the stage of desiccation, and even cicatrisation in No. 1; so that the diagnosis, the consequences of which are so important, must offer serious difficulties, especially to the practitioner who has not had the opportunity of observing similar cases. I do not hesitate to remark that it appears very difficult, not to say impossible, to recognise with certainty the nature of the eruption in question, when it is seen in a subject for the first time, in the stage of desquamation.

" But such was not the case in this outbreak.

" Having several times had the opportunity of examining mares with a vesicular eruption around the vulva, after coition (an eruption which I had been able to follow from its first appearance to complete cicatrisation, and which was shown by inoculation of the cow to be *Horse Pox*), I found myself in a favourable position to appreciate, at their true value, the symptoms which I had discovered in the above-mentioned mares. Recalling to mind what I had observed on several occasions, I asserted that it was a case of the disease which M. Bouley, in 1863, called Horse Pox, and which Auzias-Turenne proposed to distinguish by the name pustular grease (*grease pustuleux*), a malady essentially different from *la maladie du coît*, or *dourine*, but, like it, propagated during coition.

"After this inspection at Bérat I proceeded to Rieumes, to the same establishment where, twenty years previously, a sort of enzooty had appeared, which has been described in the historical records of Vaccination, and which gave M. Lafosse the opportunity of rediscovering the vaccinogenic disease of the horse, which was considered extinct, since the days of Jenner, or at any rate the greatest confusion existed as regards diagnosis. I there inspected eleven stallions, six horses, and five asses. All, with the exception of the breeding stallion *Touche-à-tout*, which at other times was readily excited, served mares in my presence, so that I was able to examine the penis of each before the act of coition.

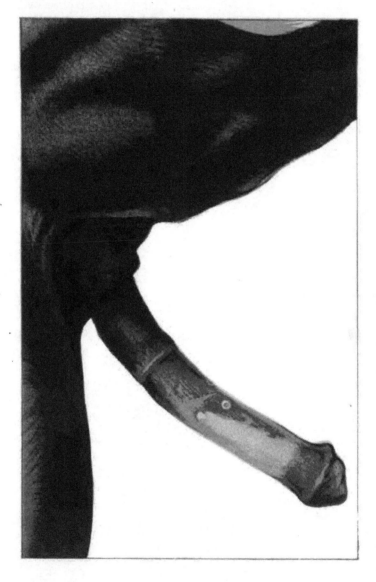

NATURAL HORSE POX (PEUCH).

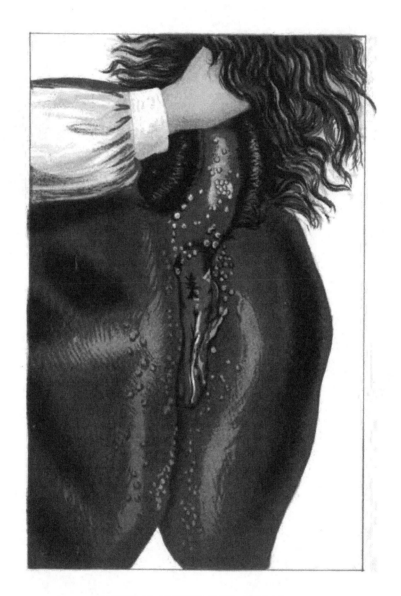

NATURAL HORSE POX (PEUCH).

"On one ass (Aramis) I observed on the right side of the penis several vesicles, scattered about from the base of the free part to the head of this organ. These vesicles, which were flattened and circular, varied in diameter from the size of a lentil, to that of a twenty-centime piece ; they had at their periphery, which was slightly in relief, a greyish colour ; at their centre, where the epidermis had been destroyed, they presented a bright rose colour and a finely granular appearance. All these vesicles were distinct from each other, and there was no infiltration or swelling of the penis. A little above the circular swelling which constitutes the base of the free part of the penis, a little dried vesicle was found with a central brownish crust. On another ass, called *Mexico*, I saw, on one aspect of the penis, a little whitish spot, circular but not in relief, on the skin, which appeared to me to be the scar of a grease vesicle. Whatever this might have been, this animal had on the external wing of the left nostril, a small pustule, which, nevertheless, showed well the characters of the vesicles of Cow Pox, or of ' grease.' I did not meet with any trace of eruption on other parts of the body, but it is not impossible that some dried vesicles may have escaped my notice; for it can be readily imagined how easy it is to overlook them in asses, with so long a coat. On the other three breeding asses I could not detect any vesicle or trace of vesicle either on the penis, the nose, around or within the lips, in the hollow of the heel, or, indeed in any part of the body, which I examined as well as I was able to considering the extreme liveliness of these animals, which fidgeted without intermission. I can say the same of the six stallions, which I examined with the greatest care without being able to find any trace of the eruptive disease, observed on the three mares and the two asses.

"But I can assert that all these stallions had coition with great ardour and without any sign of weakness, that their gait, their proud and confident bearing, their repeated and sonorous neighings, all, in fact, including their impatience, which rendered examination difficult, testified to their extreme energy and to their somewhat exuberant health. What a contrast to the *maladie du coît !* Moreover, amongst the mares which had already been served by the Rieumes stallions, and were presented to them again, I remarked two which I will designate as Nos. 4 and 5, and over which I think it useful to pause for a few moments.

"No. 4. Very old bay mare. This animal showed traces of an eruption of Horse Pox on the circumference of the vulva : here and there little dried and flattened vesicles were to be seen passing on to cicatrisation. I should mention that as the proprietor of this mare had not been alarmed by the eruption, no treatment had been employed, and the cicatrisation took place naturally and in the ordinary way.

"No. 5. A white mare, eighteen years old, was served on the 22nd and 26th of April. On the lips of the vulva there were some vesicles of grease passing on to desiccation. In addition, on the inside of the lower lip, near to the attached border, there was found, on the right side, a very fine vesicle of a pale yellow colour, of an ellipsoidal form, and of the size of a pea, not flattened or umbilicated, but well rounded, projecting, smooth, and of a pearly appearance. By the side of this vesicle or bulla a second was noticed, smaller, and not exceeding a hemp seed in volume, and with the summit slightly eroded. I may say, in passing, that an inexperienced observer might have considered these vesicles to indicate *aphthous stomatitis ;* but if we recall the remarkable observations contributed by H. Bouley to the article on *Horse Pox* in the *Nouveau Dictionnaire de médecine et de chirurgie vétérinaires,* concerning a case of an eruptive malady of the horse which was in the first place taken for *aphthous stomatitis,* but the inoculation of which produced Cow Pox, in the cow submitted to the experiment ; or if the opportunities of the *clinique* had even once brought to your notice the supposed *aphthous stomatitis* with an eruption on the circumference of the nostrils, in the hollow of the heel, or on other parts of the body, it would no longer be possible to be misled as to its nature, and to mistake Horse Pox or equine variola.

"In addition to these animals, I inspected in the commune of Labastide Clermont, a mare which had been especially brought to my notice as suffering in a very marked degree from the effects of the malady. I will speak of her as No. 6.

"No. 6. A bay mare, nine years old, served the 19th and

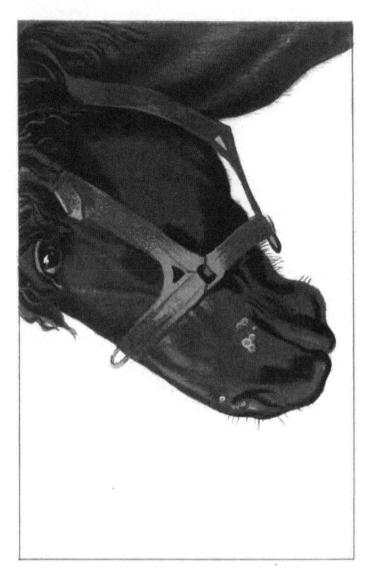

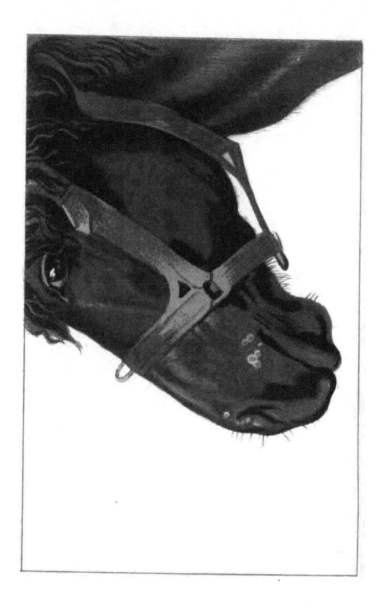

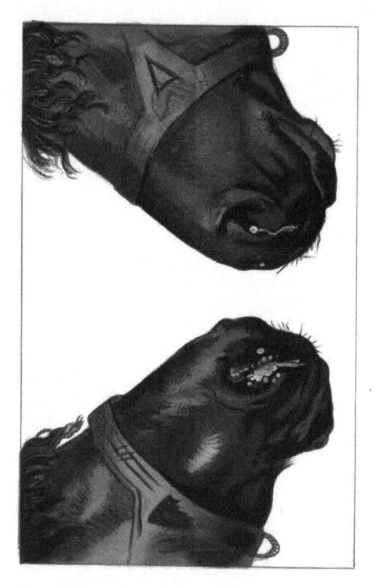

NATURAL HORSE BOY SIZES (FIGS. 12 AND ...

21st of April. I was informed that this mare was at first attended to by her master, who was a farrier; and afterwards M. Avéradère, veterinary surgeon at Bérat, was called in. On the occasion of my visit, the 11th of May, 1880, I observed traces of an eruption around the vulva; traces which were similar, but more extensive than those on subject No. 1 already described, so I need not again describe them. However, I will remark that lymphangitis existed in the right posterior limb, which was engorged, hot, and painful in its whole extent, and the animal walked at first with difficulty. I did not see the eruption in the hollow of the heel, but there was a greyish vaccinal vesicle, partly desiccated, near the lower commissure of the left nostril. I will now add that the proprietor of this mare had a vaccinal vesicle on the thumb of the right hand, excoriated and blackened, but recognisable, contracted in attending to his mare. This casual inoculation confirmed entirely the diagnosis which I had made the evening before at Bérat, although no doubt existed in my own mind, inasmuch as the symptoms observed in the asses *Aramis* and *Mexico*, and in mares Nos. 4 and 5, already demonstrated to my eyes the existence of Horse Pox. Moreover, the day after my return to Toulouse, that is to say on the 12th of May, I directed M. Cadéac, a fourth-year student, to inoculate the crusts which I had collected at Bérat two days before, from mare No. 3. This inoculation was made in the presence of the pupils, in a cow twelve years old belonging to M. Givelet, and she was placed in the hospital of the school. M. Cadéac made several punctures with a lancet on the circumference of the vulva of this animal, into which he introduced a droplet of a mixture obtained by crushing the crusts in a little water. On the 20th of May, a flattened vaccinal vesicle had formed at one of the inoculated points, having a diameter of about a centimetre; it was depressed in the centre which was occupied by a thin crust; the periphery was markedly circular, forming a sort of crown slightly in relief. The colour of this vesicle was obscured by that of the lips of the vulva; they were quite black in our experimental cow; moreover, the epidermis, which was thin, and raised by the accumulated lymph at the periphery of the vesicle, presented a greyish glistening appearance. Having taken off the crust and the epidermic pellicle which covered the vesicle, we observed after a few seconds some very fine transparent amber-coloured droplets of vaccinal lymph, welling up on the surface of the skin.

"On the 20th of May, 1880, a heifer six and a half months old, in excellent condition, belonging to M. Givelet, was inoculated with this vaccine. A great number of punctures were made around the vulva, and between the thighs, and˙on the right side of the udder, and on the teats. Several students revaccinated themselves, and on two of them vesicles formed. The inoculation on the heifer took perfectly, so that on the 26th of May each puncture was transformed into a flattened discoid vesicle, umbilicated in the centre, of a yellow-grey colour with an inflammatory areola, presenting, in one word, all the characters of the vesicles of Cow Pox. With the liquid contained in these vesicles I successfully vaccinated several children, and revaccinated some students, some of whom showed vaccinal vesicles. On the 26th of May, Dr. Salamon vaccinated children who had very fine vesicles. Lastly, two water-colour drawings were made by one of the most eminent artists of Toulouse, M. Loubat, one representing the vaccinal eruption of the heifer, and the other that of one of the vaccinated children, forming, in a way, unimpeachable evidence of these inoculations, which had been made in the presence of most of my colleagues and pupils.

"No doubt can, therefore, be raised of the exactness of the diagnosis which I made as early as the 10th of May, at Bérat, after seeing the mares which had been served by the stallions belonging to M. Mazères ; and, if I insist on this question of the diagnosis of Horse Pox, when this malady is seen on mares which have been recently served, it is because it appears to me that it has not been studied in such a manner as to furnish practitioners with really useful means of recognition.

"Some writers on pathology say that the *maladie du coït* may be accompanied by an eruption which some describe as papular, vesicular ; others, as formed of white spots or diphtheritic ulcerations. Some assert that this eruption appears sometimes in the form of herpes or of eczema, sometimes of ecthyma, with or without the *maladie du coït.* M. Lafosse has even thought that it 'would not be perhaps impossible that one of the breeding animals, male or female, through sexual connection with different individuals, might generate these varieties. Fresh observations ought to be collected to establish the possibility of these results being varied by the diverse copulations of the same animal. While waiting for these observations, it appears to us prudent to admit it in practice, from the present time, not to blindly endanger the life of the reproductive animals, and also in order to free ourselves from the heavy responsibility which would encumber us under certain circumstances if the mutability of the morbid properties of the genital secretions were to be demonstrated.'

"It is not difficult to conceive what perplexities such a doctrine would give rise to in the mind of the practitioner, and what consequences it might have, as it leads one to consider all the eruptive affections of the genital organs as originating from the same source as the *maladie du coït*, if not as manifestations of this disease. But observation pure and simple, and freed from all fantastic ideas, pronounces against this singular theory of the *mutability of morbid properties ;* in other words, the *maladie du coït* is one thing and *Horse Pox* is another. And I proved this by inoculating the cow with an eruptive illness which I had observed ; the inoculation gave rise, in the cow, to a perfectly genuine Cow Pox, which developed in the child to whom it was transmitted an eruption of irreproachable purity, a fact which allows us to regenerate the vaccine, and to procure for ourselves at any time, and in any place, a vaccine as pure and as active as that which Jenner himself employed. I do not assert that the *maladie du coït* and *Horse Pox* cannot exist simultaneously on the same subject. I own to having no information on this subject, and there is not, to my knowledge, any observation which proves it. Nevertheless, I consider that such a fact would not be in opposition to the principles of the pathology of the contagious maladies, and I am not unwilling to admit it as having been demonstrated. We should then know how the practitioner should act should such a thing occur, and how he can correctly foresee all the consequences of the disease which he has under observation.

" I have no intention here of discussing the complete patho-logical history of the *maladie du coït*. I will confine myself to remarking that cutaneous *plaques* have been mentioned as a very important symptom in the course of this affection; they form projections of three to four millimetres, of a diameter vary-ing from a centimetre to five centimetres; they appear on the neck, shoulder, flank, forearm, and some other parts. These *plaques*, are the seat of an oozing, which lasts for eight, ten, and twelve days, then they gradually become effaced without leaving any trace behind. It would be puerile to point out to the reader the great differences between this eruption of cutaneous *plaques* and that which characterises Horse Pox. They can be readily appreciated when we recall the characters of the vaccine vesicles and compare them to those of the cutaneous *plaques*, which in a way constitute the specific eruption of the *maladie du coït*. Nor will it be difficult to distinguish Horse Pox from the vesicular, papular, and other eruptions which have been the subjects of such varied descriptions, if inoculation in the cow formed for the practitioner the true criterion of the illness which he has under observation. But it is clear that having admitted the possibility of the development of the *maladie du coït* and of Horse Pox in the same subject, I ought to ascertain if there are not other points which enable the practitioner to form a well-grounded opinion about the illness under observation. The time has come to apply the data acquired by science respect-ing the etiology of *dourine* or *maladie du coït*. I cannot do better than reproduce here a passage from a clinical lecture of Professor St. Cyr of the School of Lyons. This learned and respected teacher, after having reviewed all the causes which have been invoked to afford an explanation of the development of *dourine*, formulates among other conclusions the following propositions :

" ' That the true cause of the *maladie du coït*, when we know how to look for it, will be found in the *importation of a foreign stallion.*'

" ' That *dourine* has only one known cause, *contagion ;* that all the others to which it has been thought possible to at-tribute it, are more than problematical, and that in practice, as well as in theory, there is no ground for believing in them.'

"And M. St. Cyr adds '*dourine* is not an autochthonous malady born from local influences, but is, on the contrary, an exotic illness which has been imported, and the origin of which it will be always possible to trace if the practitioner exercises in his etiological investigation the attention and the perspicacity which it requires.'

"This announcement throws light, it seems to me, on the differential diagnosis of *dourine*. Shall I add that even if this malady were mistaken at its initial period, it would not be long in declaring itself by wasting, weakness, and an exaggerated sensibility of the lumbar region; a sharp flexion of the posterior pastern joints, the appearance of cutaneous *plaques*, then of at first, partial paralysis, etc., all being symptoms which enable us to distinguish *dourine* from Horse Pox, the course of which is at the same time so simple and so mild. These are phenomena known to all practitioners who have had the opportunity of seeing the real *maladie du coït*.

"To sum up, if an eruptive malady appear after coition, inoculation of the cow furnishes a valuable diagnostic sign to the observer, which it appears to me useful to insist upon, owing to the good results which it gives.

"I now approach a question which appears to me to be not less interesting than that of the diagnosis. I wish to speak of the contagion of Horse Pox from the facts which I was able to observe at Rieumes.

"The information furnished to me by M. Mazères, the proprietor of this breeding establishment, concerns five out of the six mares which I examined. It establishes :—

"That mare No. 1 was served 'three times by different asses, 25th, 27th, 30th of April last.' Mare No. 2, 'served twice by the same ass, *Mexico*, 26th, 28th of April.' Mare No. 3 'served four times by the same ass, *Mistigry*, the 23rd, 25th, 27th, and 30th of April.' No information about mare No. 4. Mare No. 5, 'served twice by the same horse, *Sultan*, 22nd and 26th of April.' Mare No. 6, 'served twice by the same ass, *Porthous*, 22nd and 26th of April.'

"If the reader will now recall what I have already mentioned about the state of health of the stallions of the serving stall at Rieumes, he will see that, in spite of the attention with which I examined these animals, I found on only two of them—the asses *Aramis* and *Mexico*—the characteristic eruption of Horse Pox. However, in the first place, Mare No. 3, which had been served by the ass *Mistigry*, on which I did not observe any eruption of Horse Pox, exhibited a splendid vaccinal eruption which had even developed on the under surface of the tail, where I collected crusts, inoculation from which proved, as we have seen, an excellent source of vaccine; in the second place, Mare No. 6, served by the ass *Porthous*, had a very confluent perivulvar eruption with consecutive lymphangitis, although I was not able to discover the smallest vesicle on the penis of *Porthous* or elsewhere; finally the horse *Sultan* showed no vaccine vesicles and nevertheless the mare No. 5, which he had served, had been infected with an eruption which had left obvious traces on the circumference of the vulva and on the buccal mucous membrane, where the vesicles were found which I have described, and which I consider to be Horse Pox. As to mares Nos. 1 and 2, covered by the same asses *Aramis* and *Mexico*, their contamination was explained; but what are we to think of the appearance of Horse Pox on the mares served by stallions whose penis showed no vesicle? *A priori* it may perhaps be admitted that the development of Horse Pox preceded coition, and that this eruption, being at first discrete, passed unnoticed by the groom as well as by the breeder, or indeed. that there was a simple coincidence between the occurrence of this eruption and the coitus, without any connecting link. These suppositions doubtless are not improbable, nevertheless neither one nor the other appears to me to be well founded considering the special seat of the eruption on the circumference of the sexual parts and its development after coition, on five out of six mares which I examined. We must then endeavour to find out how the contagion was carried when the penis of the stallion was free from all lesions.

"Must we in this connection, admit with M. Lafosse, that the infectious agent does not exist before the coitus, that it is

formed during the accomplishment of the act of copulation,
doubtless at the expense of the male or female secretions, perhaps
of both, and under the influence of the nervous influx or force
which is accumulated in the genital organs by the friction of
copulation ?

"But I do not see on what principle or on what scientific
ground this theory rests, and therefore it is quite useless to
pause longer over it.

"Let us see if it be not possible to give a more simple and
rational interpretation from the facts which I have established.
I think, with M. St. Cyr, that it may be possible that 'without
being ill themselves, the stallions were the mediatory agents of
contagion, by carrying to healthy mares virus which they had
taken from diseased ones; in this way they would play the
part of *corps contumaces* as they say in *Sanitary Police*, and
nothing more.'

"Do we not know that Horse Pox can be communicated by
the sponge ?

"M. Arloing has explained the presence of this eruption on
the circumference of the vulva of four mares, from the habit
which the groom had of washing every morning the sexual
organs of these animals with the same sponge. Moreover, the
sponge is not the only object which can act as the agent in
transporting the virulent matter. The hobbles, the litter, the
blunt hook which is employed in the operation for *javart*, and
even the finger of the operator, have communicated Horse Pox,
as Trasbot and Nocard have observed in several cases; and it
would be difficult to understand why the penis of the stallion
should not be a means of transporting virulent matter, in the
same way as an inert body or, accidentally, the finger of the
surgeon. This being explained, I will finish this paper with
some practical considerations on the prophylaxis of Horse Pox.
In the first place, I will remark that Horse Pox transmitted by
coition is not of importance, except from the fear which it
inspires in breeders, and which immediately induces them to
regard this eruptive affection as syphilitic. And this alarm,
consequently, brings discredit upon the breeding establishment
whence the illness has spread. It is the business of the

veterinary surgeon to reassure the breeders, by acquainting them with the exact consequences of this affection, of the diagnosis which they are able to establish. And, not to put it too strongly, it will also gain him the esteem and confidence of his fellow-citizens, and, I am not afraid to assert, that in thus acting he will have done more to reconcile the interests in question, than by giving himself up at random to theoretical discussions, which are necessarily useless to the practitioner who is always endeavouring to cope with the difficulties of his art.

"The nature of the malady being perfectly recognised, is it not in all cases necessary to have recourse to sanitary precautions? I have every reason to think, from my own observations and those of various practitioners, especially, Lautour, who saw on the penis of a stallion 'a score of little pustulous tumours, the size and shape of variolous pustules,' that Horse Pox is of no more importance when it appears after coition than when it appears under any other circumstance, for example, during an attack of strangles. And then do we not know that vaccination of the horse has been considered as a measure preventive of strangles? Doctor Sacco, quoted by Gohier in 1813, reports that he had vaccinated 'eighty-three breeding mares and that none of them had ever been attacked with strangles.' Last year Professor Tasbert, of the school of Alfort, asserted the identity of strangles and Horse Pox, which he proposed to call variola of the horse, and recommended the same means for preventing the complications of strangles. Doubtless at the time when the mares are put to the stallions they have generally passed the age at which strangles appears, but it will be readily admitted that a fresh attack of Horse Pox, like revaccination, would best serve to guarantee the protection of the organism against a fresh attack of strangles, if such a guarantee exists. In this case, a mare which may have an eruption of Horse Pox around the vulva and on the teats, which is not unusual will herself transmit, the preservative virus to—I was going to say to vaccinate—the colt or the mule which she suckles, and this would be all for the best, as the young animal would be, for the future, protected from the serious effects of strangles.

However this may be, Horse Pox developed around the vulva, at the end of the nose, in the mouth, and in the hollow of the heel, is always Horse Pox; therefore, when the eruption is confluent and pruriginous, simple cleanliness is sufficient or lotions of fresh water whitened by a few drops of goulard water to accelerate cicatrisation, which is generally completed by the third week. If lymphangitis supervene, simple emollient lotions, gentle walking exercise, nitrate drinks, and green food will easily subdue it. Even if the complications are very slight it may be useful to anticipate them to a certain extent.

" With this object it will be advisable to let the stallion rest for several days when there is a confluent eruption seen on the penis, and, in the same way, mares affected with the vaccino-genic eruption must be temporally put out of use. Finally, the groom is recommended to pass a paint brush imbued with olive oil on the lips of the vulva of the mare, before she is served, as this diminishes the chances of absorption.

"After what I have written in the preceding pages it will be understood that these precautions are only of secondary import-ance, and that the practitioner ought, above everything, to be able to determine the true nature of the contagious malady which he has under observation. I shall consider myself happy if the present work should prove useful in this respect."

Horse Pox in Algeria.

About eighteen months afterwards M. Peuch met with a case of Horse Pox in Algeria. An account was published in the *Revue Vétérinaire*, July 1882.

" The 24th of last October, being at Boufarik, I, and one of my old pupils, M. Renaud, veterinary surgeon of that commune, observed a splendid example of the vaccinogenic illness in a horse, a thoroughbred Arab, four and a half years old, belonging to one of the principal colonists of Mitidja, M. Debonno. The following are the symptoms which I observed on the subject in question :—Around the nostrils there were numerous flattened discoid, umbilicated vesicles the size of a lentil; some were in

process of desiccation, others in full secretion from which, on
the slightest pressure, a limpid fluid exuded of an amber colour.
Towards the inferior commissure of the left nostril we noticed
a superficial ulceration, the size of a silver five-franc piece, with
scalloped edges, covered in part by crystalline crusts, which were
yellowish and transparent ; elsewhere the skin exhibited a bright
red colour, and a delicately areolar aspect. A yellowish serous
discharge escaped from the left nostril. The pituitary membrane was strongly injected, notably on the side corresponding to
the discharge, where on the nasal septum vesico-pustules could
be seen of the size of a small lentil, of a rounded form, and of
a whitish and yellowish colour. In the mouth, and particularly
inside the lips and on the lateral surfaces of the tongue, there were
a multitude of small bullæ or vesicles of pearly appearance and of
the size of a pea ; some were isolated and prominent, the greater
number confluent and as if eroded at their centre ; a viscous
saliva escaped in abundance, while the mouth was being ex-
.amined. The sublingual glands, especially those on the left
side, were engorged, hot, and painful on pressure. The coat
in patches on the lateral aspect of the neck, on the shoulders,
the flanks, and in the hollow of the heel, was staring, giving the
appearance of small paint brushes. On passing the hand over these
parts, small lenticular nodules were felt, which were nothing else
than the vesicles of Horse Pox—some of them dry, others
secreting. The animal appeared dejected, depressed ; there was,
moreover, slight fever, and the appetite had fallen off. Considering these symptoms, and above all the appearance of the
perinasal eruption, M. Renaud and I did not hesitate to assert,
in the presence of Dr. Chafnuis, of Boufarik, that it was a case
of the eruptive illness of the horse which M. Bouley has
proposed to call Horse Pox,[1] from two English words, horse
and pox (variola). It was decided to collect the liquid which
oozed from the vesicles, and to preserve it between pieces
of glass. Being obliged to leave, the same day, for Oran
where I was expected, I charged my old pupil, M. Renaud,
to collect the virus, and I am happy to be able to say that he

---

[1] *Vide* p. 401.

acquitted himself in the most satisfactory manner. We had also decided that inoculations should be made on cows.

In a letter dated the 4th of November last, M. Renaud informed me that, having inoculated four heifers, fifteen to ten months old, with the Horse Pox in question, he had obtained Cow Pox. In the same letter M. Renaud informed me that three horses, which had eaten from the same manger as the one which we had inspected on the 24th of October last, were attacked, the 4th of November following, with very well characterised Horse Pox. It appears to me useful to mention this fact, as it indicates a mode of transmitting Horse Pox which is generally ignored. Having said this I return to our first observation.

"On the 21st of December last I begged M. Renaud to send me some of the Horse Pox, and the vaccine which he had cultivated. In a most obliging way, for which I cannot thank him too much, my young colleague sent me on the 10th of January following, two slips of glass charged with Horse Pox virus obtained from the subject which we had visited together, and two slips with vaccine collected from the heifers which he had inoculated. I received this packet on Sunday, the 15th of January last, and the same day, with the concurrence of my colleague, Professor Bidaud, I inoculated, at the experimental farm attached to the Veterinary School of Toulouse, belonging to M. Givelet at Montredon—1st, an Ayrshire cow aged about nine years, in an advanced stage of gestation, with the dried Horse Pox previously moistened in a drop of tepid water; I made twenty punctures around the vulva and the perinæum. 2nd, another cow, seven years old, also in a state of advanced gestation, with the Cow Pox which had been derived from the Horse Pox. I proceeded in the same way as on the previous subject. The 19th of January, the fifth day after the inoculation, I observed that on these two animals, the punctures exhibited no inflammatory process, except one or two amongst them, which were slightly papular, all the others were no longer visible, so that I thought that my culture would remain sterile. I own that I was agreeably surprised on seeing on Tuesday last, 24th of January, when I was on a weekly excursion with the pupils to the farm, that the greater part of the punctures made ten days before, which were invisible on the 19th of January, were now transformed into fine vaccinal vesicles surrounded by an areola of a rose-colour. And the 25th of January last, these two cows were taken to the Veterinary School of Toulouse where, in conjunction with M. Cadeac, teacher of the Clinique, I vaccinated two fine Dutch heifers vigorous and in good health, one aged fourteen months, the other seven months. Five days later there were as many vesicles as there had been punctures, and Drs. Armieux, Jougla, Caubet, and Parant, invited by the Director of the Veterinary School to visit the vaccinated heifers, proved the perfect genuineness of the vaccinal eruptions, which had been produced on the perinæum and on the teats.

"This eruption has been the starting point of cultures of vaccine on heifers and calves up to the end of last May, and the vaccine thus kept up, has been used for vaccination of about fifteen hundred persons."

In this country, it is more than probable that some of Jenner's stocks of equine lymph are still in use ; but equination is not wittingly practised, for it is commonly supposed that all the lymph employed for the purposes of vaccination has been derived from Cow Pox. In France, on the other hand, it is extensively employed. M. Layet informed me that at the Animal Vaccine Station at Bordeaux, the lymph which gave most satisfaction was derived from the horse, and that he had been able on two occasions to renew his stock from equine sources.

CHAPTER XV.

IN a former chapter, an account has been given of Small
Pox inoculation in foreign countries. The methods
employed and the results of this practice are, historically
and pathologically, of the greatest interest; but the fact
of its having been adopted all over the civilised world,
stands in an important relation to the introduction of
vaccination. Variolation was the forerunner of vaccination, and it was the widespread adoption of the
former, which paved the way for the latter. Jenner
did not evolve an entirely new system of medical
treatment, but he proposed a different form of an
already existing, but dangerous, practice. I will now
briefly refer to the reception of his proposal on the
Continent.

The *Inquiry* was made known to the scientific world
on the Continent, through the medium of the *Biblio-
thèque Britannique*. Early in 1800, vaccine lymph
was despatched to Hanover and Vienna, and Dr. de
Carro, who particularly distinguished himself by his

zeal in employing the new inoculation, greatly assisted in diffusing a knowledge of vaccination throughout Europe.

From Vienna, lymph was conveyed by Dr. Peschier to Geneva; but there the new method received a temporary check, for all the persons who were vaccinated, afterwards contracted Small Pox, some by infection, and others by inoculation. These untoward results were explained as the result of "spurious vaccination," and the practice was not therefore abandoned. Dr. Odier was another powerful advocate of the new inoculation. He drew up a paper on the subject, which was handed by clergymen to parents when they brought their children to be baptized.

In Hanover, vaccination was introduced by Ballhorn and Stromeyer, and Jenner's work was translated by the former into German. In Prussia, the clergy were particularly active in assisting the profession to spread the "benign preventive," and in Russia, it was widely employed after receiving the patronage of the Dowager Empress. Vaccine lymph was obtained by the Empress from a physician at Breslau, and an infant was vaccinated by the surgeon to the Emperor. The child was named Vaccinoff, and a provision settled on her for life. In Sweden, though variolous inoculation had become "one of the most lucrative branches of professional practice," the subject was re-investigated by the College of Health; this learned body pronounced in favour of the "Jennerian discovery," and

vaccination was established throughout the kingdom.
In France, the Director of the School of Medicine
at Paris, received some vaccine lymph, and thirty
children were inoculated; but the stock was soon lost.
Woodville took a fresh stock to Boulogne, and proceeded from thence to Paris, and a bulletin announced
the event "of France having now got Dr. Woodville,
a learned man, animated with generous zeal, and
meriting gratitude and praise. Already he had vaccinated six thousand children with invariable success, for
the prevention of the Small Pox is a kind of prodigy."[1]

In Italy, vaccination was introduced by Sacco, who
investigated the origin of vaccine lymph, and succeeded
in raising stocks from a disease of cows in Lombardy,
from the ulcerated heels of horses, and from Sheep
Pox. Sacco was instrumental in persuading the
Milanese Government to adopt strong measures, and
we are also told that "proclamations were read from
every pulpit; vaccination was practised in every church,
and the clergy gave such effectual aid, that the professor
and his associates, in three years, vaccinated seventy
thousand persons, and extinguished the Small Pox in
Lombardy."[2]

In 1800, Joseph Marshall and John Walker "procured
medical diplomas from the indulgent university of
Leyden, and being low in fame and pocket, made

---

[1] Moore. *The History and Practice of Vaccination.* p. 254. 1817.
[2] Moore. *loc. cit.* p. 263.

application to Dr. Jenner, and obtained his sanction for a very useful project."[1] Jenner obtained a passage for them in a frigate, and they proceeded to Gibraltar, Minorca, Malta, Palermo, and Naples, teaching and practising vaccination. Having finished his vaccine tour, Marshall wrote a description to Jenner, which contained the following account of the introduction of vaccination into Palermo:—

"It was not unusual to see, in the mornings of the public inoculation at the hospital, a procession of men, women, and children, conducted through the streets by a priest carrying a cross, come to be inoculated. By these popular means it met not with opposition, and the common people expressed themselves certain that it was a blessing sent from Heaven, though discovered by one heretic and-practised by another."

Vaccination rapidly found its way to Cadiz, Seville, Barcelona, and all the principal cities of Spain; and Dr. Francisco Xavier Balmis, physician to his Majesty, still further extended the practice, for he obtained permission to diffuse the new inoculation in the Spanish American and Asiatic dominions. To defray expenses, "he obtained the rare and profitable permission of freighting a ship with a variety of goods, and of trading at every port he touched." The Canary Islands, Porto Rico, Caraccas, Lima, Chili, Charcas, Havannah, Yucatan, Guatemala, Acapulco, the Philippine Islands, Macao, Canton, and St. Helena

---

[1] Moore. *The History and Practice of Vaccination.* p. 264.

were also visited by either Balmis or his assistants, who asserted the efficacy of Cow Pox, " not merely in preventing the Natural Small Pox, but in curing simultaneously other affections of the human frame." [1]

Lymph from the National Vaccine Establishment was taken to Persia by the British ambassador. From Vienna, Dr. de Carro sent lymph to Constantinople, and thence to Bombay. In India, the new method was opposed by the natives, but their objections were overcome by an ingenious device.

" In order to overcome their prejudices, the late Mr. Ellis, of Madras, who was well versed in Sanscrit literature, actually composed a short poem in that language on the subject of vaccination. This poem was inscribed on old paper, and said to have been *found*, that the impression of its antiquity might assist the effect intended to be produced on the minds of the Brahmins, while tracing the preventive to their sacred cow."

The universal appreciation of the danger of inoculating Small Pox, the promise of everlasting security by means of a harmless substitute, and the exercise of the, so-called pious, frauds which have been referred to, explain at once the rapid acceptance of vaccination by ignorant peasants; but the acceptance of Cow Pox inoculation by the scientific world requires another explanation which however is not difficult to find.

[1] *Letter* from Doctor Edward Jenner to William Dillwyn, Philadelphia p. 16. 1818.

The principle embodied in the practice of Small Pox inoculation was, the widespread belief that in certain diseases, a mild attack would, as a rule, ward off, or modify, a second attack. Now, in the case of Cow Pox there was this initial difficulty, that it was a disease totally distinct from Small Pox. As was soon pointed out, Cow Pox and Small Pox are radically dissimilar.[1] That Jenner foresaw this difficulty, and endeavoured to meet it by the invention of the term *variolæ vaccinæ*, or *Small Pox* of the cow, is not at all unlikely; but whether there was motive or not, the designation of Cow Pox as *variolæ vaccinæ* had, without doubt, a very great effect in rendering the new inoculation acceptable on the Continent. The physicians abroad were thus led to believe that vaccination embodied the same principle of obtaining protection from Small Pox by inducing a mild attack of that disease; it was not, in other words, obtaining immunity from Small Pox by a totally distinct disease, but by another kind of Small Pox—viz., *variolæ vaccinæ*, or Small Pox of the cow.

Thus, for example, Aubert,[2] in France, in the introduction to his report on the new inoculation, wrote :—

"On a donné le nom de *Vaccine*, à une espèce de bouton, particulière au pis des vaches. Par le contact du pus qu'il renferme, ce bouton si reproduit sur l'homme, et lui ôte la

---

[1] Moseley. *A Treatise on the Lues Bovilla or Cow Pox.* 1804.
[2] Aubert. *Rapport sur la vaccine.* An. IX.

susceptibilité de prendre la petite vérole. Le Docteur Jenner, fut le premier Medecin qui, jugeant cette tradition des gens de la campagne digne d'examen, étudia la nature et les effets de cette éruption pustuleuse, appelée en Angleterre **Petite Vérole des Vaches.**"

In America, Cow Pox inoculation was introduced by Dr. Benjamin Waterhouse, who wrote an article in the *Columbian Sentinel*, March 12th, 1799, headed : " SOMETHING CURIOUS IN THE MEDICAL LINE." The disease was described as " *Cow Pox*, or, if you like the term better, the *Cow Small Pox*, or to express it in technical language, the *variolæ vaccinæ*."

The virtues of the Jennerian discovery were thus described :—

" But what makes this newly discovered disease so very curious and so extremely important is, that every person thus affected is EVER AFTER SECURED FROM THE ORDINARY SMALL POX, *let him be ever so much exposed to the effluvium of it, or let ever so much ripe matter be inserted into the skin by inoculation.*"

Waterhouse preferred the use of the term *Kine Pox* to express this " wonderful antidote."

" From *Kine*, the plural of cow; thus in the Scriptures ' and they took two *Milch Kine*, and shut up their calves at home ; ' a word equally expressive, and in the opinion of some more delicate."

Dr. Waterhouse inoculated his son, Daniel, five years old, with some of Jenner's lymph.[1]

---

[1] Waterhouse. *A Prospect of Exterminating the Small Pox, being a History of the Variolæ Vaccinæ or Kine Pox*, p. 19. 1800.

" The inoculated part in this boy was surrounded by an efflorescence which extended from his shoulder to his elbow, which made it necessary to apply some remedies to lessen it ; but the ' *symptoms,*' as they are called, scarcely drew him from his play more than an hour or two, and he went through the disease in so slight a manner as hardly ever to express any marks of peevishness. A piece of true skin was fairly taken out of the arm by the *virus*, the part appearing as if eaten out by a caustic, *a never-failing sign of thorough infection of the system in the inoculated Small Pox.*"

Waterhouse carried on some further inoculations, and became convinced that the Kine Pox was a disease not to be trifled with.

To demonstrate the alleged protective power of Cow Pox against Small Pox, Waterhouse resolved to have the variolous test applied, and enlisted for this purpose the services of Dr. Aspinwall, physician to the Small Pox Hospital near Boston. Dr. Aspinwall acceded to the proposal, and inoculated Daniel in the presence of his father

" by two punctures, and with matter taken that moment from a patient who had it pretty full upon him. He at the same time inserted an infected thread, and then put him into the hospital where was one patient with it in the natural way. On the fourth day the doctor pronounced the *arm* to be infected. It became every hour sorer, but in a day or two it dried off, and grew well without producing the slightest trace of a disease, so that the boy was dismissed from the hospital, and returned home the twelfth day after the experiment. ONE FACT in such cases is worth a thousand arguments."

The pamphlet concluded with the following statement :—

" Dr. Waterhouse informs those who have applied to him out
of Cambridge, to inoculate their families, but he declined it only
until the disorder had gone fairly through his own family, and
until some of them had been inoculated by Dr. Aspinwall, and
otherwise exposed to the Small Pox. But having now confirmed
his assertion, *that the Kine Pox protects the constitution from the
infection of the Small Pox*, by **a fair experiment**, he is ready to attend
them whenever they choose. Those who live in Boston may rest
assured, that from the proximity of his residence to the capital, he
shall make such arrangement as to be able to attend them as
punctually as if he resided there."

The new inoculation was shortly afterwards tested
on a large scale. A Dr. S. obtained lymph from a
sailor, who had arrived at Marblehead from London,
and was supposed to be suffering from Cow Pox,
but in reality had Small Pox. Dr. S. began to
use it, and produced an epidemic of Small Pox.
Previous to this accident Dr. D. had inoculated
about forty persons from the arm of Dr. Waterhouse's son, and all who had been vaccinated took
the Small Pox, either casually or by inoculation,
one excepted.[1]

According to Baron—

" The occurrences at Marblehead led Dr. Waterhouse to believe
that the vaccine virus had degenerated."

Waterhouse wrote to Lettsom, begging him to

---

[1] Waterhouse. *A Prospect of Exterminating the Small Pox*. Part II.,
p. 10. 1800.

apply to Jenner for a fresh supply of lymph, pointing out that he had gained some credit by following Dr. Jenner's footsteps, and that he turned to him for further assistance.

" A letter from him, should he allow me to publish it or any part of it, might set this benevolent business a-going again next spring. Could I likewise say to the American public that I had received matter from Dr. Jenner himself, it would have a very good effect indeed."

In the meantime the Americans were made to wait by a little stratagem.

Waterhouse wrote to Jenner—

" I gave out that the winter was an unfavourable season for this new inoculation, and by that means I suspended the practice throughout the country from that period until the arrival of fresh matter and your letter. Now we are going on again, but not with the faith and spirit of the last season. Some unlucky cases have damped the ardour of a people who received this new inoculation with a candour, liberality, and even generosity, much to their credit."

The new inoculation was not introduced without some opposition, but Waterhouse[1] succeeded in establishing the practice.

" The characters in America most distinguished for wisdom and goodness are firm believers in *your* doctrine. They are not, however, over-forward in assisting me against this new irruption of the Goths. I do not wish them to do more than make cartridges, or at least hand them. At present they leave me too much alone,

---

[1] Extract of a letter from Dr. Waterhouse to Dr. Jenner, dated Cambridge (America), November 5th, 1801. (Baron, *loc. cit.*)

and it is probable will only come openly to my assistance when I do not *want* them. Had I not a kind of apostolic zeal I should at times feel a little discouraged. The natives of America are skilful in bush-fighting."

Cow Pox inoculation was introduced into America on the strength of one doubtful experiment, and, as on the Continent, under the impression that it was variolæ vaccinæ or Small Pox of the Cow.

Thus were the scientists in Europe and America deceived. They were led to believe that this English disease was commonly known as Cow Small Pox, whereas it was Jenner who first named it Cow Small Pox. It was really known in England as "the Pox among Cows," or the "Cow Pox." I shall again refer to this subject in the next chapter.

CHAPTER XVI.

PROGRESS OF VACCINATION IN ENGLAND.

I HAVE already dealt with the life and letters of Edward Jenner, from the study of which an insight may be obtained into the history of vaccination in England up to the year of Jenner's death (1823).

Before passing on to the period which followed, I will point out how it was that after Cow Pox inoculation had been adopted by the profession in this country, the doctrine of Cow Small Pox came to be considered as essential. It will no doubt be a surprise to many to learn the origin of the theory that Cow Pox is modified Small Pox, as it is so universally regarded as the outcome of clinical observations and pathological experiments. To explain this point fully, I will again refer, and at some length, to the assumption, by Jenner, of the term *variolæ vaccinæ*.

The title of Jenner's original paper was "On the Cow Pox," but in the published *Inquiry* he inserted the words, *variolæ vaccinæ*. Whether this term was invented by Jenner himself, or whether it was suggested by one of the friends to whom he had shown his manuscript, history does not relate. At any rate, Jenner made himself responsible for it ; and it is therefore necessary to investigate his views as to the relation which was supposed to exist between the two diseases. In the first place, the statement which has been recently made, that Jenner believed that Cow Pox was derived from human Small Pox, and hence that the term *variolæ vaccinæ* was justifiable, is entirely without foundation. The facts of the case are, that Jenner believed that the Cow Pox was derived from the diseased heels of the horse ; he also believed that Small Pox and some other diseases arose from the same source. When the boy Phipps was inoculated with Cow Pox, Jenner was struck with the similarity to some cases of inoculated Small Pox, and he felt convinced that, at least, Cow Pox and Small Pox were derived from the same source. The idea that Cow Pox arose through the agency of milkers suffering from human Small Pox never occurred to Jenner.

Jenner's theory of the origin of Cow Pox from horse grease was well known to his contemporaries. According to Fraser, Woodville strongly objected to it, and recommended Jenner to omit it from his original paper.

" I deeply regret that he did not follow the advice which Dr. Woodville gave him upon being requested to peruse the manuscript of his first treatise on this subject, prior to its publication. The part which Dr. Woodville objected to, was the opinion broached relative to the origin of this disease, than which nothing can be more contrary to philosophy, analogy, and experiment."

Pearson [1] also criticised the term which Jenner had substituted for *Cow Pox*.

"For the sake of precision in language, and of consequence, justness in thinking, and considering that there is no way of disabusing ourselves from many of the errors of physic, but by the use of just terms, it is not unworthy of our attention to guard against the admission of newly appropriated names which will mislead by their former accepted import.

"*Variola* is an assumed Latin word, and its meaning will be popularly understood in the English tongue by saying that it is a name of a disease, better known by another name—the Small Pox. Granting that the word 'Variola' is a derivative from *Varius* and *Varus* used by Pliny and Celsus to denote a disease with spots on the skin, the etymological import of Variola is any cutaneous spotted distemper; but one of the most formidable and distinct of the cutaneous order is what is called the *Small Pox*, and therefore, as I apprehend, the name, *Variola* has been used technically (κατ' εξοκχην) to signify this kind of spotted malady, and no other.

"Now as the Cow Pox is a specifically different distemper from the Small Pox in essential particulars, namely, in the nature of its morbific poison, and in its symptoms,—although the Cow Pox may render the constitution not susceptible of the Small Pox,—it is a palpable *catachresis* to designate what is called the Cow Pox by the denomination *Variolæ vaccinæ;* for that is to say, in English, *Cow Small Pox*, and yet the Cow is unsusceptible of infection by the variolous poison."

It is interesting to note that after the publication of Pearson's pamphlet, and after the discovery of cases

---

Vol. ii., p. 87.

of Cow Pox arising independently of horse "grease," Jenner avoided, for a time, any further reference to the origin of the disease.

It was Fraser[1] who was led by the term *variolæ vaccinæ* to regard Cow Pox as *modified* Small Pox. After setting aside the Jennerian theory, that Cow Pox is modified horse grease, Fraser wrote :—

" My own opinion of the origin of this disease is certainly original, and I believed till lately that it was also singular ; but my learned friend, Dr. James Simms, has broached the same idea in a paper read before the Medical Society of London, and published in the last volume of their memoirs. I believe that the Small Pox and the Cow Pox are one and the same disease under different modifications ; and I have found, in course of conversation with some of the most eminent medical and chirurgical doctors in the metropolis, that after having attentively listened to many of the arguments which may be fairly adduced in favour of this opinion they have appeared often to incline to the same belief. I am aware that the proposition may be considered, by some, equally fanciful and absurd with Dr. Jenner's, but at the same time let them remember that it is at least supported by analogy, philosophy, and, of course, probability, although not in the present state of our knowledge by experiment. I do not intend to insist upon this doctrine as incontrovertible, nor even to enter largely, at present, into its merits with a view of establishing it, but shall content myself with observing that such a circumstance would answer the most important and useful purposes."

Before seeing what those useful purposes were, it is as well to mention that Fraser concluded this paper by asserting that his view was established on the " solid and imperishable foundation of truth ; " but,

[1] Henry Fraser, M.D. *Observations on Vaccine Inoculation.* 1805.

however carefully one may read his memoir, no evidence can be found in support of his doctrine. Nevertheless, he adopted the theory, and pointed out the following as the two great reasons for believing it :—

"*Firstly*, It would render the practice of vaccine inoculation general by reconciling the minds of the people who are now imposed upon and intimidated, and in fact shocked at the idea of its filthy ancestry.

"*Secondly*, It would place Dr. Jenner's discovery upon a rock by depriving the antagonists of vaccination of their only successful line of argument."

Thus the assumption that Cow Pox exercised a specific effect on the constitution, rendering it proof against Small Pox, led to the invention of an ingenious theory, which satisfied the minds of those who were willing to accept a plausible explanation, though it was opposed to all practical knowledge of the disease in the Cow.

But the great question, after all, was whether this disease did or did not protect from Small Pox ; and there were two ways in which this was put to the test. Were persons after vaccination insusceptible of *inoculation* with Small Pox, and were they proof against *exposure to infection ?* A sufficient answer to the first question is the fact that Jenner discountenanced the variolous test as unfair, and it is therefore unnecessary to detail the cases in which inoculation of Small Pox succeeded after vaccination. With regard to the test of expo-

sure to infection, evidence—especially towards the last
few years of Jenner's life—was equally overwhelming;
but the failures were attributed to the use of improper
lymph, or to badly or inefficiently performed vaccination, or the Small Pox was regarded as malignant
Chicken Pox. The reports of these failures proved
a crushing blow to Jenner. Never before was he
involved in so many perplexities; he even seemed
ready to acknowledge that the "spontaneous" Cow
Pox which Pearson and Woodville had led him to
pronounce as a source of genuine "vaccine" was,
after all, of no value; and it would appear as if he
were preparing, just before his death, to fall back upon
horse grease as the only source of the "true life-
preserving fluid," although in his earlier researches
he had satisfied himself that equine lymph was of no
value. With regard to the instances of the inefficacy
of Cow Pox which were brought to Jenner's notice, I
will give a short account of Dr. Alexander Monro's[1]
observations "on Small Pox after perfect vaccination."
Dr. Monro wrote :—

"Ever since the publication of Dr. Jenner's discovery
respecting the Cow Pox, there have been various rumours
afloat of Small Pox occurring after Cow Pox. In consequence
of the experience which I myself have had as to the anti-
variolous effects of Cow Pox, I confess I was led to
suspect that some mistake had been committed, either as to

---

[1] Monro. *Observations on the Different Kinds of Small Pox.* p. 144.
1818.

the nature of the disease, or as to the previous vaccination. At length, about nine years ago, all doubt from my mind was removed, in consequence of my having had ocular and very distinct evidence of **perfect vaccination having failed to produce the promised security.**"

Dr. Monro not only made his own observations, but he corresponded with other members of the profession. Mr. Cooper informed him that " cases of Small Pox after Cow Pox are now daily occurrences."

The statements made by Dr. Alexander Ramsay, of Dundee, were still more striking. In a letter to Dr. Monro, dated 27th June, 1818, Dr. Ramsay said :—

"Though our confidence, no doubt, is limited, yet it (vaccination) does appear to us of great value, and to possess many advantages over variolous inoculation. We are inclined to think that much depends on effecting the vaccine disease in its most perfect form, and preserving the pustule entire, which hitherto has not been the case.

" It must, indeed, be admitted that facts do not bear us out fairly in the conclusion that vaccination has resisted the attack of this eruptive disease in proportion to the perfection of its character. On the contrary, **several of the most distinctly marked cases of Small Pox have occurred in those who have been vaccinated apparently in the most satisfactory manner, and where the cellulated marks on both arms are still as perfect as possible.**

"In most cases, however, the pustules had not been preserved entire, but in several they were so ; and in those no circumstance whatever could be found, on the strictest examination, to invalidate the evidence of **Small Pox in its perfect form having succeeded to vaccination in its perfect form.**"

After this independent testimony, Dr. Monro described

the cases in his own family, and not the least striking incident in their history is the fact that they had been vaccinated by Mr. Bryce, and submitted to his test.

The first case was Dr. Monro's eldest son, aged fifteen.

"He had been vaccinated, according to my father's notes, on the left arm by Mr. Bryce with Cow Pox matter, on Saturday, October 29th, 1803."

Fifteen years afterwards, the boy caught Small Pox. The following is the full history of the case :—

"EDINBURGH, *February* 28*th*, 1818.

"A. M., æt. fifteen, was this morning seized with headache, lassitude, drowsiness, and considerable general oppression.

"He went to church, but on returning home from the morning service was still more oppressed ; his face was much flushed, and his eyes red ; had severe headache ; was very drowsy ; threw himself on the sofa, where I found him sleeping at one o'clock P.M.

"His skin was then hot ; pulse but little affected ; had no appetite, and took no dinner. In the evening, his pulse became quick ; he was more flushed ; eyes redder, and headache more severe. Got ʒi of the compound powder of jalap. Passed a very restless night ; frequently started up, and talked a great deal in his sleep.

"*Monday.*—Pulse 110. Still more flushed and oppressed ; had hot and cold fits. Had a stool from the jalap, which was natural as to colour and quantity. Was frequently sick ; 10 grains of ipecacuanha were prescribed. Vomited freely a considerable quantity of yellow-coloured fluid like bile. Passed a still more restless night than the preceding, and talked a great deal in his sleep. Was occasionally sick during the night.

"*Tuesday.*—Pulse 120. Skin hotter ; face still more flushed and swollen ; more thirsty ; tongue white ; complained of cold.

No stool. Got ʒi of compound powder of jalap and 4 grains of calomel. Complained much of coldness of the feet.

"*Wednesday* (1*st day of eruption*).—Skin hot and red ; much thirst ; had three or four stools from the medicine. He sneezed frequently. There are several small, red, round spots, like a flea-bite, on the back of the left hand, and on the little finger, and also on the forehead ; the red colour of which is not removed by pressure, and pressure is painful. Tongue white ; still complained much of cold, especially of the extremities. There is a slight moisture on the face. Pulse 120.

"*Thursday* (2*nd day of eruption*).—The number of red spots on the forehead is now much greater, and there are also a number on the cheeks, nose, ears, lips, arms, and legs ; the skin between these is of a florid red colour. The cheeks and eylids are swelled and red. Eyes slightly inflamed ; he cannot bear the light, and sneezed a good deal. Pulse 60. Passed a good night. Little appetite. Starting in sleep ; much disturbed by dreaming, and talked a great deal during his sleep.

"*Friday* (*third day of eruption*).—The red spots on the skin are considerably broader, and not of uniform size over the whole body, nor equally prominent ; those on the face and neck are farthest advanced. Each spot has a distinct red line round its basis ; in the centre of many of those on the face, neck, and breast-bone, there is a small quantity of a serous fluid, with a depression in the centre. Eyes more inflamed, and more tender. There are a number of pimples among the hair, especially on the back of the head, which are very itchy. Had a good deal of sneezing. Tried to sit up, but it produced acute headache, and he could not do so above ten minutes. Has slight soreness of his throat, which he refers to the larynx. Has no difficulty in swallowing. Several pustules on the face have run together. No stool. A tablespoonful of syrup of senna was prescribed at 11 o'clock A.M., and a second similar dose given at half-past 11 at night.

"*Saturday* (*fourth day of eruption*).—Nearly in the same state as yesterday. Had three or four loose stools from the medicine.

"*Sunday* (*fifth day of eruption*).—Passed a good night ; no thirst ; no fever. He had a free motion in the morning. Appetite improved. The pimples on the face and lobe of the ears are of different sizes, and filled by a watery fluid. The transparent vesicles have distinct necks, and are very like blisters occasioned by boiling water.

"I conceive that the transparent vesicles were formed on the top of the original pimples. Dr. Rutherford, however, holds a different opinion as to the origin of the transparent vesicles, and supposed, that in consequence of inflammation of the skin, a serous fluid was suddenly effused under the scarf skin, and formed vesicles at the side of the Small Pox pimples.

"The vesicles filled by transparent water are more numerous on the face than those filled by pus, for there are not above half a dozen of pustules on the face filled by pus, which have a manifest depression in the centre. The pimples on the breast, those on the back, arms, thighs, and legs, are exactly like the pimples of the Small Pox, and are filled with pus. The progress of the pimples on the face has been quicker than that of those nearer to the centre of circulation. The pimple over the breast-bone, which had made the greatest progress, was punctured with a lancet by Mr. Bryce, and was found to contain pus ; and Mr. Bryce said, he had no doubt but that it would, by inoculation, communicate the Small Pox.

"Skin not so itchy to-day. The vesicles which were filled by a watery fluid, in the course of four or five hours lost considerably of their prominence, were less tense, and were by no means so transparent, and seemed filled with whey, and some of them burst on turning the head and pressing on them. This day, Mr. Lizars made a drawing from the face, which conveys a more accurate idea of the appearances than verbal discription. (Vide Plate III.) Got at 12 o'clock P.M. a tablespoonful of syrup of senna.

"*Monday, March 2nd (sixth day of eruption).*—Slept a good deal yesterday afternoon ; passed a good night ; took his breakfast with appetite. The pustules on the face are not so tense as yesterday. The medicine has operated twice. No thirst ; no fever. The pimples on the arms and legs are now become pustular, and Dr. Rutherford and Mr. Bryce think them perfectly like those of Small Pox. Mr. Bryce punctured one of them, which was found to be filled with thick viscid pus. The cuticle over the pimples on the arms and legs is thicker than that of those of the face; and hence the pustules are more of a grey colour. The cuticle of those vesicles of his face which are filled with a watery fluid, is shrivelled, of a yellow colour, and in some of them there are a few opaque white spots. Many of the pimples on the leg seem to have gone back. The face and legs are now less swelled. The spaces between the pustules of the face are less red than yesterday.

"I observed about nine in the evening, that the vesicles on the face which had been filled by a transparent fluid, had shrunk very considerably. Pulse 60. Was at nine in the evening in a sound sleep, from which he did not awake though a candle was held near to his eyes. Pulse 64.

"*Tuesday, March 3rd* (*seventh day of eruption*).—Passed a good night. Pulse 60, and regular. The greater number of the larger vesicles which contained the clear fluid have burst. On some of them, the scarf-skin is much shrivelled, and these are filled by a small quantity of yellow fluid. No stool. Eyes less tender. There is now but little redness on the skin of the body between the pimples.

"The progress of the pimples has been very irregular; those on the left hand are to the touch, hard, and of a light grey colour, though they first appeared. The progress of these pimples has not been nearly so rapid as of many in other parts of the body. On one of them being opened, it was found to contain purulent matter. Many of the smallest pimples on every part of the body have gone back, and on pressing the skin, no hardness is perceptible. The pimples on the breast have not gone on to suppuration faster than those of the extremities of the body.

"There is a diffused redness between the pimples on the extremities, but it never was so great as between the pustules on the face.

"None of the pimples which resembled those of Small Pox were above a quarter an inch in diameter, and many as small as pin points.

"Mr. Syme made his drawing between 11 and 12 o'clock from the pustules on the left arm, and also of the one on the back of the hand.

" No headache, thirst, or heat of skin.

" *Wednesday, March 4th (eighth day of eruption).*—Passed a good night. Pulse 64. Skin cool; no thirst. A small crust of a deep brown colour is formed over many of the pustules; in a few on his forehead, there is no matter. The skin between the pimples of the face is now of the natural colour, and the swelling of face and lips is gone. The pimples on the left hand and fingers which appeared first are still of a grey colour, feel hard, are painful when pressed, and there is no matter now in them; but there are other pustules on the back of the hand which evidently still contain matter. Mr. Bryce opened one of them, and found it filled by very viscid yellow matter. Many of the pimples on both thighs are still filled by matter; in the centre of others, there is a slight scale, which gives the appearance as if the pustules were depressed in the middle. Skin still very itchy.

" *Thursday, March 5th (ninth day).*—Passed a very good night. Appetite to-day very keen. Pulse 60. The greater number of the pustules have now dried up; there are, however, still a few containing purulent matter upon the hands and thighs. The crusts of the pimples on the face, which resembled the blisters from burns, are of a light yellow colour, and are surrounded by crusts of a dark brown colour formed on the pustules, which resembled those of Small Pox. Many of these crusts on the face have now fallen off, but the skin under them is rough, and slightly elevated. Dr. Rutherford supposes that a little crust was formed upon the skin after the larger crusts had fallen off.

" *Friday, March 6th (tenth day).* — Passed a good night. Pulse 64. No headache; no thirst; appetite good.

" *Saturday, March 7th (eleventh day).*—All the pimples are now dry in the outer layers. A great many of the dry crusts have fallen off. On drawing the fingers along the skin, there is an evident elevation where the pimples were; for a few of the layers of the dried vesicles still remain. Pulse natural; no headache; feels himself now much stronger.

" *Sunday, March 8th (twelfth day).*—The crusts still continue on the face, and those on the thighs, arms, and hands have a considerable degree of hardness and transparency. Is in all other respects quite well.

"*Saturday, March 14th (eighteenth day of eruption).*—There are still some crusts on his face, and a great many on the thighs, arms, and hands, though he took the warm bath last night. There are three very evident pits of a triangular form on the left temple, the bottom of which is very irregular. The cuticle over the crusts on the hands has burst, and now forms a white line around the basis or rather circumference of the dried crust.

"*March 17th.*—Many of the crusts on the extremities of the body, and especially those on the arms, have not fallen off.

"*March 19th (twenty-first day since eruption appeared).*—There are still many of the crusts on the arms and legs.

"*March 22nd (the twenty-second day since the eruption appeared).*—Three pimples of different sizes, and in different states of progress, were observed to-day on the right thigh, and at no great distance from each other. One was like a flea-bite, of a pale red colour, and felt globular when the finger was drawn along. A second has a circle of a deeper red within the paler red, and there is a clear spot on the top; in a third, the crimson ring is still more apparent, and the centre of it seems filled with a liquor like whey, evidently depressed, and had every appearance of the genuine Small Pox pimples.

"*March 23rd.*—The pimples which have appeared on the thigh continue to follow the usual course of the pimples of the modified Small Pox.

"A number of crimson-coloured blotches appeared on the skin after the crusts fell off, and these were not obliterated at so late a period as the 2nd of June. During the progress of the disorder, a dish with nitrous fumigation was constantly kept in the room."

I do not propose to quote in full the particulars of the other cases in the family, but the history of the vaccination is important.

"J. M. was inoculated in his left arm on Wednesday, December 17th, 1806, when three months and three days old. A pustule has formed, about one-sixth of an inch in diameter, which is red at the edges, and its middle rises into a point, from which matter has oozed out, and, by drying, formed a yellow crust. On Monday, December 22nd, 1806, five days after the inoculation, Mr. Bryce inoculated him with matter from his left arm : instead of laying the lancet flat upon the arm, and rubbing off the matter while the point of the lancet was under the cuticle, he punctured the arm, with the point placed perpendicularly, three or four times.

"*December 23rd.*—Thirty-two hours afterwards, a pimple about one-tenth of an inch in diameter, and of a red colour, had formed on his right or last punctured arm. The vaccination was at the time considered complete."

J. M., æt. 11, Monday, March 16th, 1818, suffered from symptoms which developed into an attack of Small Pox.

The third child, K.M., had also been inoculated with Cow Pox, and tested by Mr. Bryce, and, at the time, Mr. Bryce, and Dr. Monro and his father, regarded the vaccination as perfect. On March 15th, 1818, K.M., æt. thirteen, had symptoms which proved to be those of an attack of Small Pox.

Among other cases reported to Dr. Monro, was the son of Dr. Hennen. This boy contracted Small Pox, and at first, as the boy had been vaccinated, the disease was considered as Varicella. But the source of infection was a soldier, in whom the disease was ascertained to be Small Pox. Dr. Hennen wrote :—

"This boy was vaccinated by myself when three months old, and I had every reason to be satisfied with the genuineness of the matter ; he has often been exposed to variolous contagion in Spain, France, and Portugal, and particularly last year at Portsmouth."

Another letter of great interest was received from

Dr. Smith of Dunse, 2nd June, 1818. Dr. Smith wrote :—

"I had, indeed, seen several cases of Small Pox supervening upon vaccination, which I mentioned at the time to Dr. Farquharson ; but as he seemed to think lightly of them, I judged it prudent to take no further notice of the circumstance. Even now, though I have seen a multitude of cases in which Small Pox has, in every possible shape, taken place after vaccination, I feel myself placed in the painful situation of bringing forward many facts to which gentlemen of the first eminence in the profession will probably give little or no credit. . . .

"It is now about three months since Small Pox appeared in the east coast of Berwickshire, particularly at Coldinghame, Eysmouth, and Ayton. Several young people, who had not been vaccinated fell victims to the disease. In the course of a few weeks afterwards, this pestilential malady extended itself over other parts of the country, and whole families were in consequence promiscuously laid up, whether vaccinated or not. I have seen a number of cases wherein great crops of Small Pox took place after vaccination. I attended two in particular that were confluent, and watched the progress of the disease with much anxiety. . . .

"I am perfectly sensible I may have incurred much odium in the opinion of many for having had recourse to inoculation after it has so long been exploded. . . . Vaccination either does, or it does not, resist the variolous affection. If the former, vaccination cannot possibly do harm ; but, if the latter, we are imperiously called upon to communicate the Small Pox in the mildest way we can, and not leave the rising generation to the scourge of a loathsome and dangerous disease."

Practitioners had so committed themselves to a belief in the protective power of Cow Pox that even when Small Pox occurred after perfect vaccination it was impossible for many to believe it.

The disease, they said, must be Malignant Chicken Pox. This, for example, was the view taken in the case of a boy at Inverness, two years old, who had Small Pox "after having passed through the Cow Pox in its most perfect state." But Dr. Robertson set the question at rest by inoculating a child, and the child so inoculated not only had the common Small Pox, but had it severely. Dr. Smith, of Dunse, had similar experiences, and " repeatedly practised inoculation with matter taken from those who had the Small Pox after the Cow Pox."

Dr. Monro was unable to free himself from his previous convictions in regard to the prophylactic efficacy of Cow Pox, and he concluded, that the disease was milder than might otherwise have been the case.

These were not the only outbreaks of Small Pox about this time which afforded similar experiences ; and it is not surprising, therefore, that Jenner was surrounded with perplexities.

Vaccination, it is true, was in a great measure discredited, but it still survived, and was gradually reinstated. This was due partly, no doubt, to the favourable reports of the officials of the National Vaccine Establishment ; but the revival was certainly brought about more particularly by the exertions of John Baron, the friend and biographer of Jenner.

Jenner's notes and correspondence had been placed by his executors in Baron's hands. From his intimate acquaintance with Jenner, he was regarded as the most suitable person to prepare a biography. All Jenner's early letters were bequeathed to Baron by Edward Gardner. But Baron's object was not merely to write a biography of Jenner; his work was intended to restore the shattered credit of vaccination. Thus he wrote in the Introduction :—

"The recent prevalence of Small Pox in different parts of Europe, and the corresponding diminution of confidence in the virtues of the Variolæ Vaccinæ **rendered it an object of no inconsiderable importance to endeavour to restore and increase that confidence,** by showing that Dr. Jenner clearly foresaw the deviations which have been observed ; that his doctrines, if properly understood, satisfactorily account for them ; and that nothing, in fact, has occurred which does not strengthen and confirm his original opinions both with regard to the Variola and the Variolæ Vaccinæ. I would hope that something may have been done in these respects that shall tend to promote the universal adoption of a practice capable of effecting so much good.

"Nothing, I am persuaded, can ever accomplish this object except *a real knowledge of the nature of that affection which might be made to take the place of Small Pox.* A very sincere wish to accelerate this event has led me to the discussions contained in the present volume, the publication of which at this time, I would humbly hope, may not be without its use."

No one can posssibly read Baron's *Life of Jenner* without feeling the prejudices and the strong bias displayed all through the work; and no one with any knowledge of comparative pathology, can possibly

study it without being impressed with the gross
fallacies to which Baron committed himself. His
historical investigation, as I have already pointed
out, resulted in proving to his own satisfaction that
Jenner's Cow Pox was the remnant of an outbreak
of Cow Small Pox, and thus he justified the term,
variolæ vaccinæ, and endeavoured to establish the protective power of Cow Pox. But his elaborate statement
proved to be a tissue of blunders, for the disease
described as Cow Small Pox had nothing to do with
Cow Pox; it was, in fact, Cattle Plague. At the time,
however, Baron's teachings were accepted, and thus his
blunders fulfilled his purpose. Criticised in the light
of modern information, the only value of Baron's work
is to be found in the publication of Jenner's correspondence, by which we are able to judge of the
way in which vaccination was conducted from 1798
to 1823.

Baron employed other channels for spreading his
ideas, and he so far succeeded that he misled the
medical profession. Thus he was made Chairman
of a Committee of the Provincial Medical and
Surgical Association, and in their report, signed, and
probably entirely written by the Chairman, the pathological fallacies in Jenner's biography were repeated
in a description of the affinities between Human
Small Pox and the so-called Cow Small Pox, and we
are told that, " upon a due understanding of this

portion of the subject everything that is valuable in the practice of vaccination depends." Then follows an elaborate dissertation on the disease described by Layard, in this country, and by Frascatorius, Lancisi, Lanzoni, Ramazzini, and others, in Italy, in other words, on Rinderpest or Cattle Plague. Thus was Cow Pox dogmatically asserted to be Cow Small Pox; and Fraser's theory, which obscured the great fallacy in Cow Pox inoculation, was admitted as a pathological fact.

In support of the theory, Baron related that Mr. Bree, of Stowmarket, had written to say—

"During the prevalence of Small Pox in this neighbourhood, several dairies became affected with Cow Pox ; which supports the opinion of the identity of the two diseases, the latter being probably modified by being developed in the cow."

Baron also referred to a statement made by Dr. Waterhouse, of Massachusetts, in a letter to Jenner.

"At one of our periodical inoculations, which occur in New England once in eight or nine years, several people drove their cows to an hospital near a populous village, in order that their families might have the daily benefit of their milk. These cows were milked by persons in all stages of Small Pox. The consequence was, the cows had an eruptive disorder on their teats and udders, so like the Small Pox pustule, that every one in the hospital, as well as the physician who told me, declared the cows had the Small Pox."

The whole of this anecdote was hearsay. It was probably a coincident outbreak of one of the common eruptive affections of the teats ; and so little interest was taken in the event at the time, that no inoculations were made from the cows to test the nature of the eruption. And yet Baron writes :—

" It is impossible, we conceive, to doubt the fact that on this occasion the Small Pox had been conveyed from man to the cow, just as it had been communicated, in the dairies of Gloucestershire, from the cow to man."

But though Baron succeeded in carrying the general opinion of the profession in favour of vaccination, there were individual vaccinators who, occasionally, spoke out candidly enough.[1] Thus, Estlin, in 1837, wrote to the editor of the *Medical Gazette* :—

" Allow me, in the first place, to premise that, having been engaged in vaccinating (at one time rather extensively) for thirty years, I have watched, with regret, a decided decline in the activity of the virus ; and for many years, I have been endeavouring in vain to renew the lymph from its original source. On the diminished anti-variolous power of the present stock of vaccine matter I need make no remark ; the public are too painfully aware of the fact."

Badcock[2] was led to undertake his experiments by the following occurrence in 1836 :—

" Towards the end of the year 1836, **I suffered severely from a dangerous attack of Small Pox, which happened but a few months after revaccination** ; and my mind having previously been impressed with an idea that the **old vaccine** had lost its protective influence by passing through so many constitutions

---

[1] Compare Duncan Stewart. *Report on Small Pox in Calcutta, and Vaccination in Bengal.* 1827-44.
[2] Vol. ii., p. 518.

during the long period of forty years, I was exceedingly anxious to procure some fresh from the cow, for the purpose of having my own children revaccinated."

And, again, speaking of his experiences up to 1845, Badcock wrote :—

"From whatever cause it may arise, the fact has been of late years already ascertained, that the ordinary vaccine virus has lost a great deal of its protective power against Small Pox. A greater number of cases in which that disease has occurred after vaccination are met with than formerly, and in some instances those are very severe, and occasionally even terminate fatally."

In fact, an alteration in the quality of the lymph had now become one of the stock apologetics for Cow Pox failures, and the profession was still persuaded to believe in "that most precious boon of Jenner to a suffering world." According to Badcock,[1] similar experiences were met with abroad. Out of 547,646 vaccinated, 11,773 were attacked with Small Pox, 1,294 became disfigured or infirm, and 1,379 died in consequence of the disease. Indeed, in France, vaccination was credited with having no effect over malignant Small Pox; while in England, when a less malignant variety attacked the vaccinated, the argument was used that if it had not been for vaccination the attack might have been worse.

Even Ceely,[2] one of the most accurate obervers,

---

[1] Vol. ii., p. 517.
[2] Vol. ii., p. 365.

who had convinced himself that Cow Pox arose "spontaneously" in the cow, and had never been able in all his practical investigations to find any other explanation for its origin, was nevertheless so influenced by Baron's teachings, that when he succeeded in raising a vesicle on the cow by inoculation of human variola, a vesicle which had the physical characters of the vaccine vesicle, he was led to believe that he had succeeded in producing Cow Pox by inoculation of human Small Pox. Thus, Baron's historical researches, and Ceely's misinterpreted investigations, were summed up by Baron in the words, "Vaccination is now, indeed, placed upon a rock." There was not only no hesitation in substituting the term *Cow Small Pox* for the original *Cow Pox,* but although outbreaks of Cow Pox were discovered perfectly independently of any human variola, Baron's historical researches, Ceely and Badcock's experiments, and the incidents related by Waterhouse and Bree, led to the theory of Cow Small Pox, being regarded as an established fact.

In 1857. vaccination obtained further support from the Blue Book on vaccination compiled by Simon. It would be out of place, here, to analyse that report, but it remains as evidence of the extraordinary hold which the Jennerian doctrine had upon the minds of even distinguished sanitarians. It is, however, much to be regretted that the teachings and fallacies of Baron should have been reproduced, and Jenner's *Inquiry* described as a masterpiece of medical induction—a similar comment to that of Blumenbach on Jenner's researches on the cuckoo.

Not only were Baron's blunders with regard to Cattle Plague quoted with approval, but the Cow Small Pox theory again comes to the front under cover of Ceely's variolation experiment.

> "It was not till forty years afterwards that science supplied an authentic interpretation of Jenner's wonderful discovery; he, indeed, had suspected the solution, and had hinted his meaning when he called the Cow Pox by the name of 'Variolæ Vaccinæ,' for such in fact it is—the Small Pox of the cow."

Simon also endorses the following statement to show that "a host of theoretical objections to vaccination might have been met, or indeed anticipated, if it could have been affirmed sixty years ago, as it can be affirmed now,"

> "'This new process of preventing Small Pox is really only carrying people through Small Pox in a modified form. The vaccinated are safe against Small Pox, because they, in fact, have had it. Their safety is of the same sort as if they had been inoculated under the old process, or had been infected by the natural disease. The trifling disorder which they suffer, those few tender vesicles on the arm, the slight feverishness which they show, is Small Pox of the most modified kind; Small Pox so modified by the intermediate animal organisation through which it has passed, that when thus reintroduced into the human body it excites but insignificant disturbance, and no general exhalation of infected material.'"

Thus Fraser's creed led to a pathological error, which, in turn, was officially commended on the ground that it met a host of theoretical objections. The same theory having been officially accepted, has been reproduced in our medical text-books, and the student is led to believe that Cow Pox arises from milkers suffering from Small Pox, and Cow Pox is, therefore, Small Pox modified by transmission through the cow. But the fallacy of this doctrine is too obvious; for in the numerous outbreaks in cows and horses from which "vaccine lymph" has been procured, if the source of the disease were Human Small Pox, there would have been little or no difficulty in tracing the infection. But never, in any outbreak of Cow Pox or Horse Pox, has a connection with Human Small Pox been established.

The reply may be made to this, that Cow Pox is so excessively rare a disease that there have not been sufficient opportunities for observation; and that further, the rarity of the disease harmonises with the belief that it arises from Human Small Pox. Such a statement is in direct opposition to facts. Cow Pox and Horse Pox have been met with and studied again and again. If these diseases were derived from Human Small Pox, the observation would have been established with as much certainty, as that hydrophobia in man results from the bite of a rabid dog. To emphasize this point, I will give a brief summary of the outbreaks of Cow Pox which have occurred in this and in other countries.

In England, Jenner found Cow Pox in 1770, 1780, 1782, 1791, 1794, 1796. In 1798, he raised his first stock of lymph. In 1799, Cow Pox was raging in the dairies in London, and was described by Woodville, Pearson, and Bradley. In the same year, Cow Pox broke out at Norton Nibley, in Gloucestershire, and lymph was taken for Jenner's use. Later, a fresh stock was raised from the dairies in Kentish Town. Pearson and Aikin described the prevalence of Cow Pox in Wilts, Somerset, Devon, Buckingham, Dorset, Norfolk, Suffolk, Leicester, and Stafford; and Barry described its prevalence in Ireland.

From this time onwards, for a long period, natural Cow Pox received little or no attention in this country. Fresh stocks of lymph were occasionally raised, but no further attention was paid to the disease in the cow.

In 1836, Leese met with an outbreak, and raised a stock of lymph which was introduced among the current stocks. In 1838, Estlin met with an outbreak in Gloucestershire, and raised a fresh stock of lymph. Cow Pox was observed in 1838-39 by Mr. Fox, of Cerne Abbas; and again in 1839, in Dorsetshire, by Sweeting, of Abbotsbury; and in 1838, 1840, 1841, and 1845, fresh stocks of lymph were raised by Ceely, Cow Pox being frequently met with in the Vale of Aylesbury.

From this time onwards, outbreaks of the disease in the cow have not been recorded, but several practitioners met with the disease, and raised fresh stocks.

Thus, when inquiries were made in 1857, it was found that several medical men had employed fresh vaccine lymph; Mr. Donald Dalrymple, of Norwich (on two occasions); Mr. Beresford, of Narborough, in Leicestershire; Mr. Gorham, of Aldeburgh; Mr. Alison, of Great Retford; Mr. Coles, of Leckhampton; Mr. Rudge, of Leominster, and one or two others. Mr. Sweeting had met with the disease in two instances, and had disseminated lymph obtained by the vaccination of persons from each source. Another stock of lymph was raised by Ceely in 1845, and lastly, in 1887, I investigated an outbreak of Cow Pox in Wiltshire.

In Italy, Cow Pox was found by Sacco in 1800, in the Plains of Lombardy, and by other practitioners in 1808-9. In 1812, it was observed at Naples by Miglietta; in 1830, in Piedmont; and in 1832, and 1843, at Rome, by Dr. Maceroni. Quite recently several outbreaks of Cow Pox have been encountered, and the stocks of lymph renewed.

In France, in 1810, Cow Pox was found in the Department of La Meurthe, and in 1822, at Clairvaux; at Passy, Amiens, and Rambouillet in 1836; at Rouen in 1839; at Saint Illide, at Saint Seine, and at Perylhac in 1841; in 1842, at Pagnac; in 1843, at Deux Jumeaux, where, during the previous thirty years, several fresh stocks of lymph had been raised and circulated. Cow Pox broke out in a cow belonging to M. Majendie in 1844 ; and it was found at Wasseloune in the Department of Bas Rhin in 1845 ; it occurred in three Departments in 1846; at Rheims, and in the Department of Eure et Loire in 1852 ; in the arrondissement of Sancerre, and at Beziers in 1854 ; and at Guyonville in 1863. On farms in three villages near Nogent in 1864 (the disease was introduced by newly purchased cows ; milkers were infected, and from one of these milkers a lymph stock was established) ; in 1864, also at Petit Quevilly, near Rouen ; and in April 1866, at Beaugency ; in 1881, at Eysines, near Bordeaux, and again at the same place in 1883 ; and in 1884, at Cérons.

In Germany, as soon as attention had been drawn to the disease, Cow Pox was frequently discovered. It was also ascertained that it had been referred to in a Göttingen newspaper published in 1769. The disease appears to have been well known there, and milkers who contracted the disease by milking the cows had the same tradition as the dairymaids in Gloucestershire, as to its protective power against Small Pox. In 1802, Cow Pox was met with, according to Bücholz, in different parts of Germany — in Mecklenburg, Holstein, Brandenburg, Silesia, and the neighbourhood of Gresen and Erlangen. In 1812, Cow Pox was discovered in Berlin and its suburbs by Bremer ; near Luneburg by Fischer ; and in Greifswalde by Mende; in 1816 at Seggerde in Brunswick, by Giesker ; and in other parts of Brunswick.

In Holstein, from 1813 to 1824, Luders met with five epizoötics in the farms of Büstorf, Berensbrook, Ornum, Eichthal, and Holmstein, and also a great number of isolated cases. Ritter found this disease very common in Schleswig-Holstein. It was found, in 1829, by Riss, at Neu Busach, and by Albeis, near Stralsund, in 1834.

In Wurtemberg, between the years 1825 to 1837, numerous outbreaks were reported. The great number in 1829, corresponds with the publication of a description of Cow Pox :—

1825	1
1827	5
1828	3
1829	38
1830	31
1831	31
1832	18
1833	14
1834	18
1835	19
1836	25
1837	18

In sixty-nine places the vaccinogenic property of the lymph, from eighty-four cows, was established by inoculation. One hundred and twenty-six children, and a girl twenty-two years old, were vaccinated with success, and the stocks of lymph were circulated in other countries. After 1830, fresh lymph was sent to the vaccine institutions at Stuttgart, and employed successfully ; so that in ten years many hundreds of children were vaccinated with Cow Pox lymph collected in Wurtemberg.

In Holland, according to Numann, Cow Pox was found in 1805, in 1811, and in 1824.

In Denmark, it was found by Niergaard, at Fünen, in 1801.

In Russia, in 1838, an epizoötic occurred among the cows in a village in the neighbourhood of St. Petersburg.

In North America it was found by Dr. Buett, of Massachusetts, and by Drs. Norton and Trowbridge, of Connecticut, in 1801.

In South America it was found in the valley of Ablixco, in the neighbourhood of Valladolid de Mechoacan, and in the district of Calabozo, in the province of Caraccas ; and by Humboldt in Peru, and was known, according to Pepping, among the cows in Chili.

Hence it is evident that natural Cow Pox is far from being a rare disease, as many have supposed, who are unacquainted with the subject ; and, further, in not one of these numerous outbreaks has any causal relationship with Human Small Pox been established.

To assert, therefore, the theory of Cow Small Pox on the ground of Ceely and Badcock's experience, is to substitute experimental fallacies for correct clinical observation. I must again assert that there is no proof whatever that *the disease*, Cow Pox, was produced by the inoculation of cows with Human Small Pox. After a number of trials a vesicle was produced possessing the physical characters of inoculated Cow Pox ; but, inasmuch as cattle plague, when inoculated, produces a vesicle with the physical characters of Cow Pox, that Sheep Pox and Horse Pox can also be so cultivated as to produce similar appearances, there is no more reason for supposing that Human Small Pox was transformed into Cow Pox, than there is for believing that Cow Pox, Horse Pox, Human Small Pox, Cattle Plague, and Sheep Pox are all manifestations of one and the same disease.

The practical student of Cow Pox is at once convinced, without any further evidence, that the two diseases, Small Pox and Cow Pox, are specifically distinct. Cow Pox is a disease communicable solely by contact. Small Pox is a disease which, though inoculable, is also highly infectious. Cow Pox begins as a local affection, and is followed by constitutional symptoms. Small Pox is an acute disease, characterised by sudden and severe fever, which is followed after forty-eight hours by a generalised eruption.

If we study inoculated Cow Pox in early removes from the cow, we observe the formation of a papule, a vesicle, an ulcer with surrounding induration, ·

enlargement of the lymphatic glands, and secondary eruptions or vaccinides. Cow Pox, in fact, as Auzias-Turenne [1] pointed out in 1865, is strictly analogous to syphilis, and it is only by a comparison with this disease that we can really follow its natural history. In most of our medical text-books, the description of Cow Pox is not the description of the natural disease ; it is simply an account of the appearances which result after it has been artificially cultivated on the arm of a child or the belly of a calf. The ordinary description of *vaccinia* stands in the same relation to the disease *Cow Pox* as a description of the benign vesicle of variolation to the full cycle of the natural Small Pox. It is only when we have to deal with the early removes from the cow, or when the lymph reverts to its original untamed character, that we really appreciate what the symptoms of Cow Pox are. Jenner has given many instances, which stand in striking contrast to the mitigated affection described as "tender vesicles with slight feverishness." We know that Jenner met with what, at the present day, are called vaccinal accidents ; these are manifestations of the disease in its unmitigated form ; it is then associated with violent constitutional symptoms, the development of corroding ulcers, and generalised eruptions. Bousquet met with

---

[1] Vol. ii., p. 552.

ROSEOLA OF COW POX (WILLAN).

similar experiences. Estlin has fully described the results which followed from the use of lymph recently derived from the cow, and Ceely also met with similar accidents.

In speaking of Small Pox inoculation, I have referred to the differences which resulted from taking lymph at different periods; and there can be no question that the same laws which apply to Small Pox inoculation, apply also to Cow Pox inoculation. Cow Pox lymph taken at a late stage will tend on some subjects to revert to its original virulency, or, as Bousquet calls it, *sauvagerie*, just as Small Pox lymph taken at a late period and ingrafted on a suitable soil may induce, not a transient papule or a benign vesicle, but an attack of confluent Small Pox.

I have already stated that Auzias Turenne was the first to point out that Cow Pox is analogous to syphilis; but even the earliest opponents of vaccination regarded the disease as *lues bovilla*, and it had even been suggested that the cow had derived the complaint from milkers who were affected with syphilis. There is no more ground for believing in the latter theory than there is for believing that Cow Pox is produced by milkers suffering from Small Pox. It is the course which the malady runs which brings it so closely into relation with syphilis; and I find that in Horse Pox, the parallel is still closer, inasmuch as Horse Pox is transmitted by coition. In this country,

Creighton[1] has pointed out how closely the inoculated syphilis runs parallel with the natural Cow Pox; so much so that he has a tendency to regard all cases of so-called vaccinal syphilis as truly vaccinal, being reversions to the original type of the disease in the cow. This may be too sweeping an assertion, for there appears to be very little doubt that syphilis may be transmitted by vaccination; but many cases which are attributed to syphilis are unquestionably the full effects of the Cow Pox virus; and nothing could more clearly point to the analogy between the two diseases than the difficulty in diagnosing the exact nature of these vaccinal accidents.

Again, if we study the effects of syphilis artificially inoculated on the human subject, the appearances in some cases are strikingly similar to inoculated Horse Pox. Without entering into a prolonged discussion of this subject, I will refer, as an example, to the progress in Ricord's cases of syphilisation. As in inoculated Horse Pox we have the stages of papule, vesicle, ulcer, scab, and scar; and no one can compare his plates with Jenner's (see Plates IV. and XXIII.) without being struck with the similiarity in their appearances. The results of the artificial inoculation of syphilis were unknown to Jenner, but if they had been he would scarcely have failed to have observed the likeness between them. So striking

[1] Creighton. *Cow Pox and Vaccinal Syphilis.*

Facing page 462.

PLATE XXIII.

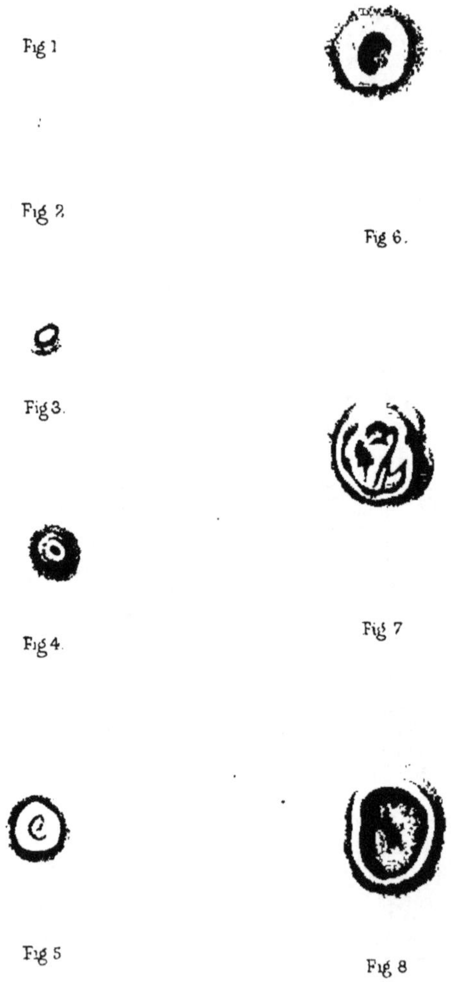
Fig 1
Fig 2
Fig 3.
Fig 4.
Fig 5
Fig 6.
Fig 7
Fig 8

INOCULATED SYPHILIS (RICORD).

COMPARE FIG. 6 WITH PLATE IV.

Vincent Brooks Day & Son Lith

indeed are the appearances, that it is possible that, by judicious selection, a strain of syphilitic lymph might be cultivated which would produce in time all the physical characters of the " vaccine " vesicle.

As the result of an investigation into the history, and especially the pathology, of " vaccination," I feel convinced that the profession has been misled by Jenner, Baron, the Reports of the National Vaccine Establishment, and by a want of knowledge concerning the nature of Cow Pox, Horse Pox, and other sources of " vaccine lymph." Though in this country, vaccine lymph is generally taken to mean the virus of Cow Pox, yet the pathology of this disease, and its nature and affinities, have not been made the subject of practical study for nearly half a century. We have submitted instead to purely theoretical teaching, and have been led to regard *vaccination* as inoculation of the human subject with the virus of *a benign disease of the cow*, whereas the viruses in use have been derived from several distinct and severe diseases in different animals.

The statement that the protective measures which have been introduced by Pasteur, such as inoculation for chicken cholera, anthrax, and rabies, are analogous to Jenner's vaccination as a protective against Small Pox, is the most recent extension of the fallacious theory of Cow Small Pox. Pasteur's system is the same in principle as the old method of Small

Pox inoculation. Variolation, though a dangerous practice, can at least claim to be based upon scientific grounds, viz., the prevention or modification of a disease by artificially inducing a mild attack of that disease. Jenner's substitution of Cow Pox inoculation was a purely empirical treatment based upon folklore, and involved a totally different pathological principle—the protection from one disease by the artificial induction of a totally distinct disease—a principle which was not, and has not been since, supported by either clinical experience or pathological experiments. The Jennerian method has for nearly a century struggled for existence with the support of the Cow Small Pox theory and the numerous and ingenious explanations of failures embodied in the assertions of spurious Cow Pox, inefficiently performed vaccination, inferior quality of lymph, deficiency in the number and quality of marks; and the misinterpretation of statistics.[1]

Inoculation of Cow Pox does not have the least effect in affording immunity from the analogous disease in man, syphilis, and neither do Cow Pox, Horse Pox, Sheep Pox, Cattle Plague, or any other radically dissimilar disease, exercise any specific protective power against Human Small Pox. Inoculation of Cow Pox, Horse Pox, and Cattle Plague have totally failed to exterminate Small Pox; and for the eradication of this disease we must in future resort

[1] *Vide* p. 163.

to methods similar to those proposed by Haygarth, which in modern times have been so successful in STAMPING OUT diseases of the lower animals, such as Cattle Plague, Foot and Mouth Disease, and Sheep Pox.

In the case of the lower animals this has been effectually performed by notification, combined with either slaughter, isolation, or muzzling. It has been stated that rabies might be stamped out of this country in twelve months by universal muzzling; with equal truth may it be said that Small Pox might be stamped out in the same time by notification and a rigid system of isolation. And if any practical benefit is to be derived from Pasteur's system of protective inoculation, I cannot see any scientific reason why nurses and other attendants upon cases of Small Pox, should not be protected by inoculation with attenuated Small Pox within the walls of a Small Pox hospital, and with due precaution to prevent the spread of infection.

There can be no doubt that ere long a system of COMPULSORY NOTIFICATION and ISOLATION will replace vaccination. Indeed, I maintain that where isolation and vaccination have been carried out in the face of an epidemic, it is isolation which has been instrumental in staying the outbreak, though vaccination has received the credit.

Unfortunately a belief in the efficacy of vaccination

has been so enforced in the education of the medical practitioner, that it is hardly probable that the futility of the practice will be generally acknowledged in our generation, though nothing would more redound to the credit of the profession and give evidence of the advance made in pathology and sanitary science. It is more probable that when, by means of notification and isolation, Small Pox is kept under control, vaccination will disappear from practice, and will retain only an historical interest.

FINIS.

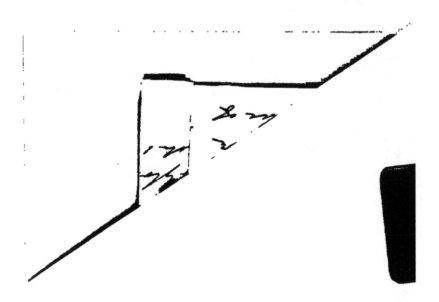

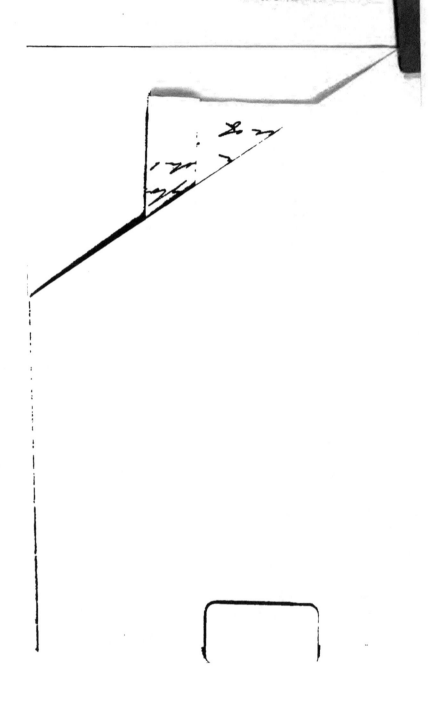

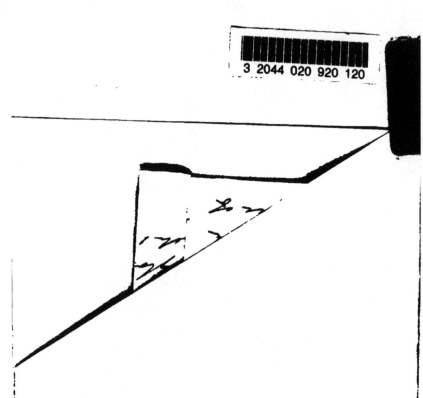

CPSIA information can be obtained
at www.ICGtesting.com
Printed in the USA
BVHW041010130720
583594BV00003B/49